AF724068

Medicine at Monte Cassino

SPECULUM SANITATIS
STUDIES IN MEDIEVAL AND EARLY MODERN MEDICAL CULTURE (500–1800)

General Editors

Iolanda Ventura, *Università di Bologna*
Karl Enenkel, *Universität Münster*

Editorial Board

Charles Burnett, *The Warburg Institute*
Michael McVaugh, *University of North Carolina-Chapel Hill*
Faith Wallis, *McGill University*

Volume 1

Medicine at Monte Cassino

Constantine the African and the Oldest Manuscript of his *Pantegni*

by

Erik Kwakkel and Francis Newton

with an introduction by

Eliza Glaze

BREPOLS

British Library Cataloguing in Publication Data

A catalogue record for this book is available from the British Library.

Cover image: Erfurt, Universitätsbibliothek, Bibliotheca Amploniana, Cod. Amplon. 4° 184, fol. 2ʳ, detail (Italy, 1147)

© 2019, Brepols Publishers n.v., Turnhout, Belgium

All rights reserved. No part of this publication may be reproduced, stored in a retrieval system, or transmitted, in any form or by any means, electronic, mechanical, photocopying, recording, or otherwise, without the prior permission of the publisher.

D/2019/0095/16
ISBN: 978-2-503-57921-4
e-ISBN: 978-2-503-57934-4
DOI: 10.1484/M.SSM-EB.5.114926
Printed in the EU on acid-free paper

Contents

LIST OF ILLUSTRATIONS

Plates

Figures

Tables

Acknowledgements

The groundwork for this project was laid during the course of a 'conversations' symposium sponsored by and held at the National Humanities Center in Research Triangle Park, North Carolina, from 30 September to 3 October 2010. This symposium, organized by Monica Green and Eliza Glaze, was entitled Excavating Medicine in the Digital Age: Palaeography and the Medical Book in the Twelfth-Century Renaissance. Here, a group of scholars — Eliza Glaze (Coastal Carolina University), Monica Green (Arizona State University), Erik Kwakkel (Leiden University), and Francis Newton (Duke University), in collegial consultation with Robert Babcock (University of North Carolina at Chapel Hill), Alison Beach (University of Cologne), Consuelo Dutschke (Columbia University), Nicholas Everett (University of Toronto), Jean Givens (University of Connecticut), Michael McVaugh (University of North Carolina at Chapel Hill), Outi Merisalo (University of Jyväskylä/University of Helsinki), and Rodney Thomson (University of Tasmania), came together as a 'Medical Palaeography Team', and subsequently continued explorations in this topic, enlisting other scholars in the project along the way and presenting preliminary unpublished findings at various conferences. We the authors of the present volume are grateful to all of these colleagues as well as the following organizations and funds for financial support in the pursuit of this project: the National Humanities Center; the National Library of the Netherlands in The Hague; Duke University; Leiden University; Arizona State University; Coastal Carolina University; the Netherlands Organisation for Scientific Research (NWO) for the Vidi grant awarded to Erik Kwakkel; and the Lawrence B. and Jane P. Clark Endowed Chair at Coastal Carolina University held by Eliza Glaze. We are also grateful to the audience of scholars and colleagues at a variety of meetings, including at the University of North Carolina at Chapel Hill, Duke University, Ohio State University, and the University of Southampton (UK); the International Congress on Medieval Studies at Western Michigan University; and the International Medieval Congress at the University of Leeds.

We are especially grateful to libraries and archives, and their staff members, who have provided us with digital photographs, films, and facsimiles: these include Leiden University Library; the Koninklijke Bibliotheek in The Hague; Duke University; the University of North Carolina at Chapel Hill; the US National Library of Medicine; the Virginia Brown Collection at Ohio State University; Gloucester Cathedral Library; Merton College Oxford; the British Library; the Wellcome Library; Cambridge University Library; the Bibliothèque nationale de France; the Staats- und Stadtbibliothek Augsburg; the Universität Erfurt's Bibliotheca Amploniana; and the Abbey of Monte Cassino. Ed van der Vlist (Koninklijke Bibliotheek, The Hague) deserves our special gratitude for his continued support, for providing high-resolution images of the full manuscript around which this monograph revolves, and for sharing his research on the medical excerpts added to its front and back.

Our greatest debt is to the colleagues who shared their insights and responded to our own hypotheses most helpfully at every turn and in every way, beginning with the distinguished colleagues named above at the initial gathering at the National Humanities Center. It was there that the idea for this book originated. But long before that meeting, Constantine, his activities as a translator, and the reception of his texts, provided a major focus for the scholarly work of several initial members of the team, in the beginning Monica Green and Francis Newton, both working at Duke, and subsequently in the 1990s their student there, Eliza Glaze. Eliza has provided signal assistance from the conception of this book until its completion. We have also benefitted from studies, both published and unpublished, of Winston Black, Iolanda Ventura, Andrew Irving, Brian Long, Outi Merisalo, and Raphaela Veit. The respective conclusions of these scholars will appear in various publications and venues aside from the present volume. As a collaborative team, we have all benefitted from fruitful conversations and speculations about what might have happened, and where, in the eleventh century, even when we have not always agreed. The present book advances the original discoveries and conclusions of the current authors only. In addition to those team members already named, our warm thanks go to Klaus-Dietrich Fischer, Mark Jordan, Outi Kaltio, Charles Burnett, Danielle Jacquart, and Robert Rodgers for their generosity in sharing texts and images of manuscripts, their scholarly perspectives, and other valuable resources. All translations in this book are the work of the authors, unless otherwise noted. Lastly, we are grateful for the editorial work undertaken by Jenneka Janzen (Leiden).

Colour Plates

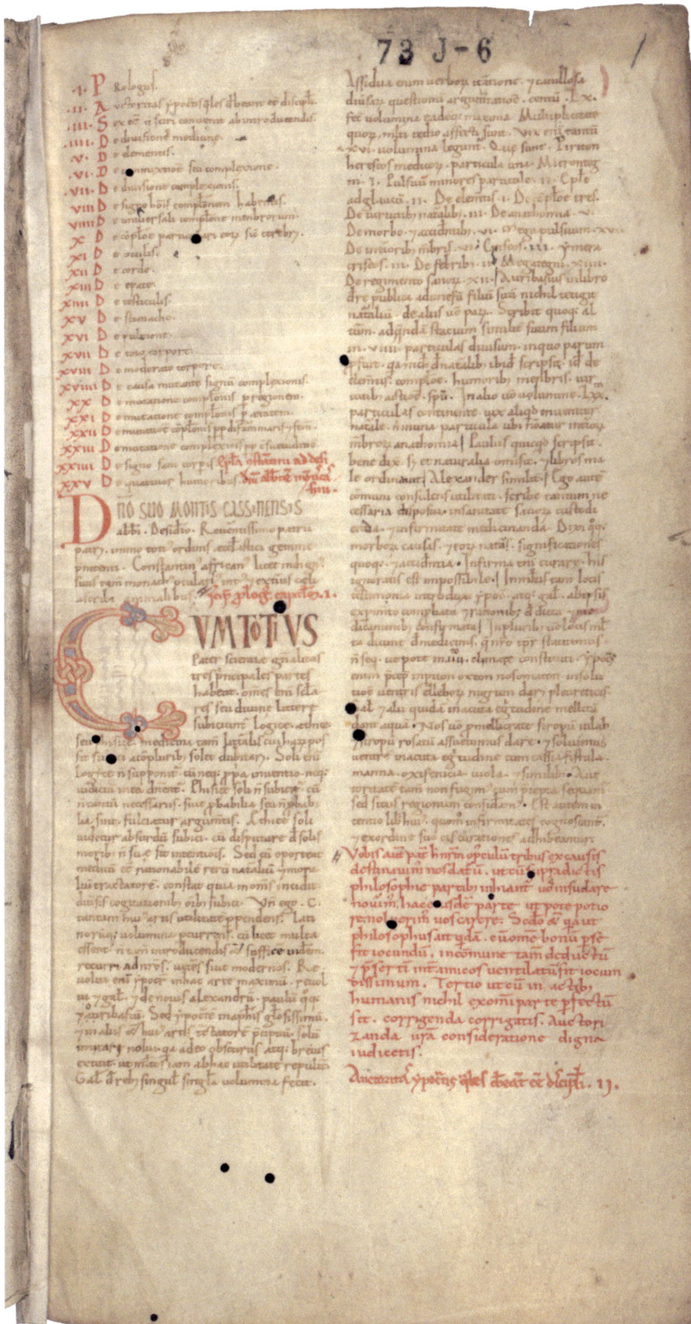

Plate I.
The Hague *Pantegni*, The Hague, Koninklijke Bibliotheek, MS 73 J 6, fol. 1r.
Late 1070s or early 1080s (before 1086).

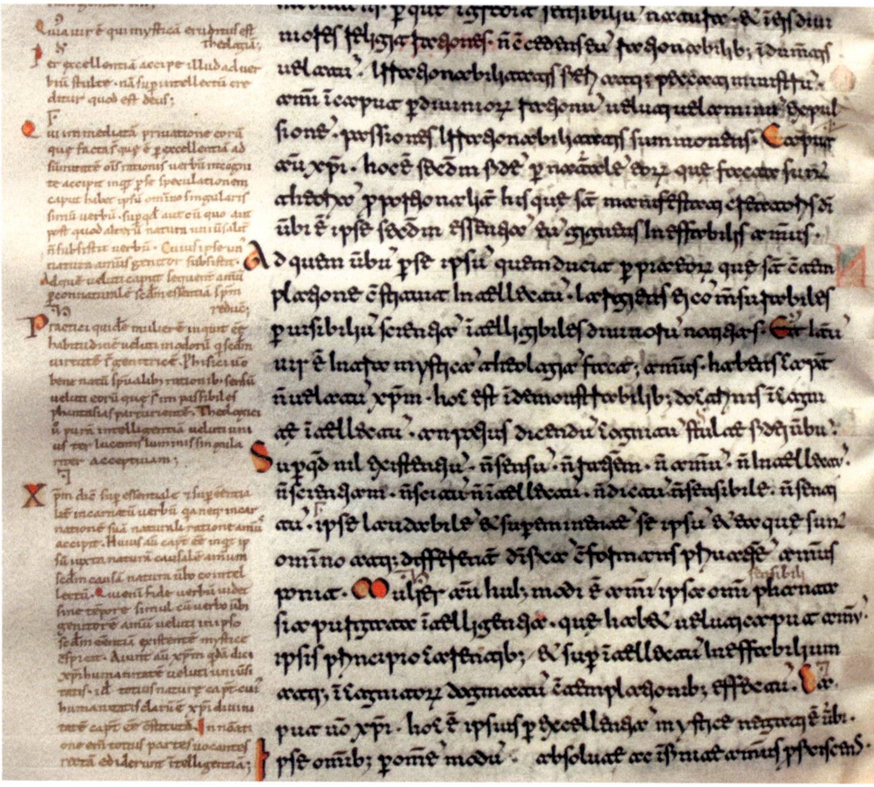

Plate II. Marginal *scholia* by Geraldus, the main scribe of the Hague manuscript, Monte Cassino, Archivio della Badia, MS 333, p. 2 (detail). 1087–1105. The text is that of Maximus Confessor's *Quaestiones ad Thalassium*.

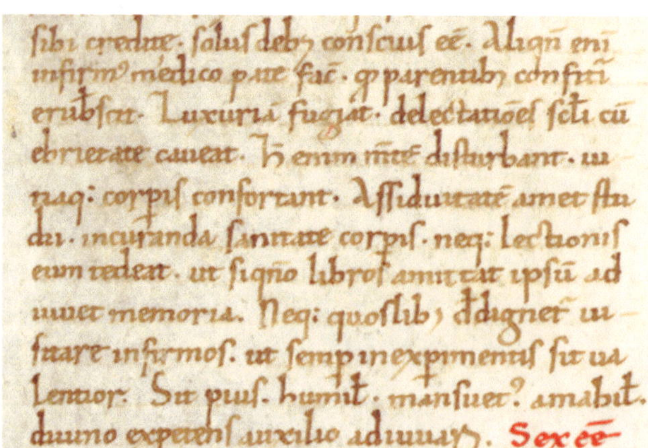

Plate III.
The Caroline script of Geraldus, here copying the chapter on deontology, describing the ideal characteristics of a medical student. The Hague, Koninklijke Bibliotheek, MS 73 J 6, fol. 1v. Late 1070s–1080s (before 1086).

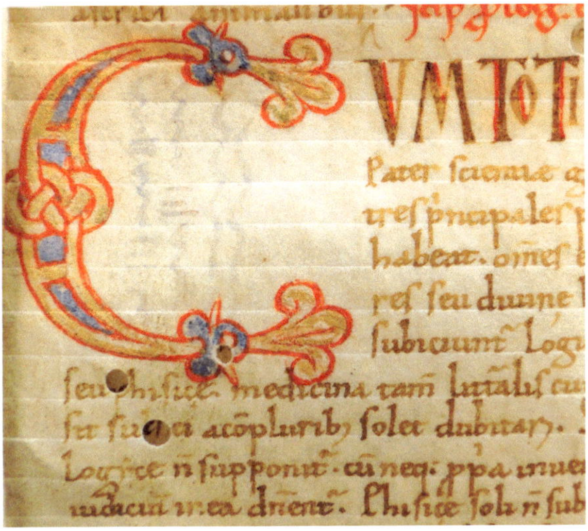

Plate IV.
Execution of the letters; the large initial C marks the beginning of the body of Prologue Part B, based upon Isidore of Seville's three types of knowledge: *logica*, *aethica*, and *physica*. The Hague, Koninklijke Bibliotheek, MS 73 J 6, fol. 1[r] (detail). Late 1070s–early 1080s (before 1086).

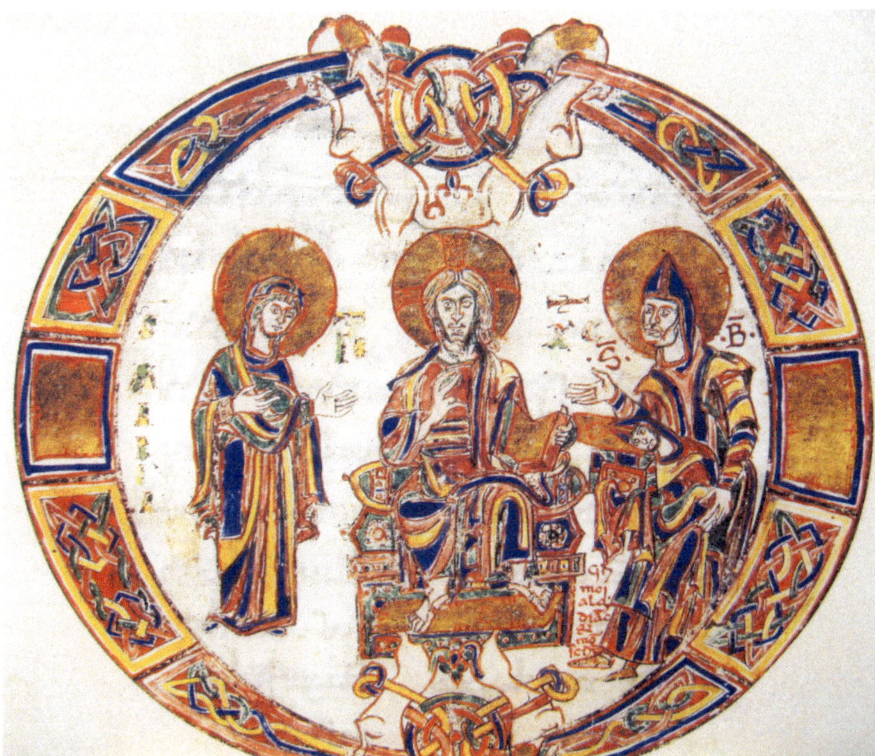

Plate V. Decorated initial O showing the enthroned Christ. Grimoald the scribe, with his golden shoes, shelters beneath the arm of St Benedict on the right. He self-identifies in the inscription, 'Grimoald, deacon and monk, the scribe'. Monte Cassino, Archivio della Badia, MS 109, p. 295. *c.* 1075– *c.* 1100.

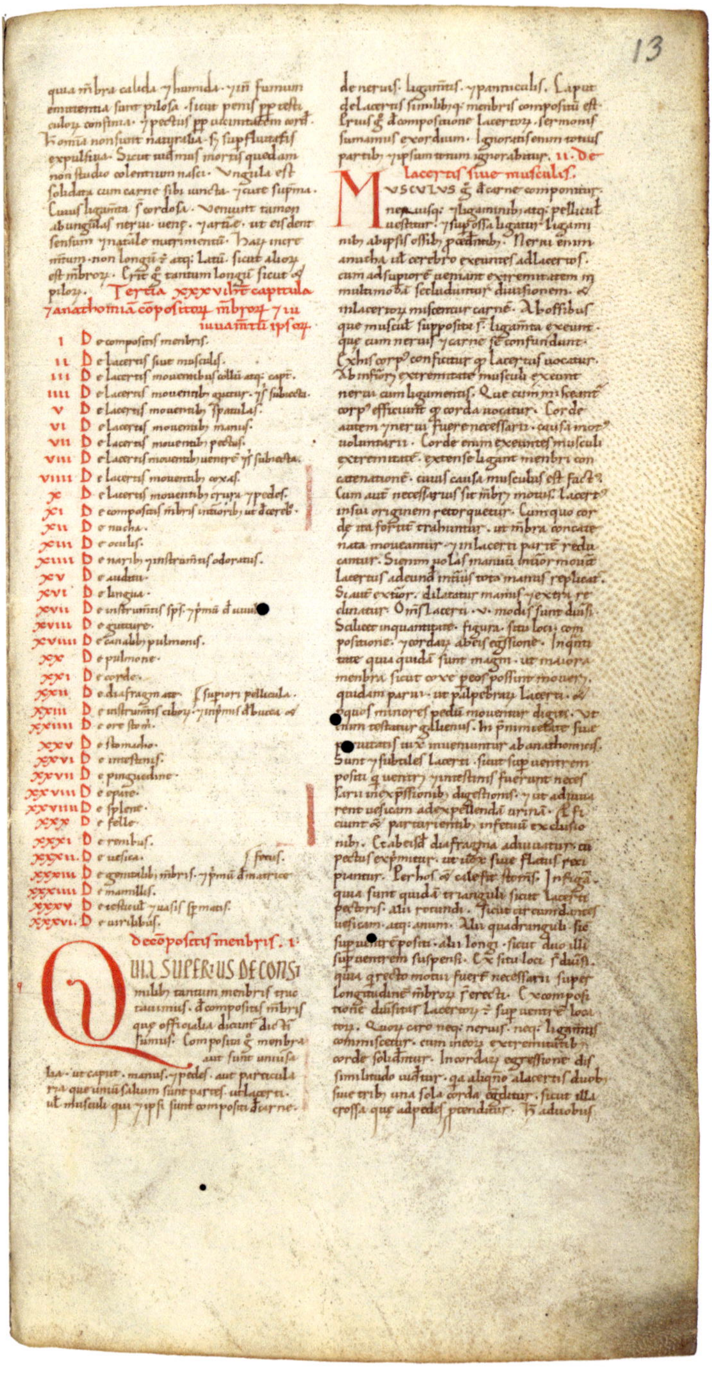

Plate VI.
Page with different types of rubrication in col. A (numbers in the *capitula* list, rubrics, initials), The Hague, Koninklijke Bibliotheek, MS 73 J 6, fol. 13r (*Theorica Pantegni*, beginning of Book III, detail). Late 1070s–early 1080s (before 1086).

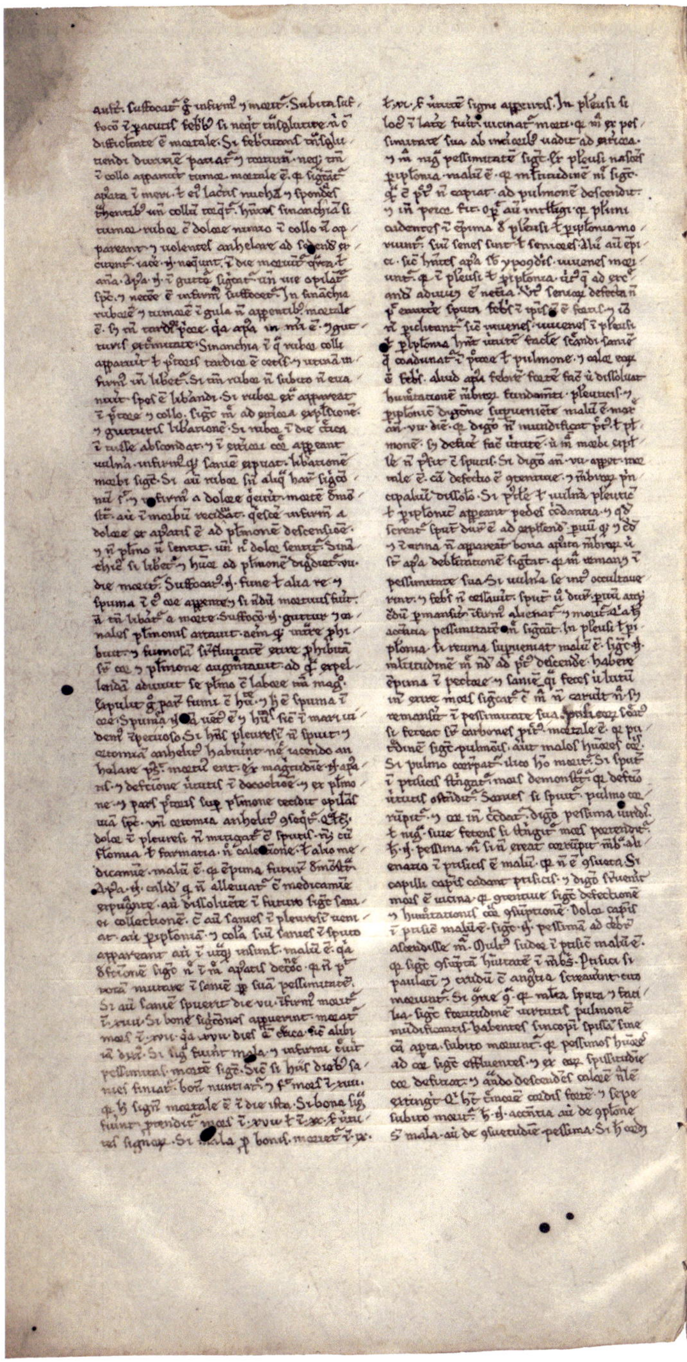

Plate VII.
First page of Scribe C, who completed this abandoned manuscript of the *Pantegni*.
The Hague, Koninklijke Bibliotheek, MS 73 J 6, fol. 85v.
c. 1150–*c.* 1200.

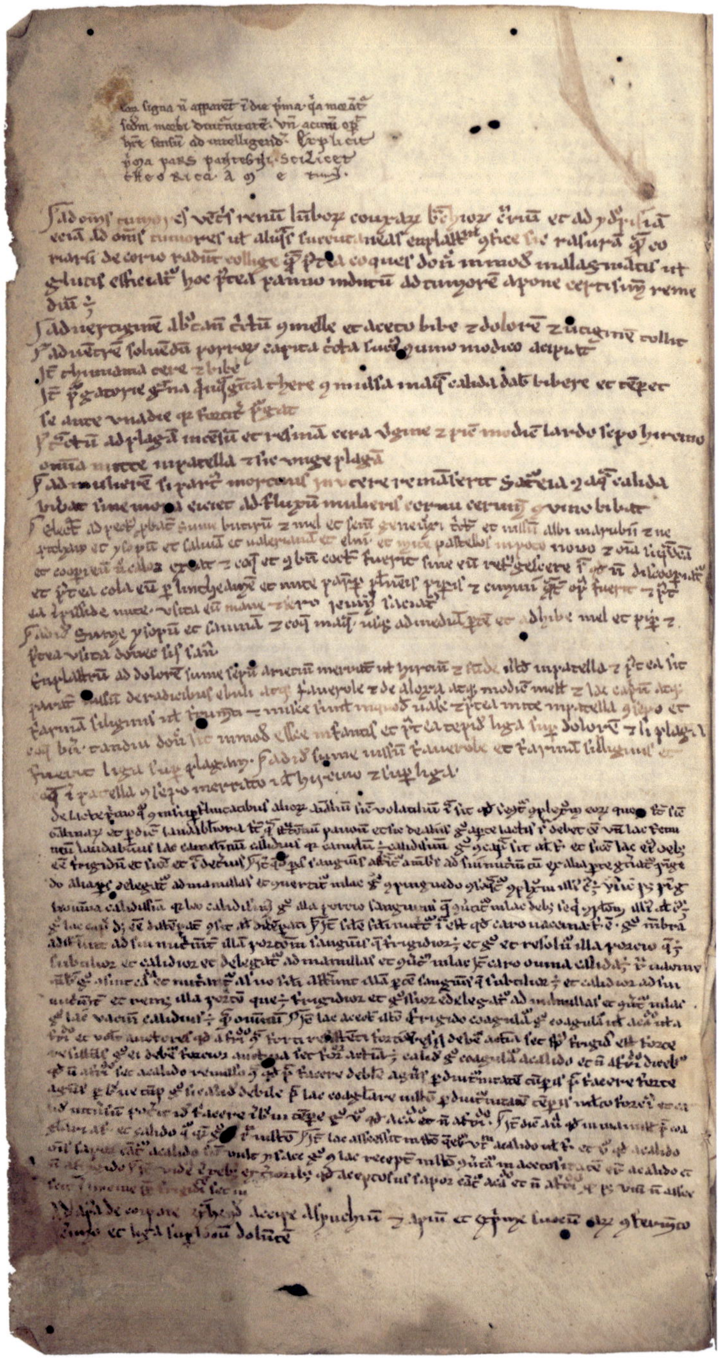

Plate VIII.
Following the *explicit* of *the* Theorica by Scribe C (top, col. A), the rest of the page is filled with excerpts by Scribe D. The Hague, Koninklijke Bibliotheek, MS 73 J 6, fol. 87v. *Explicit* and excerpts, *c.* 1150–*c.* 1200

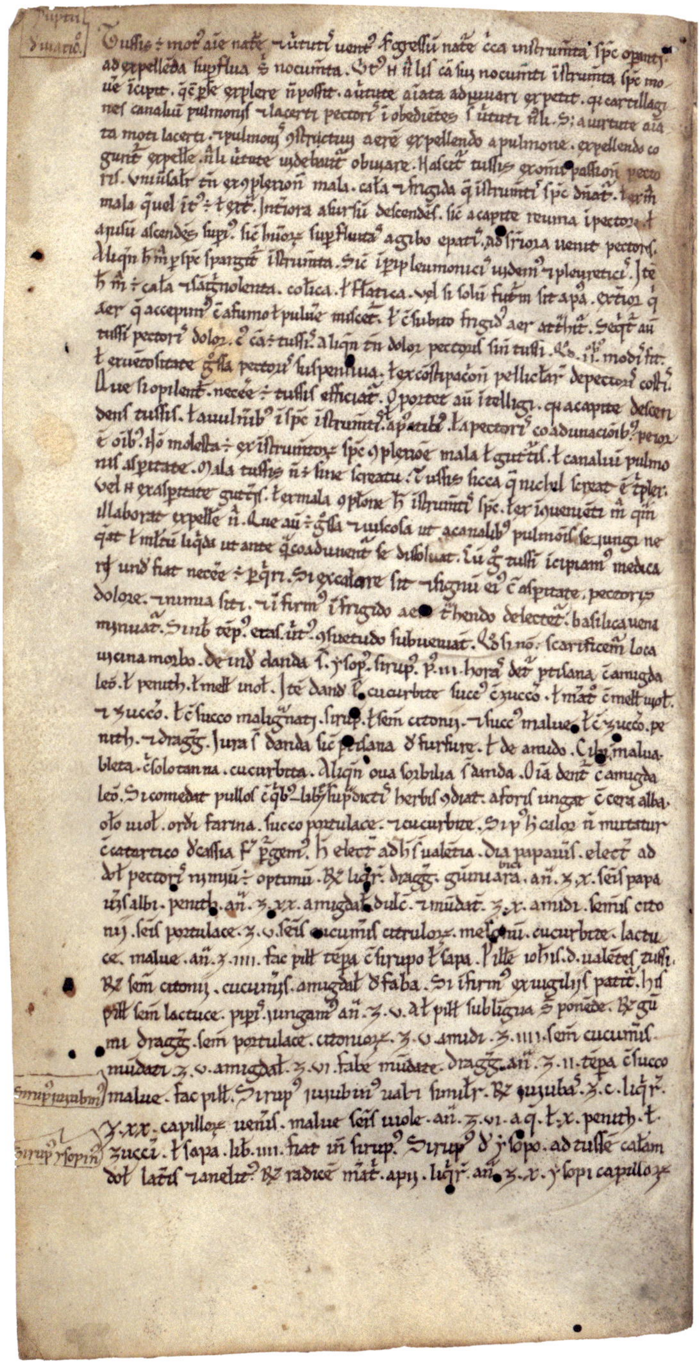

Plate IX.
Second page of medieval excerpts copied by Scribe E, containing the first part of *Viaticum* Book III, Chapter 6, 'De tussi'. The Hague, Koninklijke Bibliotheek, MS 73 J 6, fol. iv. *c.* 1150–*c.* 1175.

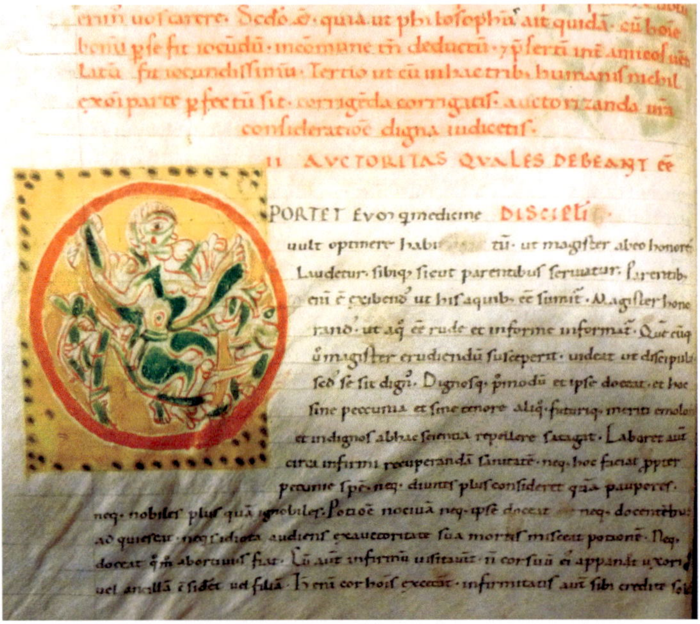

Plate X. Prologue of the Paris *Pantegni*, Paris, Bibliothèque nationale de France, Latin 6887, fol. 1[v]. *c.* 1100– *c.* 1125.

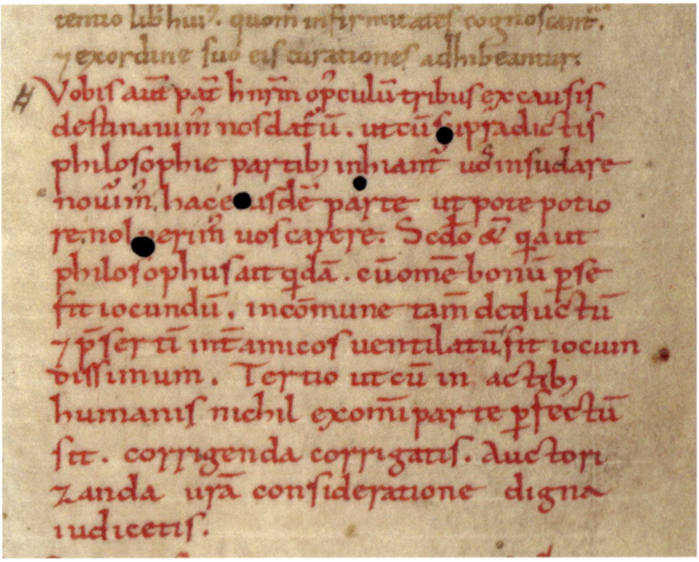

Plate XI. Script of the Hague Rubricator, a.k.a. Scribe B, writing Prologue Part C. Late 1070s–1080s (before 1086). In the lowest line, Scribe C gives the rubric to Chapter 2, the authority of Hippocrates on what type of persons medical students should be (*c.* 1150–*c.* 1200). The Hague, Koninklijke Bibliotheek, MS 73 J 6, fol. 1[r] (detail).

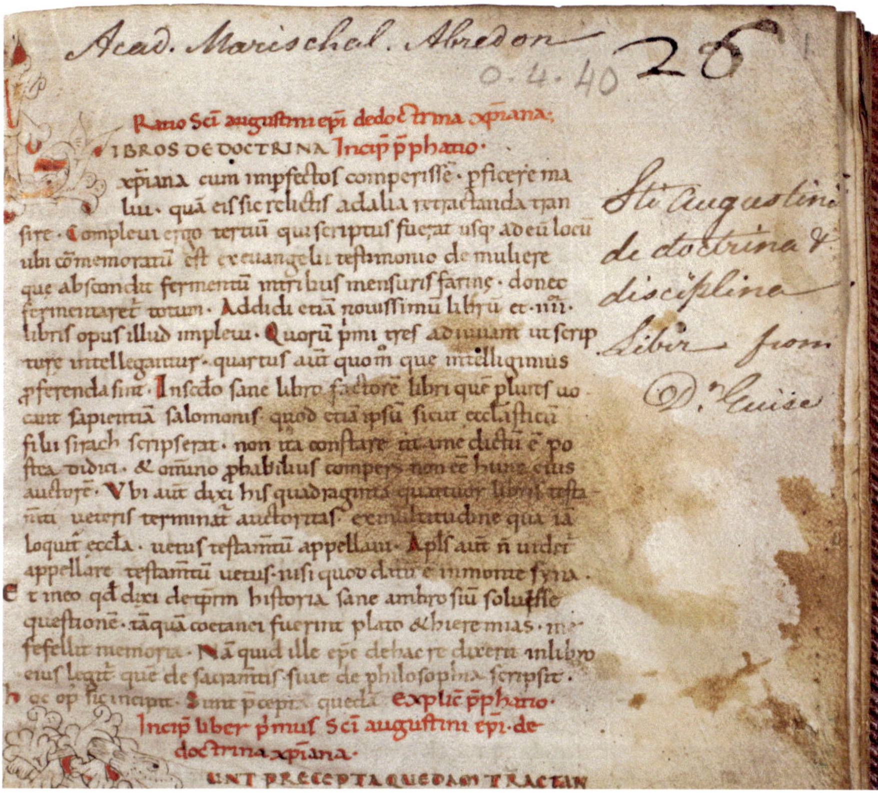

Plate XII. Hand of the Hague Rubricator, Aberdeen, University Library, MS 106, fol. 1r. *c.* 1075–*c.* 1100. Augustine, *De doctrina Christiana*.

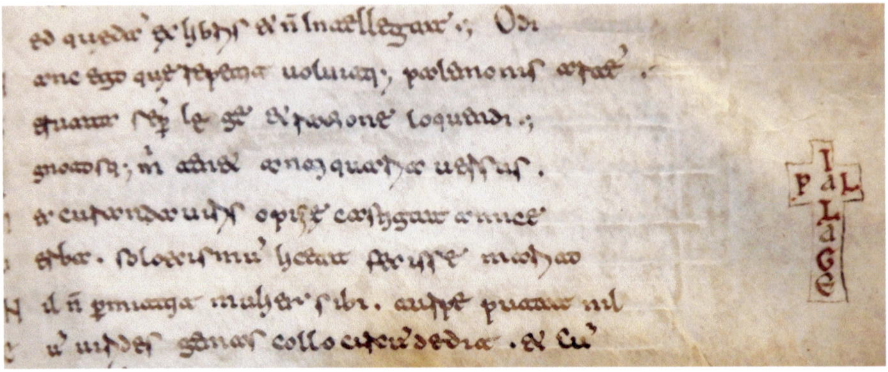

Plate XIII. Hand of the Bodleian Juvenal Scribe, entering in alternating red and black and in a cross-shape, the rhetorical figure 'IPALLAGE' (= HYPALLAGE) in the margin of Juvenal's *Satires*, Oxford, Bodleian Library, MS Canon. Class. lat. 41, fol. 23r. *c.* 1075–*c.* 1100. Reproduced with the permission of the Bodleian Library.

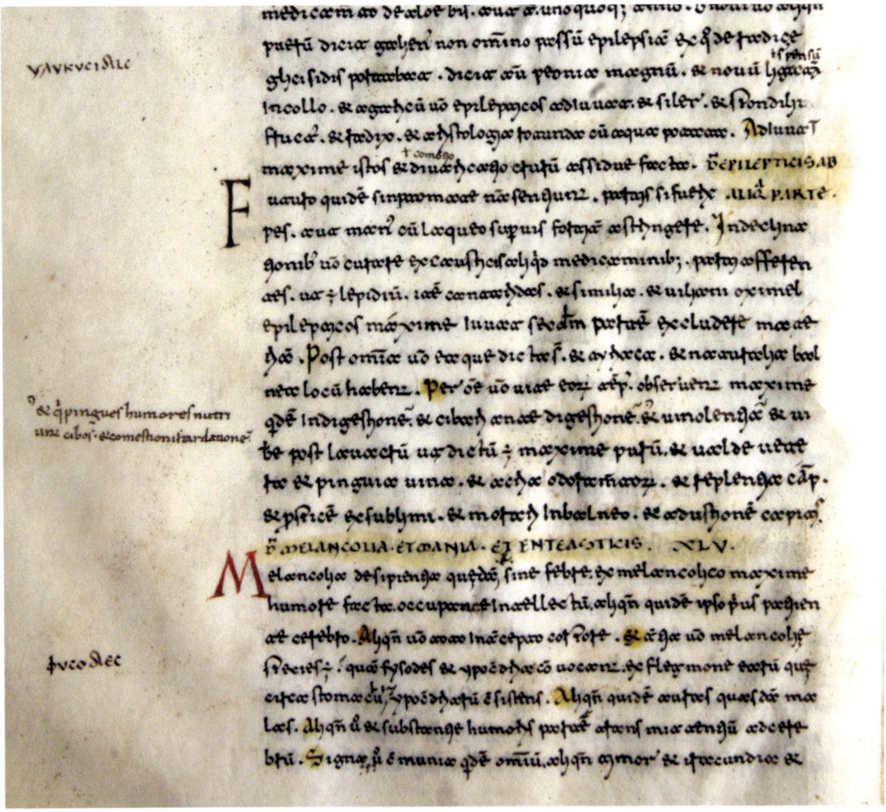

Plate XIV. Hand of the Bodleian Juvenal Scribe writing in Greek (upper and lower marginal gloss), the main text (Paul of Aegina) in Latin, and the Latin correction (left margin, centre), Monte Cassino, Archivio della Badia, MS 351, p. 19. *c.* 1075–*c.* 1100.

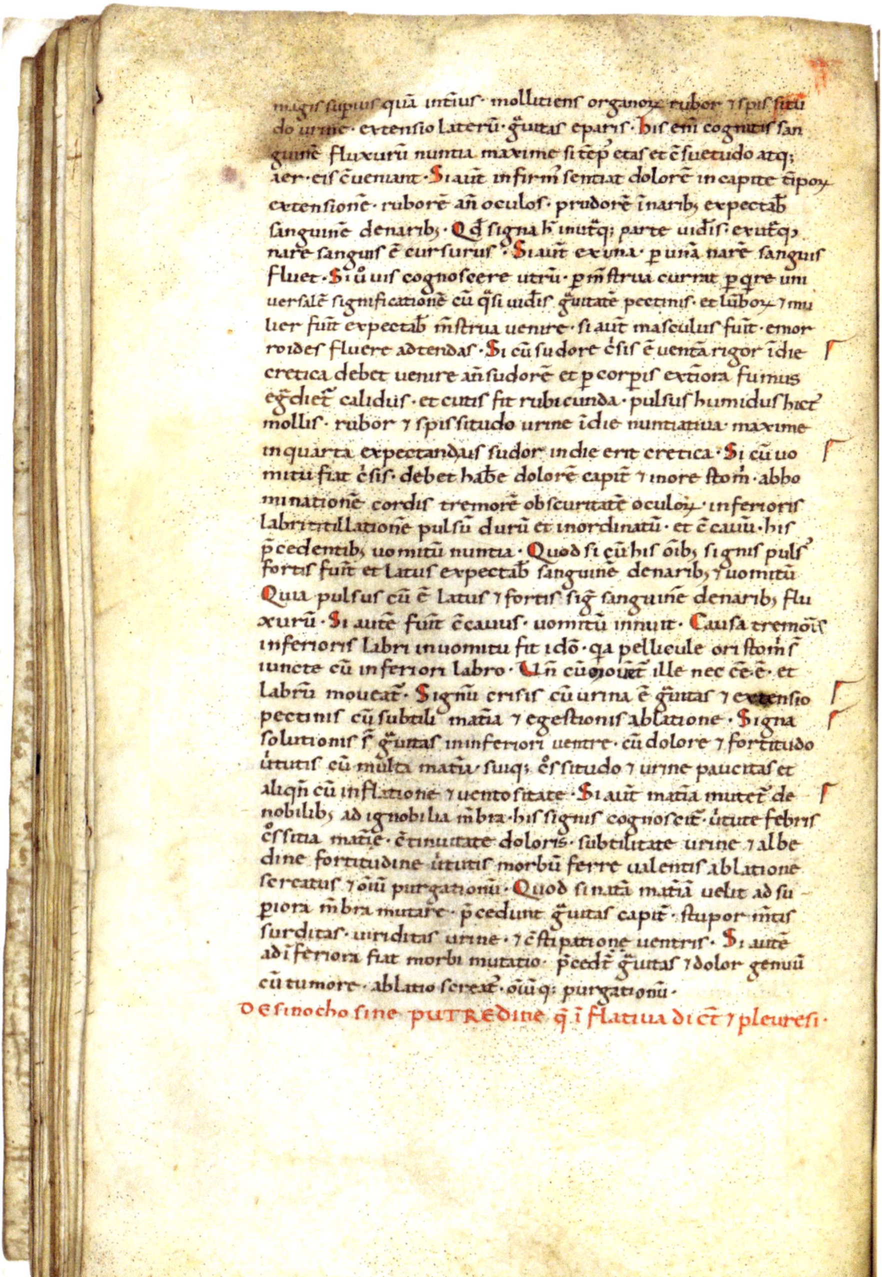

Plate XV. Hand of the Hague Rubricator, Padua, Biblioteca Universitaria, lat. 892, fol. 32v. *c.* 1075– *c.* 1100. *De febribus.*

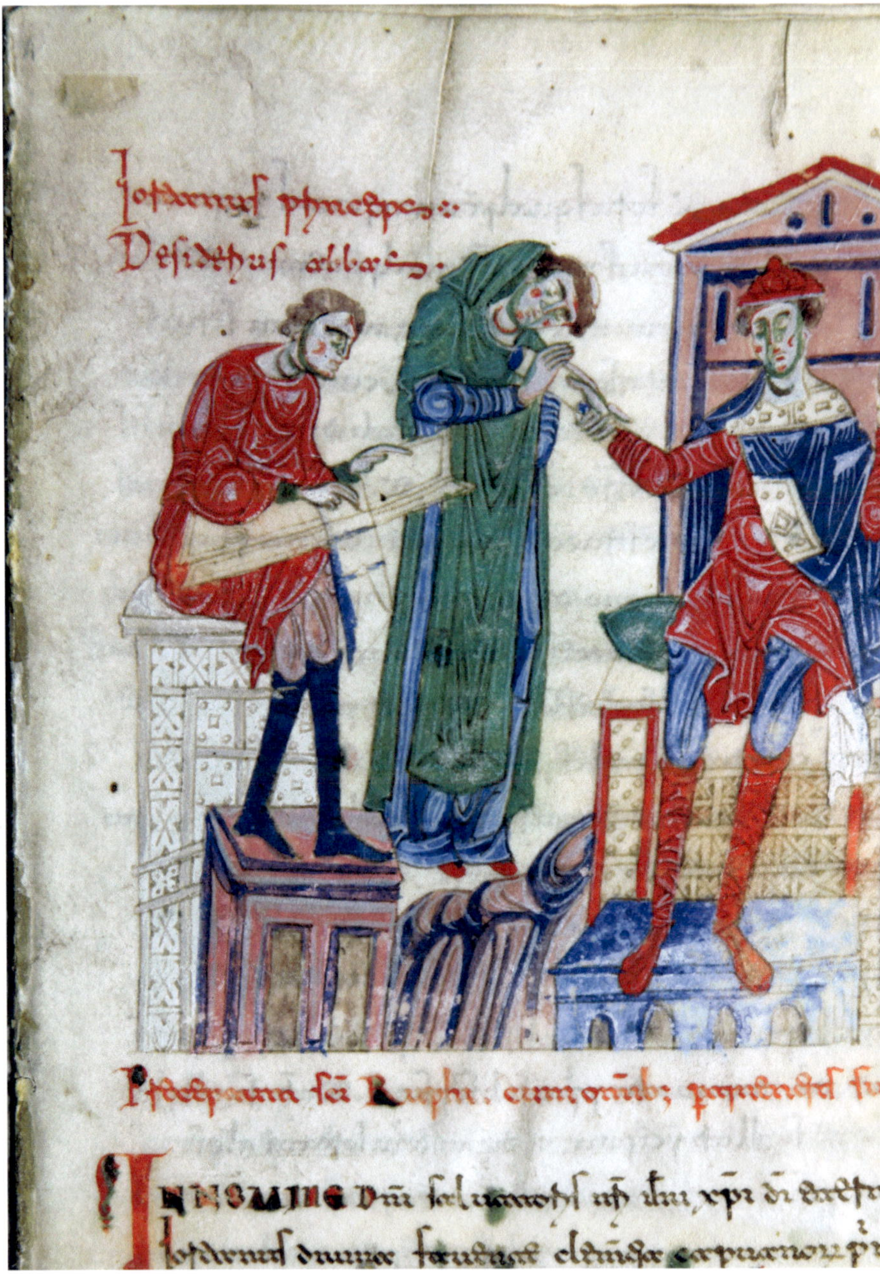

Plate XVI. In the miniature Prince Jordan of Capua (right) presents a donation to Abbot Desiderius of Monte Cassino (centre), as a lay scribe (left) takes down the terms of the gift c. 1100–1150. The Register of Sant'Angelo in Formis. Monte Cassino, Archivio della Badia, Regesto 4.

Preface

This book celebrates one manuscript and one translator. The manuscript in question is The Hague, Koninklijke Bibliotheek, MS 73 J 6 (hereafter 'the Hague manuscript' or 'MS 73 J 6'), which contains a Latin translation and adaptation of the Arabic *Kitāb Kāmil aṣ-ṣināʿa aṭ-ṭibbīya* (*Complete Book of the Medical Art*) written by the Persian physician ʿAli ibn al-ʿAbbās al-Maǧūsī (d. 982).[1] Echoing al-Maǧūsī's title, the title of the translated Latin work was *Pantegni* (Greek for *The Complete Art*). The translator and adaptor of this text was Constantine the African, who entered the Abbey of Monte Cassino in *c.* 1077 and died there before 1099 (fig. i). The text of the *Pantegni* in the Hague manuscript was copied between 1077 and 1086, and that same book, MS 73 J 6, though incomplete, is the oldest surviving copy of the text, as this monograph demonstrates.

This medical encyclopaedia, both humane and scientific, was a learned resource of a kind never before known in the Latin West. It stands in particularly stunning contrast to the medicine known in medieval Europe down to this moment in the late eleventh century. Its unique character can be seen on the first leaf of the Hague manuscript. On the recto, the central section of the Prologue discusses briefly the new, preferred pharmacopoeia including, for example, the Arabic 'iulab' (our 'julep'). On the verso, the text of the encyclopaedia proper opens with the ancient, noble words of Hippocrates, under the heading, 'Auctoritas Hippocratis. Quales debeant esse discipuli' (A passage from Hippocrates. The character that students [of medicine] should possess). It is one version of the famous Hippocratic 'Horkos' (Oath).

[1] The Hague manuscript is digitized in its entirety at <https://www.kb.nl/en/themes/medieval-manuscripts/liber-pantegni> [accessed 1 February 2019].

The Hague volume is a crucially important manuscript, a treasure in the history of medicine, the history of translation, and the transfer of knowledge. Yet it must be stated at once that this priceless volume presents a wide range of enigmas.

1. A manuscript contemporary to the lifetime of Constantine, whose home in Europe was first Salerno, and then Monte Cassino, might logically be expected to have been produced in that region. Both centres lay in the Beneventan script zone. Beneventan, the dominant type of script in South Italy from the eighth century through the twelfth century, was overwhelmingly — as far as is heretofore known — the book script of Monte Cassino in the period of Constantine's residence there. Could the Hague manuscript, in Caroline script throughout, have been produced in that house?

2. The name 'Pantegni' does not appear at the opening of the Hague manuscript. In fact, there is no title or incipit of any kind on its first page, where one should indeed stand, nor is the reader given the name of the author. Why these strange absences?

3. The Prologue to the work, on fol. 1ʳ, is in three parts. Parts A and B are in the hand of the text that follows, but Part C, for which space had been left on this first page at the bottom of the second column, is written in a different but contemporary hand, and — even more strange — in red ink (see fig. 1.1 and pl. I). Was the text then produced by more than one person? If so, who were these various individuals? And what were their respective roles?

4. In connection with the possibility of multiple authors, a close examination of the Prologue's red Part C reveals a very different style of Latin. In fact, of the three parts of the Prologue, Parts A and C are elaborate and highly rhetorical in character, while Part B is factual and straightforward. What does this tell us about the process of this text's creation? Already it appears on fol. 1ʳ that what we have before our eyes is a text-in-the-making, an accretive process captured in this manuscript.

5. The text of the *Pantegni* in MS 73 J 6 is marked by a number of blank spaces scattered throughout. There are nine of them, from the first section of the book to the last. What is the meaning of these textual lacunae?

6. At fol. 78ʳ, the original rubricator left off his work; the remaining incipits and chapter titles had to be added by a subsequent scribe. Why this interruption?

7. At the foot of the second column of fol. 85ʳ, at the end of the last line, the text of the original hand breaks off mid-sentence. As a result, for complete-

ness the text of the last five pages of the *Theorica Pantegni*, starting with the continuation of the severed sentence at the top of fol. 85^{v}, had to be filled in by another hand. This happened a century later, and none of the *Practica* was ever added. Why was the text abandoned, and so abruptly, mid-sentence?

8. The very shape of the Hague manuscript is unusual. Its long, narrow format distinguishes it as dedicated to some special purpose. What can the very dimensions tell us about the book and the intent of its makers?

9. More broadly, what do these aspects of MS 73 J 6, the oldest manuscript of the *Pantegni*, suggest about its relationship to some other early manuscripts of this text? Specifically, if this earliest, and therefore incomparably valuable, book shows the text still in process of completion, what of the next oldest manuscript? Does its text show a resolution of the incomplete aspects of the Hague volume?

10. Lastly, a parallel and paradoxical problem: at least one or two manuscripts, though younger than the Hague manuscript, preserve a version of the text that is older. As has been noted, the Hague volume contains a text that shows stages of development. A very small number of manuscripts however, while copied at least a half-century after the Hague one (such as a copy of the *Pantegni* preserved today in Erfurt), nevertheless contain a text showing an earlier stage of development than does the Hague manuscript. What can this earlier text-stage tell us about the history of the creation of Constantine's *Pantegni*?

Such are the puzzling questions that the present monograph addresses. In studying them, it is our conclusion that MS 73 J 6, while in Caroline script, was in fact produced at Monte Cassino during the lifetime of Constantine himself. In all, Constantine produced at least twenty-four and perhaps as many as thirty-four translations, and the Hague manuscript demonstrates how he managed to be so prolific.[2] It is an exceptionally important manuscript. As will become clear, the Hague codex bears evidence of a team of scribes and scholars who

[2] The lower number is that given in Peter the Deacon's *De viris illustribus*, reproduced in Bloch, *Monte Cassino in the Middle Ages*, pp. 127–34. The higher number has been suggested as a possibility by Monica Green in papers delivered at Ohio State University's Texts and Contexts conference in November 2014, and Kalamazoo's International Medieval Congress in May 2016. For a list of thirty works attributed to Constantine, including bibliography, see 'Constantinus Africanus' on SISMEL's Mirabile Web. Actually, the present study adds another work, the *Isagoge*, to the list of Constantine's translations; see pp. 92–93. Even twenty-four translations represent a considerable undertaking, especially for a mature author living in a foreign land.

helped the translator in various stages of production. To draw out this information, the present study combines textual and historical observations with physical (codicological and palaeographical) evidence from the Hague manuscript and other codices from Monte Cassino.

After the Introduction, which provides the necessary historical background as well as the known facts related to Constantine and his translation activity, Chapter 1 presents the main scribe of the Hague manuscript, Geraldus. Among surviving manuscripts from Monte Cassino, a handful of others copied by this Geraldus are identified through a comparative palaeographical study. These identifications also introduce us to some of Geraldus's fellow monks who form a team that was actively involved in the production of medical manuscripts in the scriptorium of Monte Cassino. Chapter 2 examines codicological aspects of MS 73 J 6 to shed light on Constantine's translation practices: lacunae in the text suggest that the text was left in a revision stage. Chapter 3 introduces the individuals who helped Constantine the African produce his translations. This 'Team Constantine' consists of scribes and scholars, and their activities allow us to reconstruct some of the logistics of producing such a high volume of translations. Chapter 4 focuses on a peculiar codicological aspect of MS 73 J 6: its narrow proportions. Here it is argued that the manuscript was made for use in the classroom, providing evidence that medical teaching was undertaken at the abbey at a sophisticated level.

Finally, Chapter 5 addresses the broader implications of identifying a manuscript from the 'desk' of Constantine the African. It queries how the manuscript contributes to our understanding of the professional biography of the translator. Here perhaps the most surprising implication is introduced: contrary to previous assumptions, the Hague manuscript and its unfinished text suggest that Constantine did not start working on his *Pantegni* within the walls of Monte Cassino, but rather appears to have brought a well-advanced translation with him when he entered the abbey. This earlier text, Chapter 5 shows, survives in a manuscript in Erfurt. In other words, certain observations invite us to consider that Constantine was already working on his ground-breaking text, and some further medical translations, while in Salerno.

The present book, then, proposes solutions to the enigmatic and even mysterious aspects of Hague MS 73 J 6, chapter by chapter. It shows us how known scribes, translators, and assistants, with variant drafts of texts written on different substrates and preserved in different surviving manuscripts could, in pursuit of the goal of completing what their great patrons clearly recognized was a revolutionary product in the history of Latin knowledge, struggle with an extremely challenging set of problems. The problems are complex, though the evidence is abundant, and to the eye of experts, quite clear. This book captures and explicates one stage in a process that has been widely hailed as a fundamental watershed in Western scientific knowledge: the point at which medical knowledge inherited from the Greeks, almost entirely lost to the Latin West but transmitted so faithfully by the Islamic world, reached Latin readers in Europe and became comprehensible. The history of ideas was utterly transformed.

Erik Kwakkel and Francis Newton
February 2018

Abbreviations

BAV	Vatican City, Biblioteca Apostolica Vaticana
Berlin, SBPK	Berlin, Staatsbibliothek zu Berlin –Preussischer Kulturbesitz
BM	Bibliothèque municipale
Brussels, KBR	Brussels, Koninklijke Bibliotheek van België/ Bibliothèque royale de Belgique
Copenhagen, KB, GKS	Copenhagen, Kongelige Bibliotek, Gamle Kongelige Samling
Florence, Laurenziana	Florence, Biblioteca Medicea Laurenziana
The Hague, KB	The Hague, Koninklijke Bibliotheek
London, BL	London, British Library
Monte Cassino, MS	Monte Cassino, Archivio della Badia, MS
NAL	Nouvelle acquisition latine
Oxford, Bodleian	Oxford, Bodleian Library
Paris, BnF	Paris, Bibliothèque nationale de France
SB	Stiftsbibliothek
UB	Universiteitsbibliotheek
UL	University Library

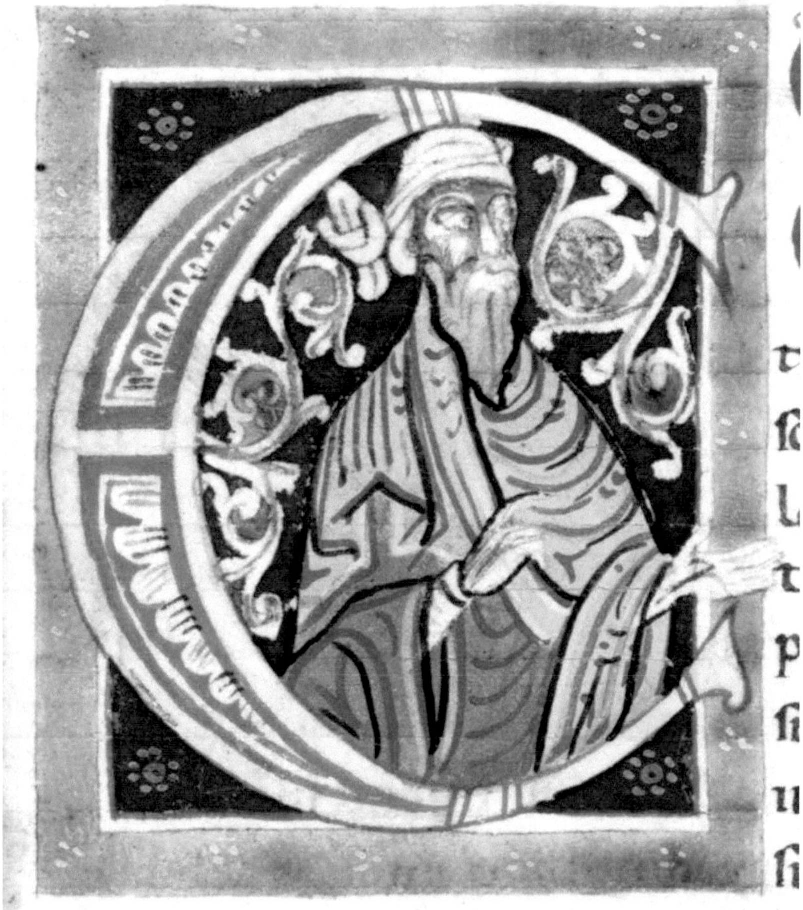

Figure i. Portrait of Constantine the African, or of the Arabic author who was his source. Erfurt, Universitätsbibliothek, Bibliotheca Amploniana, Cod. Amplon. 4° 184, fol. 2r. Italy, 1147.

Introduction: Constantine the African and the *Pantegni* in Context

Eliza Glaze*

The Career of Constantine

There are three distinct sources for the life and career of Constantine.[1] The oldest is the account preserved in the *Chronica monasterii Casinensis* (*Chronicle of Monte Cassino*) and was probably written by Guido, monk of that house, in the years just after 1100.[2] This impeccable account must be carefully distinguished from the version produced by Peter the Deacon, who was active around the middle of the twelfth century, in chapter 23 of his *De viris illustribus*. Peter's rewriting is helpful in that it contains a few additional titles in its list of Constantine's oeuvre, but it is seriously marred by romantic and even sensational elaborations, the products of Peter's fervid imagination. The second distinct source is from Salerno; it is embedded in a commentary on Constantine's translation of Isaac Israeli's *Dietae universales*, written by Magister Mattheus F[errarius] of Salerno,

* The present Introduction has, at its foundation, many years of conversations between colleagues both near and far, as well as papers, and the discussion of papers, that we have shared at meetings and conferences since 2010. Francis Newton's long-standing interest in medical texts of the Beneventan zone is manifest in his published scholarship. Much of the inspiration for the present Introduction is therefore the consequence of Professor Newton's scholarly expertise and his abundant generosity in discussing possible scenarios about Constantine, Monte Cassino, and Salerno with his colleagues. Needless to say, Constantine, his milieux, and his long-term influence has also been a topic of great interest. This Introduction, however, aims to provide a suitable context for this book's analysis of the Hague *Pantegni* and its genesis.

[1] These are found, in English translation by Francis Newton, in Appendix B of this monograph. A schematic representation of their contents is presented in table *i*.

[2] The attribution to Guido is part of the argument, based on fresh examination of the Monte Cassino sources, in Chapter 3.

and preserved in Erfurt, Universitätsbibliothek, Bibliotheca Amploniana, Cod. Amplon. 8° 62. This contains valuable information from the Salernitan perspective. The third source is the exciting and colourful account surviving in a thirteenth-century manuscript in London (BL, MS Sloane 2426), first published by Charles Singer,[3] which fancifully makes Constantine not an African but a Cordoban; as its major points of reference are Cordoba and Montpellier, it is here called the Cordoba–Montpellier tradition.

Imitating the sober style of Guido, the chronicler of Monte Cassino, we rehearse briefly the salient facts of Constantine's story. Born in Carthage (modern Tunis), he was educated in 'Babilonia', that is, Old Cairo (Fusṭāṭ). His learning included extensive medical training, and certainly encompassed detailed knowledge of the pharmacopoeia of contemporary Islamic culture of the Middle East and beyond. Returning to Ifrīqya, he encountered in his native land conditions quite unfavourable, and perhaps even dangerous, to learning and intellectual pursuits. He escaped and made his way to Salerno. There he lived in obscurity for some time before being recognized, as both the *Chronicle of Monte Cassino* and the Salernitan Master Mattheus F[errarius] assert, by one 'frater principis' (the brother of the prince),[4] who then accepted him into elite and honourable society. This 'brother of the prince' was the learned Abbot Johannes de Curte. In Salerno Constantine would have also known the famous Archbishop Alfanus. Moreover, the Monte Cassino source says that he became a friend of Robert Guiscard, who conquered Salerno and ousted the last Lombard prince, Gisulf II, in 1076/7. It seems that the first of these contacts combined, in a fashion that must have been frequent, the secular and the ecclesiastical.

From Salerno Constantine made his way to Monte Cassino, was warmly received by Abbot Desiderius, and abandoned secular life to become a monk. A stunning anomaly is that (according to the *Chronicle of Monte Cassino*) he arrived at the abbey with an endowment created for him by the rulers of Capua, Prince Richard and his son Prince Jordan, and by Jordan's wife Gaitelgrima.

[3] Singer, 'A Legend of Salerno'.

[4] The *Chronicle of Monte Cassino* account identifies 'the brother of the prince' as 'the brother of the king of the Babylonians'. Mattheus F[errarius] says that this turning point was the recognition of Constantine's medical expertise by an 'abbas', the 'brother of the prince of Salerno [Gisulf II]', who was Johannes de Curte. The two accounts tell the same story and thus confirm one another, but, understandably, the local Salernitan account provides the correct identification.

Death came to Constantine at a great age at Monte Cassino before the end of the century (specifically, no later than 1098/99).

To return to the question of sources, translations of which can be found in this volume's Appendix B, the salient features of the three biographies can be summed up in the table on the following page (Table i). It is argued here that these three biographies confirm and correct one another in discrete details, and considered together, create a coherent narrative that helps us understand the trajectory of Constantine's career. Certainly they agree upon key elements of the story: Constantine's great learning, his mastery of medical knowledge, and his enjoyment of the patronage of local elites. They also point to his arrival from North Africa at the port city of Salerno by the time of, or perhaps prior to, the conquest of that city by Robert Guiscard in 1076/7, his subsequent relocation to Monte Cassino where he became a monk, and his death.

Background: North Africa

In order to evaluate the significance of Constantine's translation programme, and his efforts to introduce into Europe Latin renditions of many of the Islamic world's most important pieces of medical literature, it is first necessary to consider what Constantine's educational experience in his native North Africa might have been. One of the surest truths about learning and literature in Muslim lands is the extent to which scholars in the Islamic world inherited and expanded upon the classical tradition of Greek literature and learning. Indeed, Franz Rosenthal has shown both the depth and breadth of these scholars, who engaged in translation programmes of astonishing richness. Rosenthal charts successive generations' efforts to transmit the classical elements of logic, ethics, metaphysics, medicine, geometry, arithmetic, optics, geography, astronomy, musicology, mechanics, and literature. Translations of medical works produced in Islamic territories emphasized a variety of valued classical sub-genres; these included the importance of students acquiring a firm grasp of medical ethics and deontology, humoral pathology and medical theory, anatomy and pharmacology. Students needed to ground themselves equally in both theory and practice.[5]

[5] Rosenthal, *The Classical Heritage in Islam*. See also Pormann and Savage-Smith, *Medieval Islamic Medicine*, chaps 1–4; Ullmann, *Islamic Medicine*, chap. 2; Jacquart and Micheau, *La médecine arabe et l'occident médiéval*.

Table i. Narrative elements in the biographies of Constantine the African.

Origin	Reason for departing North Africa	Reason for arriving in South Italy	Patronage
Monte Cassino biographies[6]			
Carthage	Fellow Africans wanted to kill him out of envy of his learning	None given	Robert Guiscard and Richard, prince of Capua
Salerno biography by Mattheus F[errarius][7]			
None given, but a 'Sarracenus' (Saracen) and a 'mercator' (merchant) who did not speak or understand Latin	None given, but travelled to Salerno 'quia mercationis causa huc venit' (for the sake of trade)	'quia mercationis causa huc venit, et multas mercationes secum attulit' (He came here for the sake of trade and brought considerable trading goods with him)	Johannes, 'abbas de curia' (abbot of the court); Archbishop Alfanus of Salerno
Cordoba-Montpellier biography[8]			
Cordoba (no mention of Africa)	Fled the consequences of his near-fatal effort to treat the king of Cordoba	Captured and enslaved by pirates; sold to a tanner	The king of Cordoba, and later, the 'princeps Salerni' (the prince of Salerno)

But how was medical knowledge and expertise acquired, and what constituted medical wisdom in Constantine's day within the great cities of his

[6] Peter the Deacon's *De viris illustribus* and the *Chronicle of Monte Cassino*: see parallel columns in Bloch, *Monte Cassino in the Middle Ages*, pp. 127–34. Of the two, the account of Peter the Deacon is the lengthier and more detailed, but also the more fantastic. See Francis Newton's translations of these two accounts in the present volume's Appendix B: I. The Monte Cassino Tradition (in Two Forms), Cas. 1 and Cas. 2.

[7] This 'Salerno biography' is found in Erfurt, Universitätsbibliothek, Bibliotheca Amploniana, Cod. Amplon. 8° 62. It is transcribed and translated by Francis Newton in the present volume's Appendix B: II. A Salernitan Tradition (see pp. 199–200).

[8] The 'Cordoba-Montpellier biography' is found in London, BL, MS Sloane 2426. See Francis Newton's translation of this account in the present volume's Appendix B: III. An Account from Cordoba and Montpellier, Sloane.

eligion	Profession
Jnclear, but became a monk fter arriving at Monte assino 'ad hunc locum erveniens sancteque habitum eligionis' (coming to this lace and donning the habit f the religious life)	'egrediens Babiloniam petiit, in qua grammatica dialectica, geometria, arithmetica, mathematica, astronomia nec non in phisica Chaldeorum, Arabum, Persarum, Saracenorum, Egiptiorum ac Indorum plenissime eruditus est' ([In] Babilonia [Old Cairo], [...] he received a thorough education in grammar, dialectic, geometry, arithmetic, mathematics, [and] astronomy, as well as in the medicine of the Chaldaeans, Arabs, Persians, Saracens, Egyptians, and Indians)[9]
onstantinus autem arracenus exstitit' (Now onstantine was a Saracen)	'mercator tamen [...] Qui per interpretes cognoscens ipsum in medicina satis valere, per interpretes eius querebat de colore de sustantia urinae, et in omnibus de urinis bene responderet.' Constantine was a merchant whom the abbot of the court (learning through the interpreters that the man himself [Constantine] had considerable competence in medicine, asked him through his interpreters about the colour and consistency of the urine; and in all respects he answered well regarding the urine specimens)
Iuslim, but in Salerno actus est et Christianus, et ostea Montis Cassinensis onachus' (he became a hristian, and afterwards a onk of Monte Cassino)	Physician-student of 'Alboansardi Cordubensis, qui *Pantegni* composuit' (Albansoardus of Cordoba, who composed the *Pantegni*). He earned recognition in Salerno as a captive by treating the prince successfully and earning widespread fame: 'curatur [...] et princeps. Deinde ubique terrarum famosus' (then a cure [...] was worked upon the prince. After that, Constantine was renowned all over the world)

native Ifrīqya? Recent studies affirm that there were two primary routes to the mastery of medical literature: apprenticeship as a student guided by a master (sometimes a senior family member), or self-mastery through independent study. It seems that formal medical training within an institutional framework like a *madrasah* was rare, and unknown prior to the thirteenth century. Such efforts could be supplemented through training within hospitals, or by attending public demonstrations and debates known as 'majālis'.[10] It is certainly pos-

[9] Peter the Deacon's account added rhetoric, music, and necromancy to his curriculum.

[10] Pormann and Savage-Smith, *Medieval Islamic Medicine*, pp. 80–85. Examples of famous physicians and medical writers who trained by these methods are explored by Leiser, 'Medical Education in Islamic Lands'.

sible that Constantine acquired his familiarity with medical literature either through auto-didacticism or by some combination of these methods.

It is no accident that many of the texts Constantine later translated into Latin were the products of North African physicians.[11] Chief among these was the tenth-century author Ibn al-Ǧazzār, who is said to have studied medicine in Qayrawān under Isaac Israeli. Constantine translated Ibn al-Ǧazzār's comprehensive medical handbook for travellers as the *Viaticum*, also producing shorter works from al-Ǧazzār's corpus on the degrees (powers) of medicines, on leprosy, and the *De coitu* on sexual intercourse.[12] Constantine also produced a number of translations from the texts of Ibn al-Ǧazzār's mentor, Isaac Israeli (Isḥaq ibn Sulaymān al-Isrāʾīlī, a.k.a. Isaac Iudaeus), a Neoplatonic Jewish philosopher and medical practitioner who originally trained in Fusṭāṭ, and became court physician to the Aghlabids in Qayrawān early in the tenth century. Isaac's medical writings combined both philosophical and scientific traditions, including medical ethics.[13] From amongst Isaac's many writings, Constantine chose to translate several, producing the *De febribus*, *De urina*, *Dietae universales*, and *Dietae particulares*. A third author active in Tunisia was Isḥāq ibn Imrān, whose treatise on melancholy was rendered into Latin by Constantine as *De melancholia*. As Monica Green points out, the vast majority of Constantine's translations were authored by physicians active in North Africa, and especially in Qayrawān, in the tenth century.[14]

The focus of the present book, the *Pantegni*, was however not based upon a work by a North African author, but by ʿAlī ibn al-ʿAbbās al-Maǧūsī, who served, it seems, in distant Shiraz at the court of ʿAḍud al-Dawla.[15] All the same, Danielle Jacquart and Charles Burnett observe that it was 'not unlikely that Constantine would have found a copy [of al-Maǧūsī's great encyclopaedia] amongst the community of renowned doctors in Qayrawān'.[16] Similarly, by-then classic texts like the *Aphorisms* of Hippocrates, and Galen's *Methodus medendi* would have been widely available across the Islamic world, as would several essential texts produced in ninth-century Baghdad by Ḥunayn ibn

[11] What follows in the present paragraph is based upon Green, 'Constantine the African'.

[12] Wack, *Lovesickness in the Middle Ages*, especially pp. 34–35 on al-Ǧazzār.

[13] Simon, 'L'éthique médicale (Moussar ha-Rofim) d'Isaac Israeli'; Altmann and Stern, *Isaac Israeli*, pp. ix–xi.

[14] Green, 'Constantine the African'.

[15] Micheau, 'ʿAlī ibn al-ʿAbbās al-Magūsī', especially pp. 12–15.

[16] Burnett and Jacquart, 'Preface', p. vii.

Isḥāq.[17] It seems very likely then that Constantine the African's education, even if he studied under a master, also included the close study of the many texts he translated into Latin after arriving in South Italy in the second half of the eleventh century.

But if Ifrīqya was so rich in medical traditions and ready patronage, why would Constantine ever have felt the need to leave his homeland to become an exile in Italy? The biographies that recount Constantine's departure from North Africa and his arrival in South Italy indicate differing degrees of distress associated with the move: either the violence of his professional enemies at home, the arrival in a city where he did not speak the language, or a near-fatal accident in prescribing incorrect medicinal dosages for a royal patron. The answer, in all probability, is that Ifrīqya was no longer peaceful; the golden age of the tenth century in which medicine had prospered had passed, and a time of troubles had descended upon the region and its peoples.[18] Charles Dalli details the series of political and military crises that brought Ifrīqya and her people such grave distress. He describes how all of Ifrīqya fell prey to the consequences of the rebellious Zirid dynasty, against whom their Fatimid overlords in Cairo sent the invading tribesmen of the Banū Hilāl and Banū Sulaym. Qayrawān was destroyed in 1057, and in the words of Ibn Khaldūn, the enemy swept across the Maghreb like 'a swarm of locusts'.[19]

Although South Italy also experienced the steady incursions and a succession of Norman conquests, the fact that the Normans were arranging shipments of grain to North African ports by 1076 and making profitable trade agreements with the Zirids of Ifrīqya might have made Italy a tempting destination.[20] Indeed, Constantine may not have been alone by any means in

[17] On the evidence for the *Isagoge* as a product of Constantine's workshop, see Newton, 'Constantine the African', and following chapters in the present volume.

[18] This argument is advanced by Hettinger in her 'Zum Lebensgeschichte und zum Todesdatum des Constantinus Africanus'. Although Hettinger's premise is convincing, her dating of Constantine the African's death cannot be accepted. On this, see Newton 'Constantine the African', pp. 19 and 22.

[19] Dalli, 'Bridging Europe and Africa'; Brett, 'Ifriqiya as a Market for Saharan Trade'.

[20] Dalli, 'Bridging Europe and Africa', p. 78; Smith, 'Calamity and Transition'. Smith's outstanding article demonstrates that while Muslim and Jewish traders dominated the Mediterranean exchange in the tenth century, in the eleventh century the tide began to turn, and as the century progressed, the Italian republics assumed the lead in this exchange. By the twelfth century the reversal was complete, and the Italians were demanding and negotiating generous terms with Islamic (and Byzantine) governors.

departing Ifrīqya for safer lands.[21] Recent analysis of documents attesting the diaspora populations' reception in one region of Sicily reveals the presence of Muslim villeins and tenants, including teachers, an apothecary, needle-makers, and weavers, many of whom identified themselves in the records by the place names from which they had come, including several 'al-Ifrīqī', 'al-Tūnisī', and 'al-Itrābulusī' (modern Tripoli). It seems that in this time of troubles, there was a considerable diaspora from North Africa to Norman lands, where refugees accepted a decreased socio-economic status.[22] This exodus from Ifrīqya apparently persisted well into the twelfth century, and in the eleventh also included other medical practitioners; documents of the Abbey of La Trinità in Cava de' Tirreni, just north of Salerno, record one 'Phillipus medicus Chartaginensis' (Phillip, a physician of Carthage) participating in the sale of property in Salerno in January 1092.[23] In light of these patterns, it is unsurprising that Constantine refers to himself in one of the opening chapters of the *Pantegni* as 'Constantinus Africanus'.[24] It is likely that he self-identified in this way from his earliest days in Salerno.

Background: Italy–Salerno

After his arrival in South Italy, Constantine, as the biographies note, managed to win the patronage of the region's elite. Patronage, of course, had long been a significant factor in the production of translations in the Islamic realm. What we know of the experiences of Ḥunayn ibn Isḥāq, his predecessors and successors, and of the role of Baghdad's House of Wisdom in general, underscores this point most thoroughly.[25] The patronage of the caliphs, and their ongoing support, played a vitally important role in the Graeco-Arabic translation

[21] Metcalfe, *The Muslims of Medieval Italy*, provides excellent analysis of this period and the movement of populations.

[22] Falkenhausen, Jamil, and Johns, 'Twelfth-Century Documents'. Although the extant documents they edit and translate date from the first half of the twelfth century, the authors note several of these were surely based upon and represented updates of late eleventh-century originals.

[23] Cava de' Tirreni, Biblioteca Statale del Monumento Nazionale della Badia di Cava, Arca XV.26. The appearance of *medici* as witnesses or agents in the documents preserved at Cava, and throughout Italy, is discussed by Larpi, 'Early Medieval *Medici* in Italian Charters, *s.* IX–XI'.

[24] The Hague, KB, MS 73 J 6, fol. 1^{v}, col. B.

[25] Pormann and Savage-Smith, *Medieval Islamic Medicine*, pp. 24–40; Ullmann, *Die Medizin im Islam*, pp. 115–18.

programme. Moreover, since this pattern of elite patronage was imitated to lesser degrees across the Islamic world in subsequent centuries, on his arrival it is unsurprising that Constantine would have expected to need the support of South Italy's leading figures, both within the Church and in secular society. All three of the biographies of Constantine demonstrate, to some degree, his interactions with members of the great elite of his day and the support they extended to him.

According to Master Mattheus F[errarius], it was because of his demonstrated expertise in urinalysis that Constantine was accepted by Abbot Johannes de Curte and his circle.[26] Here the amusingly precise parallel found in the Cordoba–Montpellier version confirms the process of recognition. It is clear from the scattered evidence of manuscripts, documents, and inscriptions, that the 'Abbas' it refers to was Abbot Johannes, the brother of Gisulf II, the last Lombard prince of Salerno, and at the same time abbot of the court chapel, today S. Pietro a Corte. He was well known in his day.[27] In addition to his position at the court chapel, he was granted by his nephew, Count Henry of Monte Sant'Angelo in the Gargano, a piece of land nearby. Here he constructed and supervised a *xenodochium* for the care of pilgrims and the infirm at the shrine of St Michael. Further, his name lived on in the history of medicine in the Middle Ages and beyond through those of his recipes preserved in Salernitan receptaries, especially the *Antidotarium Nicolai*. These recipes combined exotic ingredients from the East, such as nutmeg, pepper, and lignum aloes, with wildly expensive ingredients (which surely only the rich could have afforded) like pearl and lapis lazuli. One recipe, the *Electuarium ducis*, was created for Guiscard's own son, Duke Roger Borsa.[28]

[26] This detail of Mattheus F[errarius]'s Salerno account is confirmed obliquely by the Cordoba–Montpellier legend. In it, Constantine arrives in Salerno as a slave to a tanner, a task which he practised 'on the shore' at Salerno. According to Mattheus F[errarius], the 'Abbas de Curte' and Constantine met near the shore, at the abbot's church. As a tannery slave in the Cordoba–Montpellier version, Constantine could be said to have 'worked in urines' near the shore; as a visiting merchant expert in urinalysis in Mattheus F[errarius]'s version, Constantine 'worked in urines' near the shore. Again, the versions of Constantine's biography offer essentially the same story, though the local, Salernitan version gets the specifics correct.

[27] The full evidence is presented for the first time in Glaze, 'Salerno's Lombard Prince'; the analysis of this Salerno biography is based upon that study. On Johannes in the documentary tradition of Monte Cassino, see Bloch, *Monte Cassino in the Middle Ages*, pp. 99 n. 3, and 288, and the literature cited there.

[28] The several named remedies of Johannes are analysed closely in Glaze, 'Salerno's Lombard Prince'.

Besides Johannes 'Abbas de Curte', there was an even greater ecclesiastical force at work. Constantine benefitted also from the patronage of Alfanus, archbishop of Salerno, who was himself a translator of Greek medical knowledge into Latin, and renowned for his interest in and experience with medicinal preparations since the 1050s. This churchman, a former monk of Monte Cassino and archbishop of Salerno since 1058, was also known for his medical books and the richness of his medicine cabinet since at least 1055, when he had packed both up and departed with the young Desiderius (later abbot of Monte Cassino) to visit the court of the pope, who was in Tuscany at the time. The passage recounting Alfanus's interest in medicine, his ownership of medical books, and his cache of medicines found in the portion of the *Chronicle* composed by Leo Marsicanus, is worth citing at length:

> Interea Desiderius ob nimiam abstinentiam multasque vigilias in languorem non modicum decidens medendi gratia Salernum perrexit [...] cum ecce fama percrebruit papam Victorem ab ultramontanis partibus Romam venisse eumque ad partes istas in proximo venturum fore. [...] secumque ire orat suppliciter Desiderium. Et quoniam miram cantandi peritiam et medicine artis scientiam non parvam habebat eiusdemque artis codices nonnullos secum a domo detulerat, magni aliquid se habendum in summi pontifices curia omnimodis confidebat.
>
> Confectis igitur atque aptatis, quotquot potuit, medicaminibus [...] ad Romanum pontificem in Tusciam proficiscuntur [...]
>
> (In the meantime, Desiderius by reason of excessive abstinence and many vigils had seriously weakened his health, and in search of healing he journeyed to Salerno. [After Desiderius's removing to Benevento, and while he was at the monastery of Sancta Sophia with his friend Alfanus] word spread abroad that Pope Victor had come towards Rome from the regions beyond the mountains. [Seeking to meet the pontiff] Alfanus begged Desiderius to go with him. And since Alfanus possessed a marvellous skill in singing and no small knowledge of medical science and had brought from home several manuscripts of the same art, he had confidence that he would be regarded in every way as a person of weight in the court of the supreme pontiff. Therefore, assembling and packing as many medicines as possible [...] they set out for the Roman pontiff in Tuscany.)[29]

Alfanus translated one major work of medical anthropology from Greek into Latin, and is credited with producing two short treatises on prognosis and diagnosis.[30]

[29] Latin text and translation taken from longer citation in Newton, *Scriptorium and Library*, p. 12 and p. 12 n. 53.

[30] Nemesius, *Nemesii episcopi Premnon physicon*, ed. by Burkhard; this text is, properly speaking, more anthropological and philosophical than therapeutic. The medical texts most

He also wrote poems concerning medicine. One jesting poem discusses the ailments induced by the marshes of Chieti, including the technical names of illnesses like 'cardiacis ictericisque | et splenis vitio vindice passis' (heart disease, jaundice, and irritation of the spleen).[31] Another of these poems, addressed to Guido, another brother of Prince Gisulf II, some time before Guido's death in 1076, praised the healthiness of the Salernitan lifestyle and the quality of medical care available there in previous decades: 'Tam medicinali tantum florebat in arte, | posset ut hic nullus languor habere locum' ([In your father's lifetime] Salerno then flourished to such an extent in the art of medicine, that no illness was able to settle there).[32] Constantine evidently returned the generosity of Alfanus's patronage by dedicating to him the small treatise *De stomacho*. That tract opens with a dedication to the 'most revered archbishop of Salerno', a *reverentissimo* phrase that echoes in fundamental respects the Prologue of the Hague *Pantegni* (discussed in Chapter 3). The biography of Master Mattheus F[errarius] already mentioned confirms the identification of Constantine's dedication of *De stomacho* to Alfanus by noting that 'for Archbishop Alfanus he created independently the *Book of the Stomach*, which proved of the greatest usefulness to him. Archbishop Alfanus wished to reimburse him [Constantine] for his costs for completing the *Practica* of the *Pantegni*'.[33] The relationship between Constantine and Alfanus seems to have been a close one, and fruitful.

Alfanus was not just a medical scholar and poet, he seems to have also been the recipient of a magnificent gift from Atto of Chieti (r. 1057–74) which included an illustrated medical compendium, now BAV, Vat. Barb. lat. 160, which he evidently received while at Monte Cassino, either while in residence

often attributed to Alfanus concern the humours and pulses. There are also a series of 'experimenta' (proven recipes) that circulate under his name and/or title. See Capparoni, *Il 'De Quattuor humoribus corporis humani'*; and Creutz, 'Der Frühsalernitaner Alfanus'. Creutz mistakenly attributed another text to Alfanus, which he immediately withdrew; see his 'Erzbischof Alfanus I', and 'Nachtrag zu "Erzbischof Alfanus I, ein frühsalernitanischer Arzt"'. See also Bloch, *Monte Cassino in the Middle Ages*, p. 98. Additional attributions are listed by Thorndike, *A History of Magic*, I, 753. On the *experimenta* attributed to Alfanus, see the following discussion. A recent translation of Nemesius's Greek text is available as *Nemesius: On the Nature of Man*, ed. and trans. by Sharples and van der Eijk. On the career of Alfanus, see Acocella, 'La figura e l'opera di Alfano I'.

[31] Newton, *Scriptorium and Library*, pp. 241–42.

[32] The translation is Bloch's, *Monte Cassino in the Middle Ages*, p. 97.

[33] Erfurt, Universitätsbibliothek, Bibliotheca Amploniana, Cod. Amplon. 8° 62, fols 49^{v}B–50^{r}A; see the following discussion. On the *De stomacho*, see now *Liber Constantini De stomacho*, ed. by Cartelle.

or while visiting.[34] The lifelong friendship between Desiderius and Alfanus surely played a fundamental role in Constantine's transfer from Salerno, the princely port city and seat of government, to Monte Cassino, the venue ruled by Desiderius, the patron who oversaw the construction or reconstruction of 'the buildings [...and] many wondrous books' in honour of St Benedict, as Newton has shown.[35] The massive construction programme and impressive production of manuscript texts undertaken during Desiderius's abbacy reveal the perfect environment in which someone like Constantine, a medical scholar with a prince's former property to bestow, would have been best able to capitalize on the human and material resources available for translating and perfecting his corpus of medical texts.[36]

[34] Newton, *Scriptorium and Library*, pp. 245–47. The significance of newly-introduced exotic ingredients from the east in the antidotaries of BAV, Vat. Barb. lat. 160 and other eleventh-century manuscripts of South Italy, are addressed in Glaze, 'Salerno's Lombard Prince'.

[35] Newton, *Scriptorium and Library*, pp. 5–11, at p. 10, referring to the miniature of BAV, Vat. lat. 1202, fol. 2^{r}. The translation is adapted from Newton's, p. 10 n. 33. One centre associated both with Desiderius's building programme, and with Alfanus's poetry, is the monastic church of Sant'Angelo in Formis, near Capua, where the Desiderian basilica features a decorative scheme inspired by Alfanus's poetry. At the end of the richly decorated *Regestum* showing the patronage of the abbey by the princes of Capua, a booklist of 143 titles written in a hand of the late twelfth century records, among other titles, a series of medical books, including the *Isagoge* and a *Lapidarium*. The *Isagoge* as a production of Constantine and his 'translation kitchen' with a team of scribes at Monte Cassino is discussed by Newton and Kwakkel in subsequent chapters. The analysis of the lapidary tradition is examined by Halleux, who postulates the simultaneous or contemporary construction of the alphabetical *Dioscorides* often attributed to Constantine and his workshop, and a *Lapidarium* of Damigeron preserved in its earliest manuscript witness (late eleventh century), Cava de' Tirreni, Biblioteca Statale del Monumento Nazionale della Badia di Cava, 3. He does not demonstrate the overlap of the two texts, but merely asserts that the correspondences are overwhelming; see Halleux and Schamp, eds, *Les Lapidaires Grecs*, pp. 193–290, especially pp. 193–228. The list of medical titles copied into the Sant' Angelo *Regestum* includes 'Aphorismus Ypocratis I, Glose cum libro herbarum I, Lapidarium I, Liber medicinalis I' and a 'Liber ysagoge Johannicii de rebus naturalibus I'. Might this list, copied down rather late, represent the early circulation of Constantinian and other medical books to a house under the heavy influence of Monte Cassino? The absence of authors popular in twelfth-century monastic collections, including Bernard of Clairvaux, Anselm of Bec, and Peter Lombard is striking. The list is reproduced in Becker, *Catalogi bibliothecarum antiqui*, no. 120 at pp. 246–47. See also the facsimile produced at Monte Cassino, *Il Regesto di Sant'Angelo in Formis*, fol. 108^{v}/p. 216. We are grateful to the late Don Faustino Avagliano for having provided a copy of the facsimile some years ago; the date of the cataloguer's script is offered by Erik Kwakkel.

[36] It is perhaps noteworthy that no major scriptorium or manuscript workshop at Salerno has yet been identified for the period *c.* 1050–*c.* 1200, in spite of that city's fame as a medical

Background: Monte Cassino

The patronage afforded Constantine is even more marked and better documented in the accounts of his arrival at Monte Cassino. The *Chronicle of Monte Cassino* states explicitly that Constantine received the church of St Agatha in Aversa, which was given to him by Prince Richard of Capua prior to his death in the spring of 1078, a gift subsequently confirmed by his son and heir, Prince Jordan of Capua and his wife Gaitelgrima (sister of Prince Gisulf II and of Sikelgaita).[37] The *Chronicle* also acknowledges in a less specific fashion the 'honour' shown to Constantine by Duke Robert Guiscard.[38] The shared support of these two leaders, the prince of Capua and the duke of Apulia, must have made a significant difference in Constantine's ability to engage in the kinds of activity he clearly pursued. That this same team pooled their efforts and sponsored the rebuilding of Salerno's cathedral in a magnificent style worthy of the apostle St Matthew's relics and of Archbishop Alfanus's increasingly influential dignity is no surprise. They were the powerhouses of the secular world in this region.[39] Their contributions to the cathedral's reconstruction is visually recorded in the architrave's inscription above the main processional entrance to the cathedral's atrium or *paradisus* (figs ii and iii). Jordan and Robert Guiscard are named in leonine hexameters across the lintel, and two fierce lions guard below; this visual pun (of the two lions of Norman South Italy) is rounded out by also alluding to Alfanus as a patron, since, as Lentini concludes, Alfanus was the author of the poetic inscription, which reads in full:

centre and, in the twelfth century, as an educational centre. Monte Cassino, on the other hand, was a veritable production centre, especially during Desiderius's abbacy.

[37] *Chronica monasterii Casinensis*, ed. by Hoffmann, pp. 411–12. The document of Prince Jordan and Gaitelgrima confirming the donation, which is still preserved in the Archivio at Monte Cassino, is discussed and reproduced in Newton, 'Arabic Medicine and Other Arabic Cultural Influences in Southern Italy in the Time of Constantinus Africanus'. See the discussion of his gift in this volume's Chapter 5.

[38] Bloch reveals that both Monte Cassino accounts of Constantine's arrival, one from the *Chronicle of Monte Cassino* begun by Leo Marsicanus, and the other from Peter the Deacon's *De viris illustribus*, testified to Robert Guiscard's support: 'ac in magna honorificentia aput Robertum ducem habitus est' (p. 128). The texts are given in parallel columns by Bloch, *Monte Cassino in the Middle Ages*, appendix 4, pp. 137–44.

[39] Ramseyer analyses Archbishop Alfanus I's efforts to reform, reorganize, and centralize the archiepiscopal see without entirely destroying local traditions of lay and consortial patronage in *The Transformation of a Religious Landscape*, especially chaps 4 and 5.

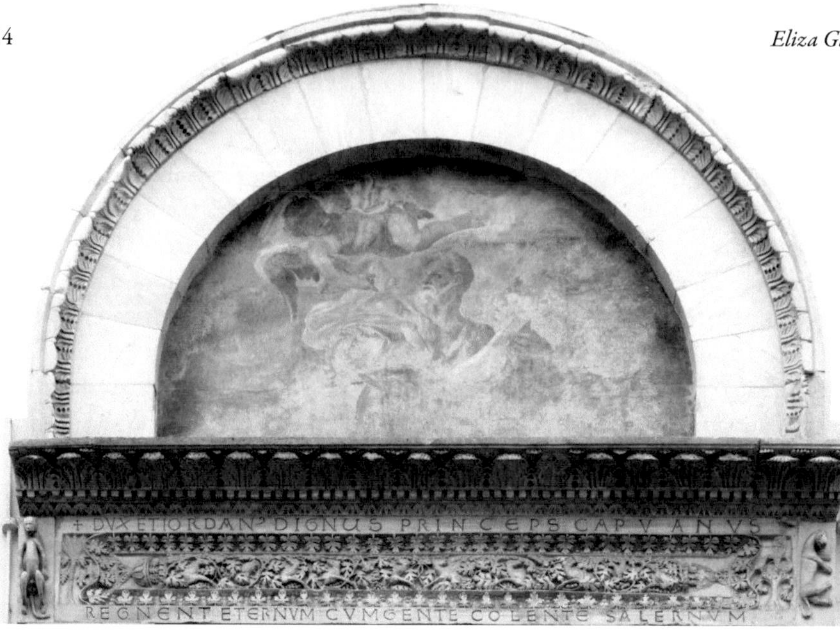

Figure ii.
The architrave of the portal to Salerno Cathedral, showing the inscription with Alfanus's leonine hexameters. After 1077.

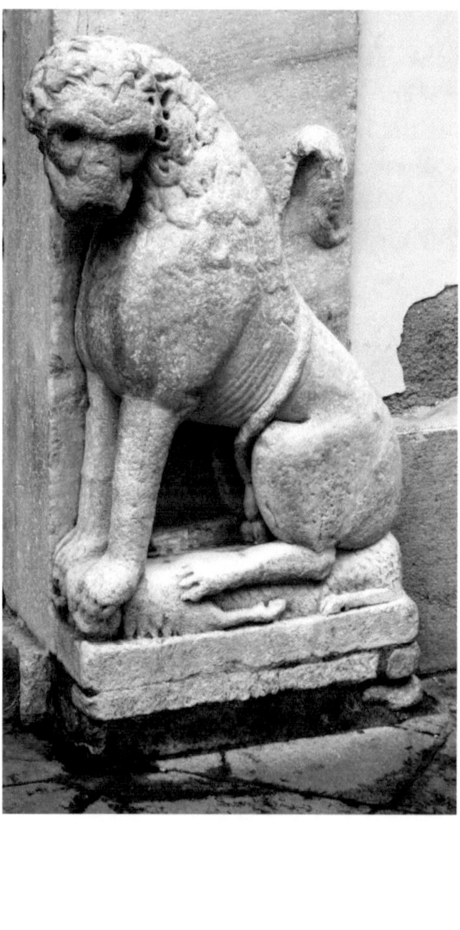

Figure iii.
One of the lions of the portal to Salerno Cathedral. After 1077.

DUX ET IORDANUS DIGNUS PRINCEPS CAPUANUS
REGNENT ETERNUM CUM GENTE COLENTE SALERNUM.[40]

(May the duke [Guiscard] and Jordan, worthy prince of Capua,
Reign forever with the people who inhabit Salerno.)

The importance of influential patrons cannot be overstated. As fig. iv clearly indicates, two generations of the most powerful secular and ecclesiastical leaders of South Italy were closely linked to Constantine as patrons: in Salerno, Abbot Johannes de Curte and Archbishop Alfanus, in Salerno and Monte Cassino, Robert Guiscard and his wife Sikelgaita, and finally, in the younger generation, Prince Jordan of Capua and his wife Gaitelgrima.[41]

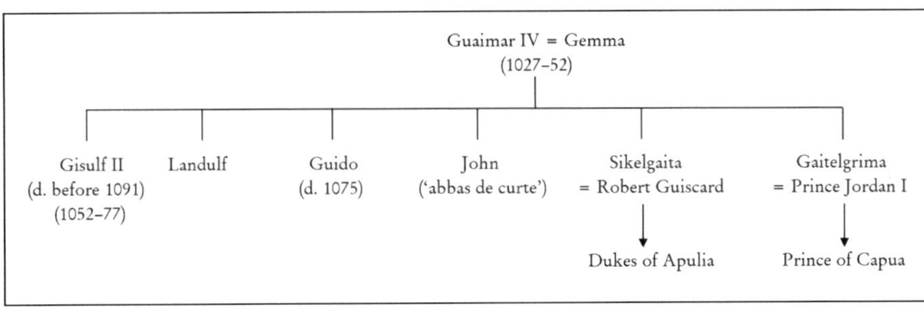

Figure iv. The last princely family of Longobard Salerno.

According to the *Chronicle*, Constantine 'was held in high honour by Duke Robert [Guiscard]'. Furthermore, the *Chronicle* tells us that it was Prince Richard who endowed Constantine with the church of St Agatha in Aversa, which Constantine, on his departure from Salerno, in turn presented to the Abbey of Monte Cassino when he entered as a monk sometime prior to Richard's death in April 1078. In 1086 Prince Jordan, Prince Richard's son, confirmed the gift in a document still preserved at Monte Cassino; Jordan states

[40] On Alfanus as author, see Lentini and Avagliano, *I carmi di Alfano I Arcivescovo di Salerno*, pp. 38–39. In his examination of *spolia* reuse in Salerno, McNeill asserts that 'for its patrons Salerno Cathedral might have represented the restoration and renewal of the building through reference to the past'. See his '*Veteres statuas emit Rome*', pp. 8–11.

[41] Genealogy of the family of Gisulf II, the last ruler of Salerno (until 1077). Table taken, with revision, from Loud, *The Age of Robert Guiscard*, by permission of the author. See also Newton, 'Arabic Medicine and Other Arabic Cultural Influences in Southern Italy in the Time of Constantinus Africanus'.

that he acted 'per interventum' of his wife Princess Gaitelgrima. The intervention of the princess perhaps points to gratitude on her part for some specific medical intervention by Constantine to the benefit of herself or her family. If this was the case, the evidence is echoed in the repeated healings of princely personages performed both in Cordoba and in Salerno by Constantine in the (admittedly legendary) Cordoba–Montpellier narrative.

At Monte Cassino, in the factual account of the *Chronicle*, Constantine translated 'a great number of medical texts out of the languages of different peoples'; Bloch's excellent edition of the Monte Cassino tradition lists twenty-three separate titles (counting those added by Peter the Deacon). Among those that may have been the earliest translations, the work on urine — this was, after all, the field in which the Salernitan and Cordoba–Montpellier traditions spoke of Constantine's expertise — explicitly speaks of the author as a 'monk of Monte Cassino'; of the two oldest (eleventh-century) manuscripts of the *Isagoge*, both were produced by scribes active at Monte Cassino before the end of the eleventh century.

Perhaps realizing that his greatest potential was as a translator poised to deliver a tremendous body of literature unknown in Latin Europe, Constantine withdrew from Salerno and proceeded to Monte Cassino. Perhaps life in Salerno during the era of Norman military action, including the prolonged siege and conquest of the city itself, created an environment too turbulent to foster fruitful intellectual activities.[42] It is likely, too, that there was some realization by both Constantine and his patrons in Salerno that the enormous task of translating so many texts, in terms of both materials and labour, would be best undertaken in Abbot Desiderius's very well-supplied, organized, and productive scriptorium at Monte Cassino.[43] Certainly Monte Cassino had resources far beyond the scriptoria of Salerno; Desiderius's scriptorium was already well into the pursuit of a programme designed to recover the texts of the *artes*, as

[42] In his *History of the Normans*, Amatus of Monte Cassino (no fan of the Lombards, and particularly opposed to the memory of Prince Gisulf II) describes in book VIII the long and bitter siege of the city initiated in summer 1076 by Guiscard and Prince Richard of Capua's forces, and the hunger experienced by the citizens of Salerno who languished within the badly-damaged city from June to December. He contends that the starving Salernitans were reduced to eating their horses, dogs, and cats, an account echoed in the *Chronicle of Monte Cassino* and in William of Apulia's *Deeds of Robert Guiscard*. The siege lasted at least six months, and the citadel did not fall until May 1077. See Amatus of Montecassino, *History of the Normans*, trans. by Dunbar, rev. by Loud, pp. 186–205.

[43] See Chapter 5 of the present volume.

well as producing handbooks for teaching. Archbishop Alfanus of Salerno's own history as a monk of Monte Cassino, and his long-standing friendship with Abbot Desiderius, surely eased the transfer of Constantine from the archiepiscopal city to the great abbey. From the beginning of his abbacy in 1058, Desiderius had undertaken a massive programme of *renovatio* that launched Monte Cassino into a golden age of artistic, architectural, and literary distinction.[44] Desiderius renewed the fabric of the great abbey's holdings (the 'terra S. Benedicti') and its intellectual products in rich styles harkening back to classical designs, but with strong Byzantine and Islamic motifs.[45] With the wealth of the scriptorium and library, and in terms of cultural receptivity, Desiderius's great abbey would have provided an ideal opportunity to support a vast translation programme like Constantine's.

What the present book shows, but with the newest pioneering developments also represented, is that substantial recovery efforts were being effected similarly in the field of medicine. The state of medical knowledge at the time of Constantine's arrival in Italy provided, to a significant degree, Constantine's motivation for undertaking his impressive and unprecedented translation programme. In Italy, Constantine found a real deficiency of medical literature compared to what he knew in Ifrīqya.[46] In Late Antiquity, Greek medical literature had been only partially rendered into Latin, and was transmitted in the early Middle Ages in guises often quite distinct from the Galenic and Hippocratic corpora of the ancient world.[47] Plagued by fragmentation and

[44] Newton, *Scriptorium and Library*. The decorative features of the manuscripts are analysed by art historian Giulia Orofino, *I codici decorati dell'Archivio di Montecassino*; see especially vol. III: *Tra Teobaldo e Desiderio*.

[45] Newton, 'Arabic Medicine and Other Arabic Cultural Influences in Southern Italy in the Time of Constantinus Africanus'. On the Byzantine mosaics and the bronze doors, see Bloch, *Monte Cassino in the Middle Ages*, pp. 40–71.

[46] In addition to an absence of literature suitable to the training of beginners (*introducendi*) in medicine, or on specific diagnostic and prognostic methods, Constantine must have realized that most of the texts attributed to Galen and Hippocrates remained unknown in the Latin West. Similarly, Alfanus writes in his *Premnon physicon* of the poverty of texts in Latin, a 'latinorum cogente penuria' (compelled by the poverty of the Latins). See the following discussion, and for Alfanus, *Nemesii episcopi Premnon Physicon*, ed. by Burkhard, p. 2, section 9 of the Prologue.

[47] On the late antique to early medieval Latin traditions, and the diminished corpus of Galenic-Hippocratic treatises available, see Beccaria, 'Sulle tracce di un antico canone latino di Ippocrate e di Galeno. I., II., III.' (1959), 1–56; (1961), 1–75; and (1971), 1–23. For a broad analysis of the state of early medieval medicine see Glaze, 'The Perforated Wall', with substantial

corruption over centuries of transmission, the state of medical literature at the time of Constantine's arrival was far from glorious. Already just before mid-century Gariopontus of Salerno, a learned practitioner and friend of Lawrence of Amalfi (formerly a monk of Monte Cassino) had endeavoured to bring order and terminological renewal to a large ensemble of texts that had circulated in Italy and across Europe since Late Antiquity. Rearranging a disparate set of texts into one synthetically ordered head-to-foot manual, and (in general) cleaning up the Latin of his sources as well as the corrupt Greek technical terminology, he introduced his *Passionarius*, hailing it, in his rather flowery prefatory statement, for its utility in aiding the physician, and thereby helping him earn everlasting fame.[48] Although the text became immediately popular, it did not suffice to resolve the deficiencies of the Latin tradition inherited from antiquity, nor to introduce the kinds of philosophical medical theory that so saturated Arabic medical literature.

An understanding of the varieties of medical literature that Constantine would have found following his arrival in Italy can perhaps be reached most effectively through consideration of the medical books either produced at or associated with Monte Cassino prior to the new translations from Arabic that Constantine introduced. Two manuscripts in particular, Monte Cassino, MSS 69 and 97, represent the broad variety of treatises Constantine the African would almost certainly have encountered when he first reached the great abbey and set out to survey written medical knowledge in the Latin West. Monte Cassino, MS 69, dating from the late ninth century, was identified by E. A. Lowe as one of the 'duo codices medicinales' from Abbot Bertarius's booklist (r. 856–84), which described a volume containing 'innumerable useful remedies'.[49] Indeed, MS 69 is a massive volume at 582 pages, and preserves a series of

expansion and analysis as *Medicine, Sister of Philosophy: Rational Medicine in the Latin West, c. 500–1200* (unpublished). The epistolary tradition into which key aspects of ancient medical knowledge were refashioned and known throughout the early Middle Ages is discussed as a typology by Langslow, 'The *Epistula* in Ancient Scientific and Technical Literature, with Special Reference to Medicine'. On medical practices in early medieval Italy, see Pilsworth, *Healthcare in Early Medieval Northern Italy*, and Glaze, 'Authority'.

[48] Glaze, 'Gariopontus and the Salernitans'. For a close analysis of one short segment of the text, on gout, in its pre-Gariopontean form and the version produced by Gariopontus, see Knight, 'The *De podagra*'.

[49] See the description and list of contents in Beccaria, *I codici di medicina*, pp. 293–97. Jeffrey Doolittle is currently completing an analysis of this manuscript for his doctoral thesis at Fordham University under the supervision of Professor Richard Gyug.

receptaries listing medicinal preparations and antidotes. An alphabetical glossary of plant materials, short tracts on weights and measures, a dietary calendar, and a few other minor works round out the volume. The whole is copied in two neat columns, and employs Greek majuscules to distinguish many of the technical terms throughout.

Monte Cassino, MS 97, produced in the ninth or tenth century and also stretching over five hundred pages, contains, along with a miscellany of shorter works, a mixture of late antique texts: the *Therapeutica* of Alexander of Tralles in three books; two treatises by Vindicianus Afer; an anatomical synopsis known as the *Sapientia artis medicinae*; a commentary on the *Aphorisms* of Hippocrates often attributed to Oribasius; the *Alphabetum Galieni*; the *Herbarium* complex that includes the work attributed to Apuleius Platonicus; Pseudo-Dioscorides' *Ex herbis femininis*; *De taxone* by Pseudo-Apuleius; and Sextus Placitus's *Medicina de quadrupedibus*.[50] Technical terms of Greek derivation are also treated with care in MS 97: they are written in majuscules and set apart by a long black suprascript line, a sort of extended macron, in several of the treatises preserved in this massive volume.

MS 97 provides several examples of medical epistles, a genre of scientific writing that originated in antiquity and enjoyed a pronounced popularity in the early Middle Ages.

Such letters attributed to great medical authorities like Galen, Oribasius, Cassius Felix, or Cleopatra were addressed either to family members (sons, daughters, brothers, or nephews), or to colleagues who had requested that the author produce a useful guide, or to the author's famous patrons. In some cases, medical epistles functioned as prefatory contextualizers of the therapeutic manuals they introduced, while in others they made up an entire, brief medical communication.[51] Frequently, such letters addressed the recipient of the text with rhetorical flourishes and superlatives; for instance, Monte Cassino's copy of Vindicianus Afer's *Epistula ad Pentadium*, a brief treatise on

[50] On these contents, see Beccaria, *I codici di medicina*, pp. 297–303; Langslow, *The Latin Alexander Trallianus*, especially pp. 45–46; *Theodori Prisciani Euporiston libri III*, pp. 425–66 and pp. 484–92; Wlaschky, '*Sapientia artis medicinae*'; Kibre, *Hippocrates Latinus*; Everett, *The Alphabet of Galen*. On the *Herbarium* complex, which is illustrated in Monte Cassino MS 97, see Collins, *Medieval Herbals*, and Grape-Albers, *Spätantike Bilder aus der Welt des Arztes*. Further discussion and a plate showing the size of the two early volumes vis-à-vis the other medical books of the abbey can be found in Glaze, 'Authority'.

[51] Langslow, 'The *Epistula* in Ancient Scientific and Technical Literature, with Special Reference to Medicine', pp. 211–34.

the humours, begins, 'Licet te scire, karissime nepos', while the *Gynaecia* attributed to Cleopatra opens, 'Desideranti tibi, filia karissima'.[52] Monte Cassino thus already possessed before Constantine's arrival at the abbey abundant examples of the kinds of dedicatory epistles Constantine would later employ in the Hague *Pantegni* and other translations, where he addresses his patron Desiderius as 'most revered father', and both Atto and Johannes, his assistants, as his dearest sons.

When Constantine arrived at Monte Cassino, probably in 1077, we might well ask which of these many medical texts Constantine would have considered most useful as communicators of ancient medical wisdom. It is difficult to know. However, as the authors point out in the following chapters, at least one manuscript that subscribes to this 'pre-Constantinian' model of anthologized late antique and early medieval texts was produced in the period immediately prior to Constantine's arrival. Moreover, they show that one of the scribes active in the Hague *Pantegni* also copied part of Copenhagen, KB, GKS 1653 4°, copied at the great abbey in the decade prior to Constantine's arrival. That manuscript offers further important insights into the versions of Latin medical knowledge that he likely encountered.

Copenhagen, GKS 1653 4° is one of the grand early medieval medical anthologies preserving sometimes derivative and pseudo-epigraphic medical literature. Although remarkable in every way, one of the most striking aspects of this manuscript is the works that it does contain. Amidst other texts, including another copy of the *Sapientia artis medicinae*, it holds a Monte Cassino-produced copy of Oribasius's *Synopsis*, a series of receptaries and antidotaries, and a unique 'Medicamentarium, quod continet dicta Uribasii doctoris per alphabeta'. This last treatise, a hitherto unstudied work not preserved in any other known manuscript, stands as an antidotary of remedies apparently extracted from the texts of Oribasius, organized alphabetically, and occupying twenty-six folios. The focus on the works of Oribasius, the great Byzantine encyclopaedist who had served as court physician to the emperor, is noteworthy, and particularly the interest in pharmacy fit for an emperor (or perhaps a prince of the Church). This manuscript, one might well argue, was designed to preserve for Monte Cassino a copy of the Byzantine authority's works, as well as other uncommon texts like the so-called *Gynaecia* of Muscio (here ascribed to Soranus), and other rare but important late antique sources on

[52] Monte Cassino, Archivio della Badia, MS 97, p. 4, and Copenhagen, Kongelige Bibliotek, Gamle Kongelige Samling, MS 1653 4°, fol. 28^{r}, respectively.

dietary substances, *materia medica*, phlebotomy, weights and measures, and prognostics.[53]

Given the Monte Cassino monks' ownership of the works of Oribasius and Alexander of Tralles, it is no great surprise that Monte Cassino came to own a text by Paul of Aegina, thus completing the triad of great early Byzantine medical authorities in Latin form. Part of Paul's encyclopaedic *Pragmateia* survives from Monte Cassino's literary collection in an extant manuscript contemporary with Constantine's activities there. This manuscript, Monte Cassino, MS 351, produced after *c.* 1070 in Beneventan by a Monte Cassino scribe, preserves book III of the seven-book treatise. It is the earliest surviving Latin translation of any segment of Paul's work, and as such deserves much greater study. It is notable, among other things, for the use of yellow washes in the Greek style, and for marginal and interlinear glosses in Greek majuscules that attempt to identify technical terms.[54]

It is curious that by *c.* 1080 Monte Cassino appears to have possessed manuscripts preserving significant portions of the textual output of the abovementioned three great Byzantine medical authorities. It is noteworthy that, as is discussed at greater length in the following chapters, although the deficiencies of each of the three Byzantine encyclopaedists' texts were noted by al-Maǧūsī in his Prologue, and that of the Latin translation produced by Constantine and his team, Monte Cassino's bibliophilic collection-developers were apparently eager to acquire all the representative portions of the Byzantines' texts that they could. That none of the Byzantine authorities' known works provided the kind of coverage Constantine (following al-Maǧūsī) desired, especially in regard

[53] For a description of the manuscript, see Beccaria, *I codici di medicina*, pp. 119–24. The apparent popularity of the *Sapientia artis medicinae* in South Italy was substantial. In addition to the copies at Monte Cassino, another copy appears in a teaching anthology compiled by Lawrence of Amalfi, according to tradition, student of Gerbert of Rheims and teacher of Hildebrand (later Gregory VII); Lawrence had taught at Monte Cassino in the 1020s, and subsequently also in Rome. This anthology is now Venice, Biblioteca Nazionale Marciana, Lat. Z. 497 (1811). On this important manuscript, see Newton, 'Tibullus in Two Grammatical Florilegia', pp. 275–80. Newton notes three such copies in Beneventan script, and that the Venice manuscript uses Beneventan abbreviations. There is another copy in Beneventan not hitherto noted: Cava de' Tirreni, Biblioteca Statale del Monumento Nazionale della Badia di Cava, 3, in which the *Sapientia* begins at fol. 151. The text was edited by Wlaschky in '*Sapientia artis medicinae*', but Wlaschky did not know of either the Venice or Badia di Cava manuscripts. An English translation now appears in *Medieval Medicine*, ed. and trans. by Wallis, pp. 17–22.

[54] Described in Beccaria, *I codici di medicina*, pp. 305–06. For the relationship between scribes of Monte Cassino, MS 351 and the Hague *Pantegni*, see Chapter 3.

to 'natural things', helps explain the extraordinary undertaking that the Latin *Theorica Pantegni* represents in the history of ideas.[55] The careful accumulation of the works of late antique and Byzantine authorities is entirely in keeping, however, with the vogue manifest at Abbot Desiderius's Monte Cassino for ancient, Greek, and even Arabic cultural products.[56]

Constantine as a Translator of Medicine

Our understanding of the order and priority of Constantine's translation programme is far from clear, but there are some indications of these. For a number of reasons, it seems that Constantine's treatise *De urina* was composed early, and probably in Salerno. It is also possible that *De stomacho*, which is dedicated to Alfanus, dates from this period or from Constantine's first years at Monte Cassino. It may well be that the *Isagoge* was also begun in his early years at Salerno, but it was certainly completed (in a perhaps imperfect form) at Monte Cassino, as discussed in Chapter 3. It is argued in Chapter 5 that the work on the *Pantegni* was begun before Constantine's arrival at Monte Cassino, and it was at least in a semi-finished state by April 1086 when Abbot Desiderius, to whom the Prologue dedicates it, was named Pope Victor III.

It is certainly clear that Constantine was interested in introductory texts, that is, texts for those undertaking their initial medical studies (*introducendi*). He was also interested in supplying translations in subjects for which there was a dearth of medical literature available in Latin. In translating Isaac Israeli's treatise on urine, Constantine made a point of stressing the Latins' poverty with respect to treatises on that topic. He was right: there was relatively little prior literature in Latin dedicated specifically to the topic of diagnosing from urine.[57] As noted already, Isaac's book on urine was likely one of Constantine's first translations. According to Mattheus F[errarius]'s colourful Salernitan biography, Constantine's ability in urinalysis was key to his good fortune in

55 It is perhaps significant that although al-Maǧūsī offered a longer list of authorities whose works he considered deficient, the *Theorica Pantegni* Prologue, apart from its criticisms of Galen, reduces that number to just 'the Byzantine three'; see Chapter 3.

56 The vogue for Greek products, including bronze doors and mosaics, is explored by Bloch's splendid *Monte Cassino*. On the early evidence for this taste for Arabic materials, see Newton, 'Arabic Medicine and Other Arabic Cultural Influences in Southern Italy in the Time of Constantinus Africanus'.

57 There are eight treatises on urine listed in Beccaria, *I codici di medicina*, from amongst 153 surviving manuscripts; all eight are quite short, at most a few folia.

Salerno. Indeed, he reports, when Constantine arrived in Salerno and walked up to the piazza before the court chapel, he found Abbot Johannes de Curte giving a public demonstration of the analysis of urine. In discussion with Constantine (via Muslim interpreters), Johannes observed that his own wisdom in urinalysis was due to long experience, rather than the accessibility of any extensive textual guides on the subject.[58] The *Isagoge* is yet more foundational, offering Constantine's translation of some version of Ḥunayn ibn Isḥāq's *Masā'il fī ṭ-ṭibb*. The *Isagoge* is helpfully brief (less than twenty pages in Monte Cassino, MS 225) and, more importantly, rich in succinct definitions of basic medical concepts ranging from the four elements (water, fire, earth, and air) and the humours to the principles of diagnosis and therapy.

The Pantegni

The very title of the text examined in this volume telegraphs just how valuable it would have been to have one volume, one text, that encompassed 'the complete art' of medicine, both theoretical and practical. Although based upon the Greek 'Pasa techne', the title effectively conveys the meaning of al-Maǧūsī's original Arabic source, the title of which meant the 'Complete Book of the Medical Art'.[59] Surely Constantine envisioned the prospect of a complete text, with ten books of theory matched to ten books of practice, as the highest accomplishment of his translation programme. On fols 1^{v}–2^{r} of the Hague manuscript, Constantine tells us what his 'complete art' would have contained:

> Liber igitur iste totus in duas partes dividitur. Prima continet rerum scientiam naturalium, et non naturalium, et earum quae extra naturam sunt. Hec autem pars appellatur theorica. Secunda pars continet scientiam custodiendi sanos, et sanandi egros [egrums *H, emend. FN*] cum dieta, et potione, et chirurgia, quae vocatur practica. Theorica decem habet particulas, quarum prima xxv habet capitula. Secunda xvi et anathomiam [anathomium *H*] compositorum membrorum et iuvamentum ipsorum. Tertia xxxv et anathomiam compositorum et [*illegible*]. Quarta xx quae continent scientiam virtutum, actionum, et spirituum. Quinta pars xxxv habet capitula, scientiam rerum naturalium continentia, quae sunt aer, motus, et

[58] Diagnoses through pulses and urine were both under-represented in the Latin literature produced and circulating before 1075; it is surely no coincidence that two of the core texts of the early *Articella*, that is, Theophilus's *De urina* and Philaretus's *De pulsibus*, provided substantially more extensive translations of these essential diagnostic methods that had held sway since the time of Herophilus and Galen.

[59] Burnett and Jacquart, 'Preface', pp. vii–ix.

quies, cibus et potus, somnus, et vigiliae, inanitio et continentia, anime accidentia. Sexta xxxv res extra naturam habentia, morbos scilicet et morborum causas, eorumque accidentia. Septima xv, quae morborum universalem significationem, et eorum causas continent. Octava pars xxii, quae morborum investigationem et causas eorum habent. Nona xli habentia investigationem interiorum morborum et suarum causarum. Decima pars xii de signis prognosticorum infirmitatum ad salutem sive mortem attinentium. Secunda pars huius libri, id est practica, similiter x habet particulas. Quae prima xxxi habet capitula custodiendi sanitatem in sanis, et diete in infantibus et senibus et egritudinem exeuntibus. Secunda lxiii capitula ad morborum simplicem medicinam attinentia, et eorum [eorum *in wormhole but decipherable*] comprobationibus iuvamenta. Tertia xxxiiii ad febres medicinandas et apostemata. Quarta xiii medicande superficiei corporis attinentia. Quinta l ad interiorum membrorum medicamenta, et maxime animatorum ut cerebri, medullarum, spondulium, nervorum, v sensuum. Sexta xv homoribus [*sic*] membrorum spiritualium attinentia, id est faucium, canalium, pulmonis, cordis, diagfragmatis, panniculi qui est super pectus. Septima li est capitulorum membris cibalibus pertinentium, quae sunt stomachus, epar, fel, intestina, vesica, renes. Octava xxxv habet capitula morbis genitalium medicandis attinentia, quae sunt testiculi, virile membrum, matrix, et mamille. Nona cx chirurgiae operationem continentia. Decima xxv compositioni antidotorum attinentia. Unicuique tamen particule debemus competentibus locis sua capitula disponere.

(Therefore this book in its entirety is divided into two parts. The first contains the knowledge of natural things and of non-natural ones, and of those that are contranaturals. Now this part is called 'theorica'. The second part contains the knowledge of the maintenance of health, and of healing the sick with diets and drink, and surgery, which is called 'practica'. 'Theorica' has ten sections ['particulas']. The first of these has twenty-five chapters ['capitula']. The second [has] sixteen chapters, and the anatomy of compound members, and the supporting of them ['iuvamentum ipsorum']. The third [has] thirty-five and the anatomy of compound ones and the [helping of them]. The fourth [has] twenty chapters, which contain the knowledge of virtues/powers, actions, and spirits ['virtutum actionum et spirituum']. The fifth part ['pars'] has thirty-five chapters, containing the knowledge of natural things, which are air, motion, and rest, food and drink, sleep and wakefulness, evacuation and retention, and accidents of the soul. The sixth [has] thirty-five [chapters], having things that are outside nature [extra- or contra-naturals], namely diseases and the causes of diseases, and their accidents. The seventh [has] fifteen [chapters] which contain the universal signs of diseases and their causes. The eighth part has twenty-two [chapters] which contain the investigation of diseases and their causes. The ninth has forty-one [chapters], containing the investigation of the interior diseases and their causes. The tenth part [has] twelve [chapters] on the signs of prognostics of disease pertaining to health or death. The second part of this book, that is the 'practica', similarly has ten sections. The first of these has thirty-one chapters

> on the maintenance of health in people who are well, and diets, and diet in infants, and the old and those who are leaving sickness [i.e., recovering]. The second [section contains] sixty-two chapters pertaining to the simple medicine of diseases, and [lacuna/wormhole in the MS] aids for the determining [of their degrees]. The third [has] thirty-four [chapters] for treating fevers, and abscesses ['apostemes']. The fourth [has] thirteen [chapters] pertaining to medicating the surface of the body. The fifth [has] fifty [chapters] on medicating the interior members, and especially of the animate organs like the brain, the marrow of the vertebrae, of the nerves, of the five senses. The sixth section [has] fifteen [chapters] pertaining to the humours of the spiritual members, that is, of the throat, canals, lungs, heart, diaphragm, [and] of the panicle which is over the chest. The seventh consists of fifty-one chapters pertaining to the nutritive members, which are the stomach, the liver, the gallbladder, intestines, the bladder, the kidneys. The eighth has thirty-five chapters pertaining to healing diseases of the genitals, which are the testicles, the virile member, the matrix, and the breasts. The ninth [has] 110 [chapters] containing the operation of surgery. The tenth has twenty-five [chapters] pertaining to the composition of antidotes. Yet to each individual section we must set out its chapters in the proper places.)[60]

But certainly the *Pantegni* as we have it in the Hague manuscript is far from 'complete'. It lacks the ten books of the *Practica* entirely, and book x of the *Theorica* breaks off at chapter 11 in mid-sentence and is unfinished. Moreover, as Monica Green, Mary Wack, and Mark Jordan have demonstrated in the vol-

60 *Theorica Pantegni*, book i, chap. 3 (excerpt), taken from The Hague, KB, MS 73 J 6, fols 1v–2r. The manuscript uses ordinal numbers for both of the 'parts', the *Theorica* and *Practica*, and for the ten 'particulas' (sections/books) which should make up each. However, in a few cases, the book being enumerated here is called 'pars'. This is reflected in our translation. The scribe uses Roman numerals for each chapter ('capitula'), even though he does not always supply the implied 'habet' and 'capitula'. Given the incomplete nature of the Hague manuscript, the confusion of the incomplete *Pantegni* in subsequent manuscripts, and its later reconstruction, this distinction seems worth mentioning here. On the reconstruction, see Green, 'The Re-Creation of Pantegni'; Wack, 'ʿAlī ibn al-ʿAbbās al-Maǧūsī and Constantine on Love'; Jordan, 'The Fortune of Constantine's Pantegni', and the catalogue of *Pantegni* manuscripts in Burnett and Jacquart, *Constantine the African*, pp. 319–51. On the three types of spirits — the animal, spiritual/vital, and natural — and their functions described in the various translations of Constantine, see Newton, 'Constantine the African', and Burnett, 'The Chapter on the Spirits'. It is possible, based upon study of the earliest manuscripts, that Constantine and his team had a difficult time bringing the terminologies of the *Pantegni*, *Viaticum*, and *Isagoge* in line with one another, especially if, as now seems likely, final versions of several translations of different Arabic authors were in process at the same time. This accounting and enumeration of contents must be compared to the *Theorica*'s account of the curriculum in Galen that was taught in late ancient Alexandria, and as Constantine knew it through the tradition of Hunain; this is recounted in Constantine's translation/adaptation of the *Isagoge*; see Chapter 3 and Appendix B of the present volume.

ume on the *Pantegni* edited by Burnett and Jacquart, the translation remained in a state of serious incompleteness for more than a century.[61] The list of extant manuscripts provided in the same volume carefully notes what portion of the text is contained in each manuscript, and reveals that the most complete version of the *Pantegni* circulating prior to the thirteenth century contained, at most, *Theorica* books I–X, *Practica* book I, and parts of books II and IX. Does this evidence validate or at least reflect a fundamental truth (retold perhaps fancifully) in the Salerno biography regarding Constantine's arrival in that city? In that account, Constantine was shipwrecked off Cape Palinuro (just south of Salerno on the Cilentine coast), and several of his books were lost, including the *Practica* of the *Pantegni*. Certainly the incomplete book IX of the *Practica*, the *Chirurgia*, corroborates the fragmentary nature of the Ur-text, and efforts by Constantine or his successors to complete it: a rubric in the manuscripts of the *Chirurgia* reports that Constantine produced what there is of book IX only up to a certain point, but that it was completed by 'a certain Saracen'.[62] Moreover, Mattheus F[errarius], after recounting the shipwreck reports that 'Archbishop Alfanus wished to reimburse him [Constantine] for his expenses for the completion of the *Practica* of the *Pantegni*'; this implies that Constantine's efforts at producing the *Pantegni* date from the period of his stay in Salerno, and continue the pattern of Salernitan patronage.[63]

[61] Green, 'The Re-Creation of *Pantegni*'; Wack, '"al-Magūsī and Constantine on Love'; and Jordan, 'The Fortune of Constantine's *Pantegni*'.

[62] The manuscript, now Monte Cassino, MS 200, fol. 2^{v}, includes an abbreviated and error-filled version of the rubric in the table of *capitula*, 'hunc usque translata sunt per Constatinum hinc in antea per quedam sarracenum' (up to this point the chapters were translated by Constantine; from here on by a certain Saracen). This late manuscript was not produced at Monte Cassino; we are grateful to the late Don Faustino Avagliano for providing us with photographs of the manuscript and permitting us to study it in person. In Berlin, SBPK, MS lat. fol. 74, fol. 260^{v}, the continuators are identified as 'Johannes agarenus' (Johannes, a Saracen) and Rusticus of Pisa, son of Bella, a professional physician, during the Pisan siege of Majorca: 'Dehinc in expeditione ad obsessionem maioricae, Iohannes quidam, Agarenus quondam qui noviter ad fidem Christiane religionis venerat, cum Rustico Pisano Bellae filius ac professione medicus, hanc nonam particulam *Practicae* ad finem usque ad principium decimae particulae *Practicae* in latinam linguam Deo adiuvante transtulerunt'. (From this point, while on expedition to the siege of Majorca, a certain Johannes, formerly a Muslim, who had recently come over to belief in the Christian faith, with Rusticus of Pisa, son of Bella and by profession a doctor, [they] by God's help translated this ninth section of the *Practica* to the end, all the way to the beginning of the tenth section, into Latin.)

[63] Erfurt, Universitätsbibliothek, Bibliotheca Amploniana, Cod. Amplon. 8° 62, fols 49^{v}B–50^{r}A: 'Archiepiscopus Alfanus pro integratione practicae pantegni expensas ei errogare

Indeed, it is possible that the Arabic copy of al-Maǧūsī's work available to Constantine may have been imperfect.[64] This is corroborated by other evidence, including the two surviving independent copies of the completion of the surgical portion of the *Pantegni*. It is, first, interesting that Alfanus is connected with the project of translation of the *Pantegni*. It is here argued in Chapter 5 that the project was in fact begun in Alfanus's Salerno. Secondly, the significance of the financial basis for the project is intriguing. The need to better appreciate the difficulties of producing even an interim draft, and the team of scribes it took to do so, are problems explored in the chapters to follow.

Conclusion

Incomplete though the *Pantegni* may have been, it was a howling success. Burnett and Jacquart list more than thirty-five manuscripts of the *Pantegni*, or some portion of the *Pantegni*, produced over the course of the 'Long Twelfth Century' (*c.* 1075–*c.* 1225), and there are certainly quite a few more that can be added to that roster.[65] Although more copies of Gariopontus of Salerno's *Passionarius* and Macer's *De viribus herbarum* survive from the same period, more than thirty-five is still a staggering number of manuscripts, especially for so long a text.[66] The evidence of the reception of the text by scholars, philoso-

voluit' (Archbishop Alfanus wished to reimburse him for the completion of the *Practica* of the *Pantegni*). See for further discussion, pp. 184–85.

[64] The tale of a shipwreck suffered by Constantine and consequent loss of a part of some of the *Practica* of the *Pantegni* is most probably fictional. An aetiological tale, it would have been created to explain why Constantine's *Pantegni* was incomplete. Students of literature and history are familiar with a classical parallel: Suetonius in his *Life of Terence* (a manumitted slave of North Africa) quotes Quintus Cosconius as saying that the dramatic poet 'died at sea as he was returning from Greece, [lost] together with plays he had translated from Menander'. In this case, the tale explains why so few (only six) of Terence's comedies had survived. This is a precise parallel: missing literary works or parts of works demand a dramatic narrative explanation.

[65] Burnett and Jacquart, in *Constantine the African*, pp. 316–51. Quite a few manuscripts in this list dated 's. xiii' based upon catalogue evidence, have been effectively re-dated by Erik Kwakkel as part of the work of the Medical Palaeography Team's collaboration, and thus now fall within the Long Twelfth Century. Additionally, an English manuscript from the second half of the twelfth century now in a private collection in New York City was included in this count courtesy of Eliza Glaze. Both Outi Merisalo and Iolanda Ventura secured information about the manuscript Hamburg, Staats- und Universitätsbibliothek, Cod. med. 228, which was produced at the middle of the twelfth century, according to Hans-Walter Stork, at St Pantaleon, Cologne. We are grateful to Professors Ventura and Merisalo for sharing their findings with us.

[66] The number of manuscripts of Macer's text has been traced by Winston Black, who

phers, and authors of the twelfth century points similarly to the *Pantegni*'s well-recognized merits in communicating a rigorously philosophical view of the medicalized human body in health and illness. As Jordan has demonstrated, the *Pantegni* soon played an important role in medical education, as its introductory *accessus* pattern guided Salernitan *magistri* in their own formulations of philosophical medicine, and the texts of the early *Articella* on which they commented.[67] This *accessus* pattern was applied also by medical teachers' lectures on other texts, including the pre-Constantinian *Passionarius*.[68] Further afield, and already before 1130, the Chartrian philosopher William of Conches relied heavily upon the *Theorica Pantegni* while producing his *Philosophia mundi*. The *Pantegni*'s inclusion of Plato proved especially valuable to him, as the portion of Plato's *Timaeus* describing the creation of the 'homo microcosmus' was not yet available in Latin.[69] Shortly after William of Conches's work appeared, one of his respondents, William of St Thierry, writing in the 1130s, utilized the *Pantegni* in his efforts to dispute William of Conches's ideas in his own *De natura corporis et animae*.[70] Moreover, the evidence of medieval manuscript inventories also attests to the popularity of the *Pantegni*. Monasteries as far-flung as Bury St Edmunds, Affligem, Peterborough, and St Amand all recorded copies of the *Pantegni* in their collections before 1168;[71] one of the Bury *Pantegni* manuscripts survives (*c.* 1125–*c.* 1150), and it was probably at Bath that the London, BL, MS Additional 22719 copy was produced (*c.* 1100–*c.* 1150). Around mid-century Hamburg, Staats- und Universitätsbibliothek, Cod. med. 228 (*c.* 1135–*c.* 1165) was copied at St Pantaleon in Cologne.[72]

joined the Medical Palaeography Team in the 'second wave'. We are grateful to him for sharing his preliminary findings with the group in advance of publication. See his '"I Will Add What the Arab Once Taught"'. On Gariopontus, see the table of twelfth-century manuscripts in Glaze, 'Gariopontus and the Salernitans', pp. 185–90 (with additional copies now identified).

67 Jordan, 'The Construction of a Philosophical Medicine'; Jordan, 'Medicine as Science'.

68 Glaze, 'Gariopontus and the Salernitans'.

69 For reference to Plato in the *Pantegni*, see *Theorica* I, chap. 3. For an edition of the *Philosophia mundi*, noting sources used by William (not just the *Pantegni*, but also the *Isagoge* of Johannitius, Alfanus's *Premnon physicon*, Theophilus's *De urina*, Macer, and Dioscorides), see William of Conches, *Philosophia mundi*, ed. and trans. by Maurach with Telle. On the use of the *Timaeus* and its transmission, see Gibson, 'The Study of the *Timaeus*'.

70 For William of St Thierry, see McGinn, *Three Treatises on Man*.

71 The *terminus* of St Amand's booklist, the latest medieval booklist of this group, is 1168. Desilve, 'De schola Elnonensi Sancti Amandi'.

72 An inventory of medical texts appearing in medieval library catalogues and booklists

Cathedral priories and libraries at Durham and Hildesheim constructed catalogues of their collections, including donations received from *magistri* and learned, well-travelled bishops offering the same testimony: Bishop Bruno of Hildesheim, for example, left his itemized collection to the cathedral when he departed on pilgrimage to the Holy Land.[73]

The Hague *Pantegni* reveals the early stages of work on the text at Monte Cassino. The other manuscripts, products of the long twelfth century, and beyond that contemporary scholars' citations of the *Pantegni*, reveal the manner and form in which the text and its influence spread across Europe. Within less than a century of his arrival in Salerno, the spread of Constantine the African's *Pantegni*, along with his other translations, to the farthest geographical reaches of Latinate Europe marked a great departure from earlier medical traditions in Latin.[74] Constantine's attempt to introduce 'the complete art' of medical theory and practice as offered by the *Pantegni* was in truth a watershed moment in the history of medicine.

across Europe is found at Glaze, 'The Perforated Wall', table 1, pp. 268–92 with substantially expanded analysis to come in *Medicine, Sister of Philosophy*, chaps 5 and 6. The Bury *Pantegni* is Cambridge, Trinity College Library, MS R.14.36, with double collations in a contemporary hand. The copy from Bath is discussed by Burnett, 'Physics before the *Physics*'.

[73] On the testimony of dated or datable library catalogues to chart the dissemination of Salernitan and Constantinian texts, see Glaze, 'The Perforated Wall', and 'Salerno's Lombard Prince'. Bishop Bruno's list appears in Sudhoff, 'Die medizinischen Schriften', pp. 348–56. Bruno's surviving *Pantegni* is Hildesheim, Dombibliothek, Hs 748. We are grateful to Alison Beach for travelling to study the manuscript and securing images for the Medical Palaeography Team.

[74] This is not to say that the new medical literature replaced older texts entirely; indeed, there seems to have been a revival of select late antique Latin medical literature, as well as eleventh-century adaptations based upon it.

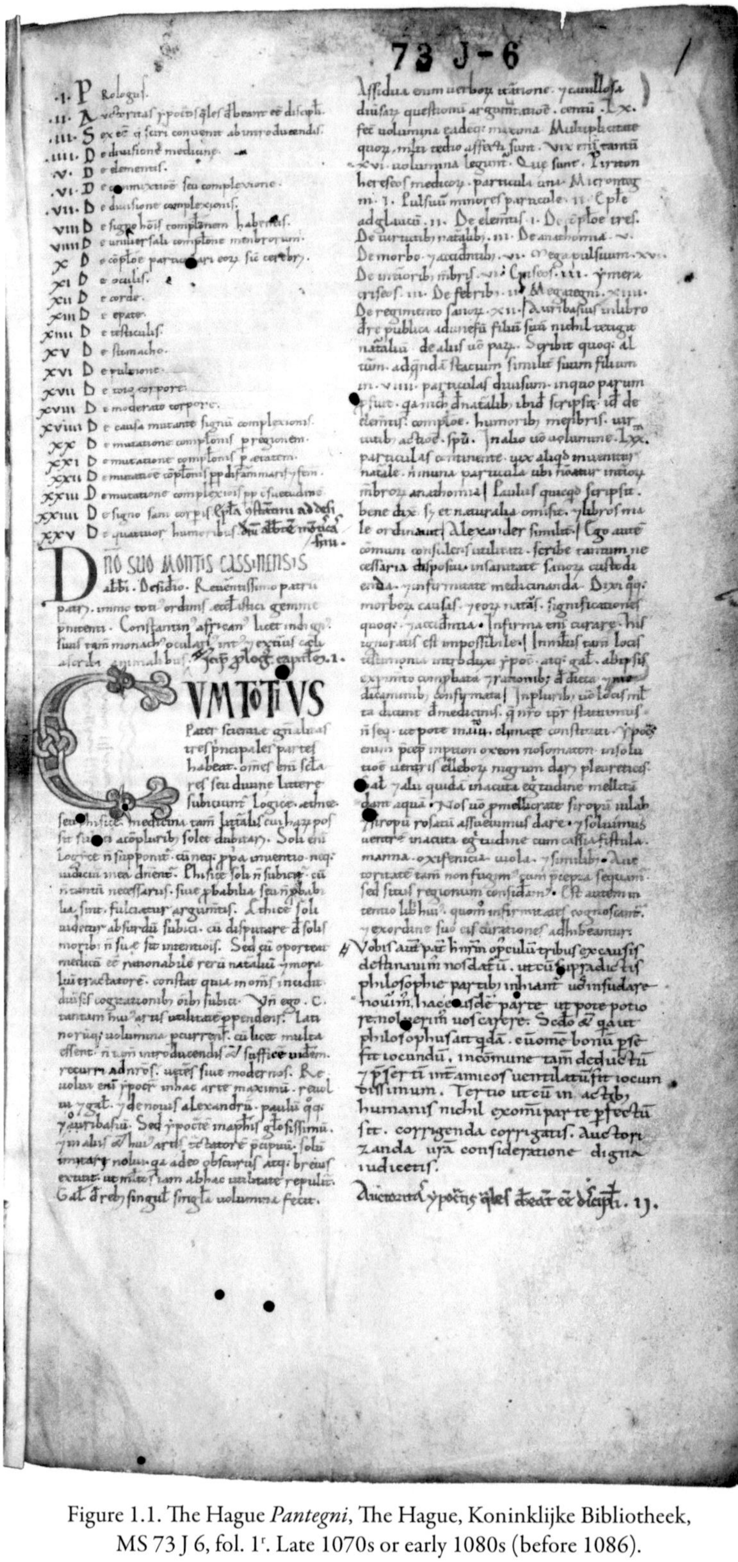

Figure 1.1. The Hague *Pantegni*, The Hague, Koninklijke Bibliotheek, MS 73 J 6, fol. 1[r]. Late 1070s or early 1080s (before 1086).

Chapter 1

The Dossier of the Scribe

The leading role in this monograph is played by The Hague, Koninklijke Bibliotheek, MS 73 J 6. The manuscript contains the *Pantegni*, a translation or adaptation by Constantinus Africanus (that is, Constantine of Ifrīqya)[1] of the *Kitāb Kāmil aṣ-ṣināʿa* of ʿAlī ibn al-ʿAbbās al-Maǧūsī, the great tenth-century encyclopaedia of medical knowledge (fig. 1.1 and pl. I).[2] It contains, however, unlike a large number of the other manuscripts, only the first part of the *Pantegni*, the *Theorica*; the parts of the *Practica* that Constantine is thought to have translated are missing.[3] In the past, the Hague manuscript has generally been assigned to the twelfth century; it is only in the last nine years that it has been recognized instead as a product of the last quarter of the eleventh century.[4] More specifically, the date of this manuscript can be set between the years 1058 when Desiderius became abbot and his death in 1087, as will be discussed.

Tradition has it that the translation of the *Pantegni* was produced at Monte Cassino, and was dedicated to the brilliant Abbot Desiderius.[5] Moreover, the Hague manuscript was itself copied at Monte Cassino. At first glance, that identification is astounding. The script from eleventh-century Monte Cassino

[1] For the recognition of Constantine's work as both translation and adaptation, see the Introduction. From this point forward, this volume addresses the *Pantegni* as a translation.

[2] Burnett and Jacquart, eds, *Constantine the African and ʿAlī ibn al-ʿAbbās al-Maǧūsī.*

[3] For the known manuscripts, see the lists in Burnett and Jacquart, eds, *Constantine the African and ʿAlī ibn al-ʿAbbās al-Maǧūsī*, pp. 319–51.

[4] The manuscript was re-dated by Erik Kwakkel during the workshop Excavating Medicine in the Digital Age: Palaeography and the Medical Book in the Twelfth-Century Renaissance organized by Eliza Glaze and Monica Green from 30 September to 3 October 2010 (National Humanities Center, North Carolina). During the same conference the date was confirmed by Francis Newton, who also noted Beneventan traits in the script (see the following discussion). An eleventh-century date (see Geyl, 'Zwei lateinische Handschriften') was not previously accepted by scholars.

[5] See the Introduction.

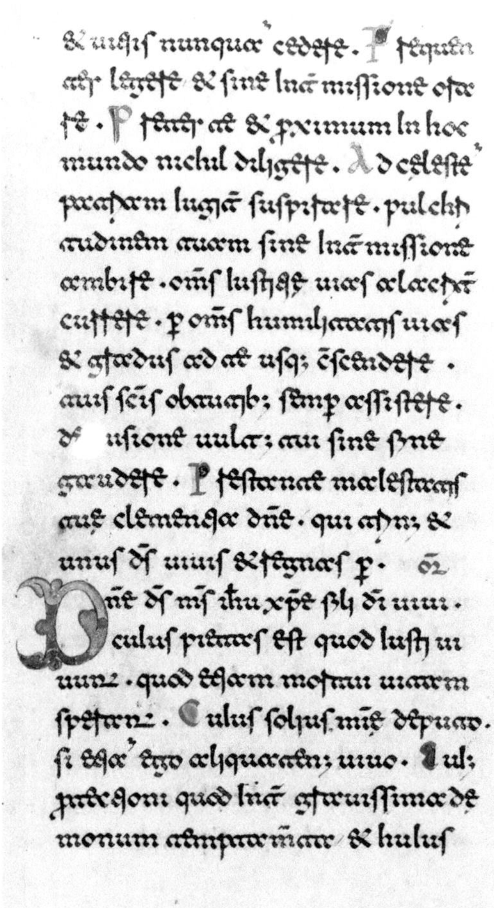

Figure 1.2.
Typical Beneventan script of Monte Cassino, Archivio della Badia, MS 442, p. 305. This text presents liturgical prayers.

is a handsome, classic, broken Beneventan (fig. 1.2),[6] while the Hague volume is written in Caroline minuscule (fig. 1.3). The task of this chapter is to demonstrate that the unexpected origin of MS 73 J 6 is the famous South Italian abbey, and to explain the manuscript's context there. In fact, the present discussion aims to identify each of the manuscripts in which the same Caroline minuscule hand appears; some are preserved at Monte Cassino itself, while others are as

[6] The classic study of the script is that of Lowe, *Beneventan Script*. A study focused specifically on the classic Monte Cassino type of the eleventh century is that of Newton, *Scriptorium and Library*. On the Desiderian gospel books, see the important contribution of Irving, '(Not) Identifying a Desiderian Evangelistary Fragment'.

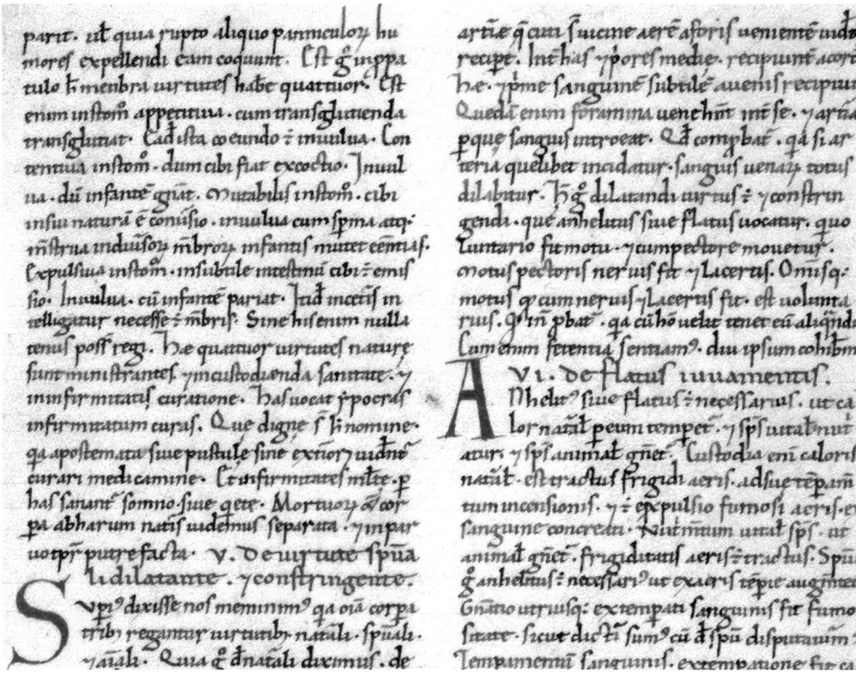

Figure 1.3. Caroline minuscule of the main scribe, Geraldus. The Hague, Koninklijke Bibliotheek, MS 73 J 6, fol. 23r (detail). Late 1070s or early 1080s (before 1086).

far removed today from their home as the Hague volume, found in libraries in cities as distant as Paris and Copenhagen. Following the brief catalogue which follows is a more detailed discussion of the character of this hand that they share, the presence of Caroline minuscule in tenth- and eleventh-century South Italy and its place in Beneventan culture, and our scribe's position in the late eleventh-century scriptorium of Monte Cassino.

The Key Manuscripts

The Hague, KB, MS 73 J 6: Constantinus Africanus, *Pantegni*

Not only is it written in Caroline minuscule, but this *Pantegni* manuscript (in contrast to the finest products of the Monte Cassino scriptorium) is, as Flannery O'Connor would say, 'plain, plain'.[7] No handsome gold initial is found on the

[7] O'Connor, 'Parker's Back', p. 510.

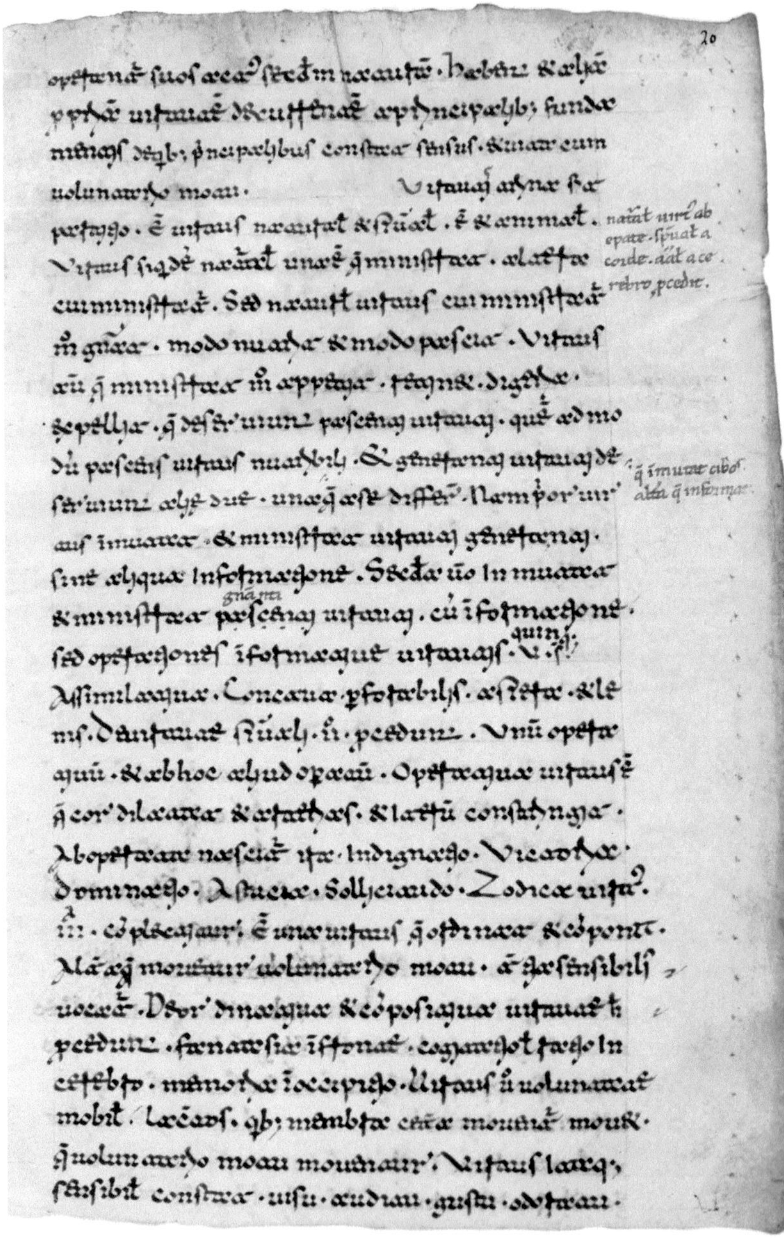

Figure 1.4. *Isagoge* in Beneventan script by the Bodleian Juvenal Scribe with marginal additions and interlinear corrections in Caroline minuscule by Geraldus. Note the blank space left for a chapter heading, but never filled in. Paris, Bibliothèque nationale de France, Nouvelle acquisition latine 1628, fol. 20r. *c.* 1070s–1080s.

opening page; there is only one decorated initial at the beginning (pl. IV), a simple **C** outlined in red, filled with saffron yellow, and with detail in blue and green. For the smaller initials at the head of each chapter, there is only the barest outline in red *capitalis*: there is no generous module of script or layout of text, only a tiny hand on an extraordinarily long, narrow page (fig. 1.1, pl. I, and the manuscript description in Appendix A).[8] Most striking of all to the palaeographer, there is no hierarchy of scripts. Some of the manuscripts discussed in our catalogue have text in handsome, even bold, Beneventan script accompanied by marginal, small Caroline minuscule in a subordinate position. The Hague *Pantegni*, however, is written entirely in that latter tiny and simple script.

Paris, BnF, NAL 1628, fols 19–26: *Isagoge*

This single gathering bound in a modern miscellany contains the *Isagoge* of Johannitius,[9] the text that was to become the opening treatise of the famous *Articella*, the fundamental curriculum of six texts that from the twelfth century served as an introduction to the subject in medical schools across Europe. The text is written in an idiosyncratic, inky Beneventan hand (fig. 1.4). What is most remarkable, however, is that there are frequent textual additions or supletions in contemporary Caroline minuscule in the margins. The original text, therefore, represents an early stage in the translation process. As evidence presented in this chapter shows, modern readers can see before their eyes the translator's second thoughts and additions.

It has been clear for some time that this Paris volume should possess great authority: it is one of two manuscripts of this seminal little book written (a) in Beneventan script, and therefore from the region of the earliest translations of Arabic medical texts into Latin; and (b) in Beneventan script of the eleventh century, therefore from both the region and the period of those earliest translations, and in fact from the lifetime of Constantine the African.[10] Additionally,

[8] More on the significance of module and layout is found in Chapter 3.

[9] Beccaria, *I codici di medicina*, p. 181. See also Jacquart, 'À l'aube de la renaissance médicale'; and Newton, 'Constantine the African', pp. 27–40, and figs 1 and 5.

[10] It is in keeping with the general neglect of these Arabic-to-Latin texts by modern researchers that there has not been a scholarly edition of the *Isagoge*; these two Beneventan manuscripts would be found central to such an edition. The only modern edition of the Latin *Isagoge* does not make use of these two; see Maurach, 'Johannicius: Isagoge ad Techne Galieni'. Maurach's edition was never intended to rest on any large number of manuscripts or on a critical examination; it was meant as a 'working text'. For further bibliography, see Newton, 'Constantine the African', p. 16 n. 1.

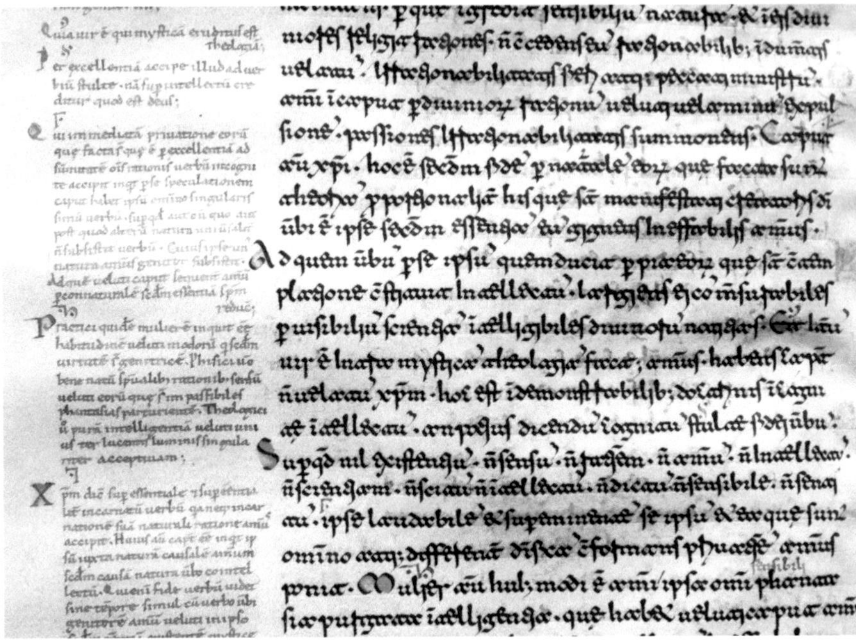

Figure 1.5. Marginal *scholia* by Geraldus, the main scribe of the Hague manuscript, Monte Cassino, Archivio della Badia, MS 333, p. 2 (detail). 1087–1105. The text is that of Maximus Confessor's *Quaestiones ad Thalassium*.

the hand responsible for the suppletions in the Paris manuscript is the same hand as the main text of the Hague *Pantegni*. It is the same fine Caroline minuscule, unshaded for the most part, with a free, somewhat irregular base line of script, ascenders (as of **d**) that may have a subtle bend, and both a distinctive ampersand and the 7-shaped symbol for *et*.

The identification of this single Caroline minuscule hand in two medical texts leads to a valuable conclusion. The scribe, resident in the Beneventan zone, wrote in Caroline minuscule, yet the scriptorium found work for him to do. Specifically, he was called upon in the case of the Hague manuscript to create a 'fair copy' (that is, a fair-enough copy) of the *Pantegni*, with space left on the first page for a supplement to the work's Prologue and, on subsequent leaves, with space left for insertion of further text in certain passages. Both, as we will show, clearly reflect an interim stage in the translator's work. In the case of this Paris manuscript, the substantial number of marginal and interlinear suppletions marks an even earlier stage in the production process followed by the translator. Was the translator perhaps standing by and orally dictating to his

Caroline minuscule-writing scribe? In any case, this scribe, rather than a type of drudge, was part of the team engaged in the cutting-edge project of transmitting Arabic medical culture to the Western world, as this book shows.

Monte Cassino, MS 333: Maximus Confessor, *Quaestiones ad Thalassium*

There is another late eleventh-century manuscript in which this scribe's hand appears prominently in the margins.[11] It is Monte Cassino, MS 333, containing Maximus Confessor's *Quaestiones ad Thalassium*. This text of a Greek Father, translated into Latin by John Scotus Eriugena in the ninth century, must have been relatively rare in Western Europe. It survives in only two Latin copies, and of those the Monte Cassino manuscript preserves the 'infinitely superior' text.[12] In this volume the text (fig. 1.5 and pl. II), presented in a single column, is written in a fully developed, heavy, and monumental Beneventan of the classic Monte Cassino type of the end of the eleventh century. Alongside in the outer margin are the ancient *scholia* also translated by Eriugena; these are in the fine, distinctive Caroline minuscule of our scribe. The contrast in the scripts of the main text versus *scholia* could hardly be greater.

The manuscript is not of the highest quality, yet it has a dignity not always accorded to ordinary patristic texts at Monte Cassino. Details of the book proclaim that it does honour to the Byzantine confessor-saint who was the original author: in the handsome gold initial **S** at the opening of the text; in the smaller capitals coloured in combinations of red, green, yellow, and blue for the beginning of every sentence throughout, even in the *scholia*; and with a yellow wash running through the letters, with a black line drawn above them, in the Greek manner. The two abovementioned medical manuscripts that our scribe had a hand in have Greek titles, *Pantegni* (The Complete Art) and *Isagoge* (Introduction), and promised to make available in Latin, from Arabic, the wisdom of Greek medical authorities. Monte Cassino, MS 333 was translated directly from Greek into Latin. All three manuscripts represent the Desiderian and Oderisian project of recovering ancient Greek learning.

[11] Newton dates Monte Cassino, MS 333 to the late eleventh or early twelfth century. Newton, *Scriptorium and Library*, p. 374.

[12] The identification of John Scotus Eriugena's translation is owed to Meyvaert; see his 'The Exegetical Treatises of Peter the Deacon', and 'Eriugena's Translation of the *Ad Thalassium* of Maximus'. See also the edition of the Greek text, with the Latin translation of Eriugena, in Maximus Confessor, *Quaestiones ad Thalassium I*, ed. by Laga and Steel, especially pp. xci–cix; on the superiority of the Monte Cassino manuscript, see p. xcii.

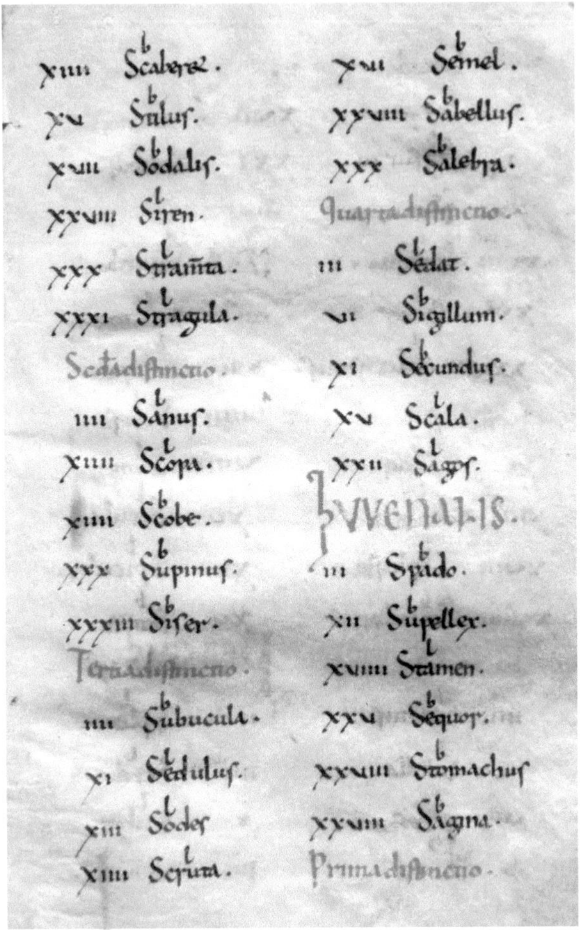

Figure 1.6.
Lexicon prosodiacum copied by Geraldus, the main scribe of the Hague manuscript, Monte Cassino, Archivio della Badia, MS 580, p. 55. 1060s–early 1070s. Geraldus writes Caroline minuscule here.

As Danielle Jacquart and Francoise Micheau have stressed (in special reference to Constantine's works), this recovery was what the monks understood Constantine was giving them.[13]

Monte Cassino, MS 580: *Lexicon prosodiacum*

The scribe of the Hague manuscript was active in the early abbacy of Desiderius (r. 1058–86) as well. Among the treasure of manuscripts from the first part of his abbacy still preserved at Monte Cassino, one of the most remarkable

[13] This point is particularly stressed by Jacquart and Micheau, *La médecine arabe et l'occident médiéval*, pp. 99–101.

is the little volume Monte Cassino, MS 580 (fig. 1.6). This manuscript was first studied by Henry W. Willard in a piece that appeared in 1929.[14] It is the earliest surviving copy of a work which Willard called 'Lexicon Prosodiacum', a handbook to illustrate the metrical quantity of the first syllable in a long series of Latin words. Its purpose was to serve as an aid in the composition of Latin verse. In more recent studies, Diane Warne Anderson provided an edition and assessed the handbook's importance.[15] In fact, she convincingly identifies its creator as the illustrious hagiographer and *grammaticus* Albericus, the scholar who aided Abbot Desiderius in the composition of his *Dialogi*, and who in 1078–79 led the decisive attack upon Berengar of Tours's teaching on the Eucharist. Alberic's treatise on the controversy still survives, and modern scholars can study Alberic's accomplishment as a controversialist.[16] It is also clearly demonstrated by Paul F. Gehl that in addition to the *Lexicon prosodiacum*, Alberic wrote the treatises on prosody that stand beside it in BAV, Ottob. lat. 1354 (*c.* 1100).[17] It is no exaggeration to argue, as Anderson and Gehl have shown, that his work was revolutionary.

The *Lexicon prosodiacum* in Monte Cassino, MS 580 is not only the earliest copy of this work. Because of one stunning aspect, it also bears unmistakable signs of representing a stage in the original creation of the treatise. Like the Paris *Isagoge*, it is written in a mixture of Beneventan script and Caroline minuscule, but with a key difference: the scribe began the text in Beneventan script down to page 11, but changed to Caroline minuscule from that point onward.[18] After, when he returned as rubricator (it is the same hand) to add the headings, he maintained Beneventan script for only the first page. The result is that for about ten pages, the main text is in Beneventan script and the headings in Caroline minuscule.[19] This mixture is an indication of a scholar's work-in-progress. A fair copy (that is, a fairly good, or reasonably good, replica) was all that was required at this stage of composition. Besides, this was a 'technical' treatise to help students compose Latin poetry, for use only in the schoolroom.

14 Willard, 'Codex Casinensis 580T'.

15 Anderson, *Lexicon prosodiacum*; and 'Medieval Teaching Texts'.

16 Radding and Newton, *Theology, Rhetoric, and Politics in the Eucharistic Controversy*, especially pp. 40–85.

17 Gehl, 'Vat. Ottobonianus lat. 1354'.

18 The reader is reminded that Monte Cassino manuscripts are paginated, and so always cited as such.

19 Lowe, *Beneventan Script*, p. 91; Newton, *Scriptorium and Library*, p. 113.

For this purpose, the combination of Beneventan and Caroline minuscule script presented no difficulties.

This scribe is that of the Hague manuscript with which the present discussion began. The rich poetic *exempla* in hexameter lines drawn from the classical and early Christian poets Virgil, Horace, Juvenal, Persius, Lucan, Statius, Sedulius, Prudentius, Prosper, Arator, and Ovid, provide a palaeographical bonus in the small capitals with which each line begins. Like the remainder of the lines, these evidence the same distinctive majuscule/minuscule hand on view, from the opening page, in the Hague *Pantegni*. The *capitalis* has its closest *comparanda* in documents.

Copenhagen, KB, GKS 1653 4°: Medical Works

There is a third medical manuscript that must enter the discussion: Copenhagen, KB, GKS 1653 4°, containing works derivative of Soranus, Hippocrates, Oribasius, and others (fig. 1.7).[20] This manuscript preserves an important collection of gynaecological texts.[21] It is also famous for its fifteen figures in black ink depicting foetal positions *in utero* (fols 17ʳ–19ᵛ). GKS 1653 4° is important to the present discussion because it also contains the hand of the Hague *Pantegni*'s scribe. He is seen, for example, on fol. 71ʳ at the bottom from the *Dieta Ypocratis*, and on fol. 148ʳ in the treatise called *Antibalomenon*.

The script here is somewhat crowded and laterally irregular, presumably in order to accommodate the text in the space available. It may, in fact, have been the case that the major texts were already written when these lesser texts were inserted, in spaces left blank, by our contemporary Caroline minuscule hand. In any case, the scribe of the Hague *Pantegni* is here seen contributing textually to another medical manuscript of great significance. With the Hague *Pantegni* and the Paris *Isagoge*, it is clear that he was called upon to take part in the copying of some of the most valuable scientific texts that Monte Cassino was acquiring under the rule of the bibliophile Abbot Desiderius. They are technical books, and Monte Cassino appears to have deliberately and purposely fostered the advance of medical knowledge in this way.

[20] Beccaria, *I codici di medicina*, pp. 119–24; Lowe, *Beneventan Script*, p. 36.

[21] Hanson and Green, 'Soranus of Ephesus', p. 1030 n. 229. According to these authorities, Copenhagen, GKS 1653 4°, though the latest of the three manuscripts used by editors, is the only one that gives Soranus's name.

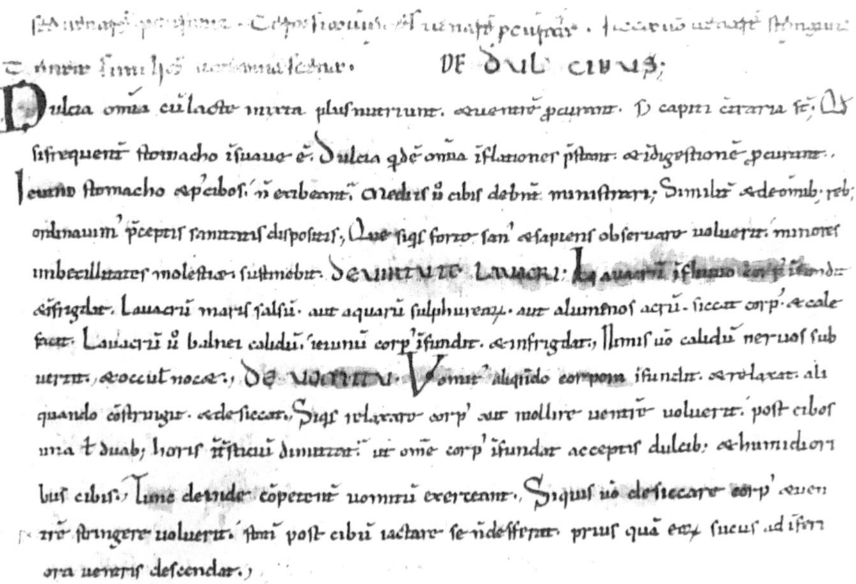

Figure 1.7. Medical manuscript that includes excerpts copied by the Apuleius Rubricator, Copenhagen, Kongelige Bibliotek, Gamle Kongelige Samling, MS 1653 4°, fol. 71^{v}. 1060s–early 1070s. The first two lines shown here are in Beneventan, the remainder in Caroline minuscule.

This identification sheds new light on another manuscript: Florence, Laurenziana, MS Plut. 68.2, part II (fols 104^{r}–191^{r}), containing Apuleius's *Apologia*, *Metamorphoses*, and *Florida*.[22] This copy of Apuleius's works is a famous product of Monte Cassino in the second half of the eleventh century, but can now be assigned, more specifically, to the first decade or fifteen years of the Desiderian period. The Copenhagen manuscript can be placed in the same period, that is, in the 1060s or the early 1070s. Like the Monte Cassino *Lexicon prosodiacum* and the Paris *Isagoge*, both Beneventan script and Caroline minuscule are present together. This means that, like those two, as a volume of technical treatises GKS 1653 4° did not need to meet the higher standards of patristic or classical volumes, not to mention books intended for liturgical use.

[22] Newton, *Scriptorium and Library*, pl. 54 and description on p. 347.

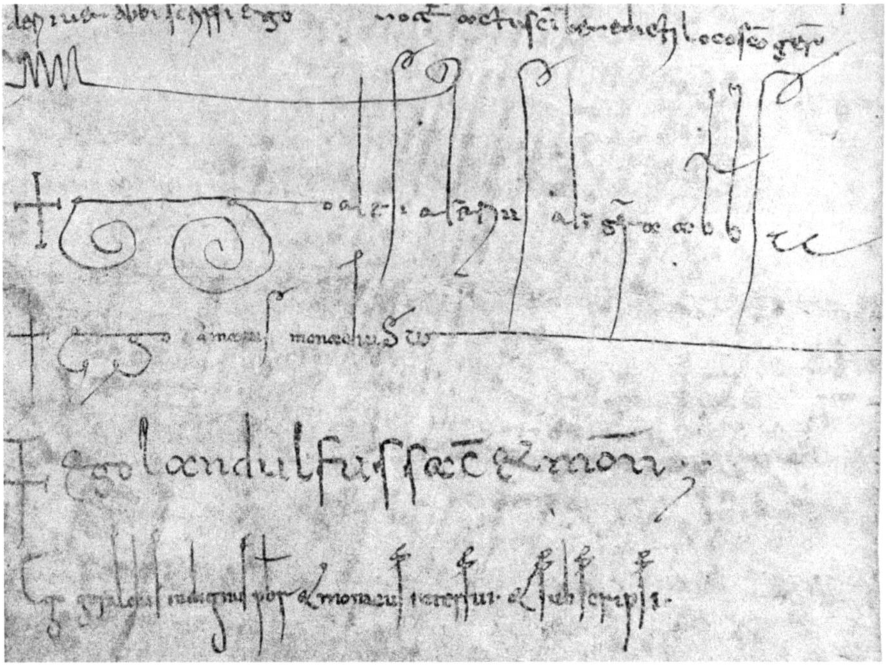

Figure 1.8. Geraldus signing his name (bottom row) in Caroline minuscule with documentary hand features: 'Ego Geraldus indignus presbyter et monacus interfui et subscripsi'. Monte Cassino, Archivum, Aula II, Caps. CIII, Fasc. II, no. 10. June 1061.

The 1061 Document for Traetto

Amazingly, we can give a name to this scribe who occupied such a vital place in Monte Cassino's scriptorium of the period. The charter Monte Cassino, Archivum, Aula II, Caps. CIII, Fasc. II, no. 10 is a document written in June 1061, in favour of Traetto (fig. 1.8). It is signed by Abbot Desiderius with, to borrow Herbert Bloch's expression, his 'tremendous *ego*',[23] then by Amatus, the

[23] Bloch, *Monte Cassino in the Middle Ages*, II, fig. 52; at I, 93, Bloch discusses Desiderius's signature and how the 'extraordinary *ego*, which dominates the entire document, literally bespeaks "a tremendous ego"'. At I, 182, Bloch also treats the immediate background of the document, and its historical significance as 'one of the great landmarks in the history of the growth of communal independence in Southern Italy'. Here, we call attention to another surprise in the Traetto document: careful examination shows that in his own signature ('Desiderius Dei gratia abbas') Desiderius began to incorporate the divine name within his own; instead of the third syllable of 'Desiderius', he first wrote the syllable 'de' as the abbreviation for 'dei' with the form of the traditional *nomen sacrum* (in writing 'desidei' he was anticipating the next word 'dei').

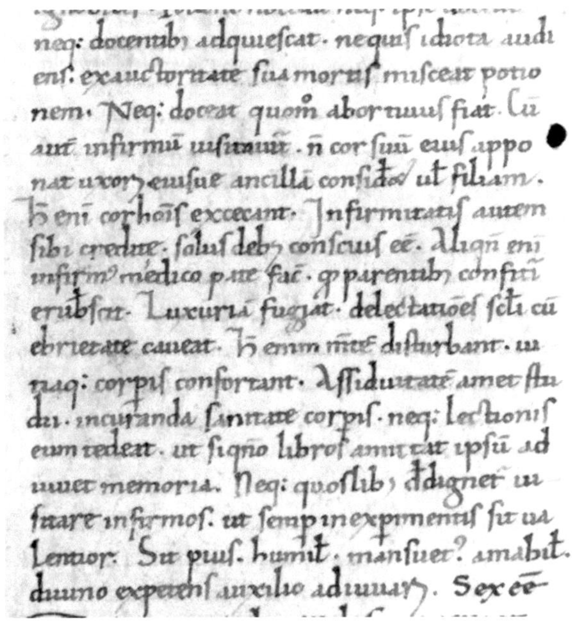

Figure 1.9. The Caroline script of Geraldus, here copying the chapter on deontology, describing the ideal characteristics of a medical student. The Hague, Koninklijke Bibliotheek, MS 73 J 6, fol. 1v. Late 1070s–1080s (before 1086).

poet and author of the famous *Historia Normannorum*, and by one 'Landulfus sacerdos et monachus'. These three signatures are in Beneventan. The fourth and final signature is in Caroline minuscule, in the hand of the manuscripts discussed above, and it gives us the scribe's name: 'Ego Geraldus indignus presbyter et monachus interfui et subscripsi' (I Geraldus, unworthy priest and monk, was present and signed my name).

Before, we knew that our scribe was a writer of Caroline minuscule, a practitioner of the minority script in a region that had its own dominant, centuries-old writing system.[24] Now we know the name of the scribe of the Hague *Pantegni*, the *scholia* in the Monte Cassino Maximus Confessor, the textual suppletions in the Paris *Isagoge*, the Monte Cassino *Lexicon prosodiacum*, and of short sections of the Copenhagen volume containing Soranus and other gynaecological works. The document also tells us that Geraldus was 'priest and monk', that is, an educated monk, which is also significant: it is important, after all, when building a picture of the scriptorium to know that the scribes have a high intellectual level.

See Newton, *Scriptorium and Library*, pl. 194 and discussion at p. 156 n. 147.

[24] The document for Traetto demonstrates in its signatures the extraordinary contrast between the scripts.

The Hand of Geraldus

In general appearance, the Caroline minuscule script of Geraldus is fairly bold, with great clarity, even where written quite small, as it is especially in MS 73 J 6 (fig. 1.9 and pl. III). It is flowing and softly stroked, with very little contrast between thick and thin strokes; instead, the moving line traced by the pen is rather uniform in breadth, unlike the broken Beneventan of Monte Cassino (fig. 1.2). It has few sharp angles, again in contrast to the Beneventan of Monte Cassino. What may have been most striking for readers in the eleventh century is the legibility of Geraldus's text.

The line of writing, when scrutinized, reveals itself to be wobbly and irregular, with a free and natural flow (again see fig. 1.9 and pl. III). Close examination of the letters that stand on the base line shows this freedom. The head line is perhaps even more informal. In sum, the Caroline minuscule is a type that one could almost call 'anti-Cassinese', with rounded, somewhat irregular, treatment of all elements.

In orientation, the script of these books is a decidedly vertical hand. The shaft of **r** leans toward the right, but most letters are patently upright; even the back of **a** conforms to this orientation. Also characteristic are the round shapes: between head line and base line the loops are relatively large and noticeable, as in **b**, **d**, **e**, **g**, **o**, **q**, and even the smaller loop of **a**.

On the horizontal plane, Geraldus takes great care to separate the letters, allotting each its own space. This is especially true of the rounded letters; any hint of lateral crowding is avoided. It is visible from the time of the document of 1061 and throughout the scribe's career; the same 'clean' look is present (except in the crowded text of the Copenhagen medical pieces he has inserted into that manuscript), in obvious contrast to the 'knitted' appearance of classic Beneventan script.

In regard to specific strokes and letters (fig. 1.10 and pl. IV), **a**, as noted, has a rather upright back with curve at top and bottom. The **d** is distinctive, and has no bend at bottom right; its ascender, however, may sway a little, probably the result of the flag at top being applied in a separate motion. Usually **e** has an angled cross stroke, or *sagitta*, often near the head line. The shaft of **r** leans right (like / but often bent) and typically curves toward the shoulder stroke. The lobes have a characteristic round, generous, flowing shape in **o** and **g**, and in the smaller lobe of **a**; this is particularly marked in **b** and **d**. The **u** is wide and equally flowing. The first minim of **n** and the first two of **m** are simple, unbent, and of uniform thickness. Ascenders, as those of **b**, **d**, and also **l**, are greatly lengthened, often bent a bit, and endowed with flags at the top. Descenders

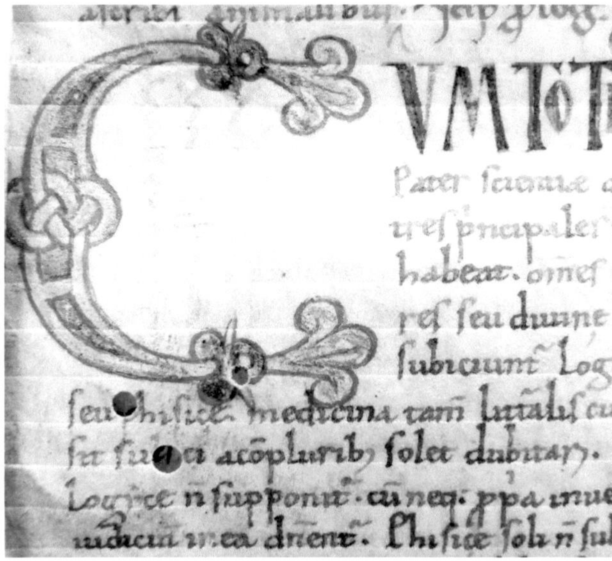

Figure 1.10.
Execution of the letters; the large initial **C** marks the beginning of the body of Prologue Part B, based upon Isidore of Seville's three types of knowledge: *logica*, *aethica*, and *physica*. The Hague, Koninklijke Bibliotheek, MS 73 J 6, fol. 1r (detail). Late 1070s–early 1080s (before 1086).

are especially varied; in the Hague *Pantegni* tall **s** tends to end on the base line, because in this compressed script it is essential to prevent descenders from entering the letter space of the line below. Geraldus writes the body of certain letters consistently, but varies their extremities considerably: for example, **g** has an identical body in each instance but its tail has a range of expressions, and the wide body of **x** remains the same while the stroke on the lower left sometimes stretches far below the base line.

The divergence in certain letter forms must be emphasized. The script of the minuscule is identical in the *body* of the lines: by this we mean the strokes and letter forms, or parts of letter forms, that lie between the head line and the base line. It is also true that the ascenders and vertical strokes that rise above the head line are very much the same. It is in the descenders or tails, as in the above-mentioned examples of **g** and **x**, that inconsistency occurs. In these letters, and a few others like them, the body remains the same, but the tail varies and is more formalized in the Hague volume. This is apparently not due to development in his style or skill across the variously dated specimens. In his first known work, the Traetto charter of 1061, Geraldus makes use of two, or perhaps three, forms of **g** with substantial tail variations in the opening words of his signature.

Two other letter forms are particularly notable. In the Hague manuscript, Geraldus adopted the Beneventan **ri** ligature for almost every occurrence of this letter combination (fig. 1.10 and pl. IV, *dubitari*, third line from bottom). It is shaped like the same ligature in his Beneventan minuscule, as seen for example in the *Lexicon prosodiacum*. This is not found in the instances of his Caroline minuscule in other manuscripts; perhaps he revived it especially for the script of the *Pantegni*. Furthermore, for the Hague manuscript Geraldus added the 7-shaped abbreviation for *et* (fig. 1.3, column B, lines 2–4) to his arsenal, while still retaining a form of his old *et*-ligature or ampersand, as seen in the 1061 document. By the time of the later Monte Cassino, MS 333, the ampersand, it seems, has disappeared and the 7-shaped form preferred.

When we turn from Geraldus's Caroline minuscule to his rather simple display script, we are again struck by the contrast with the formal Beneventan script used all around him. His characteristic *capitalis* is observable at the opening of the Hague manuscript. The first words of the *Pantegni* address Constantine's abbot as: 'DOMINO SUO MONTIS CASSINENSIS abbati Desiderio' (fig. 1.1 and pl. I). The simple elongated *capitalis* of these words (with **a** and **n** in tall but minuscule form), is written in brown ink with a rare and quiet yellow wash. An identical *capitalis* appears in the headings of Geraldus's script in the *Lexicon prosodiacum*, where these very distinctive majuscule-in-minuscule forms run down the left margin at the beginning of each hexameter line cited from the eleven poets (fig. 1.6). In general, it may be said that the execution of these forms is rare in codices: their home is in documents. The chancery effect they have in the opening of the *Pantegni* is surprising. It shows, firstly, that Geraldus was used to writing documentary materials. It could be that the documentary features in the Hague manuscript represent where the scribe fell into his chancery habits. It may also be, however, that he conceived of Constantine's work in adapting and translating al-Maǧūsī's great medical encyclopaedia as a gift on the same plane as the gifts of land and buildings made to Monte Cassino and its abbot attested in numerous chancery documents of the era. We know from the charter for Traetto, moreover, that Geraldus was a scribe of such documents.

The hand is not overall a grand calligraphic success, nor did the scribe aim for that. The interior space (between head line and base line) varies in height, and in fact there is no sense of uniformity, whether at the base or the head. Vertical shafts are unaligned. Yet, the hand has an unmistakable look, conveyed by the fluid movement, generous lateral spacing of letters, upright stance, and characteristic letter parts like the rounded **e**, **o**, and **b**, and the angular head of **r**. From the example of 1061 on, Geraldus's script demonstrates a certain clarity and simplicity.

We conclude that all these specimens, document and codices, whether of greater or lesser formality, were written by a single scribe: 'Geraldus [...] presbyter et monachus'. Although trained originally in Caroline minuscule, he

Table 1.1. Chronology of Geraldus's currently identified scribal activity.

	Date	Manuscript	Content
1	1061	Monte Cassino, Archivum, Aula II, Caps. CIII, Fasc. II, no. 10	Document for Traetto
2	1060s–early 1070s	Monte Cassino, MS 580	*Lexicon prosodiacum*
3	1060s–early 1070s	Copenhagen, KB, GKS 1653 4°	Ps.-Soranus, Oribasius, et al.
4	1070s–80s	BnF, NAL 1628, fols 19–26	*Isagoge*
5	Late 1070s or early 1080s (before 1086)	The Hague, KB, MS 73 J 6	*Pantegni*
6	1087–1105 (Oderisian)	Monte Cassino, MS 333	Maximus Confessor

had learned both the document script and the book script of the Beneventan zone and was a trusted servant of Desiderius by the third year of the famous abbot's rule; in June 1061 he wrote, in a fluent, dashing Beneventan, the text of the historic document for Traetto that is still preserved at the abbey, and in a stately Caroline minuscule with chancery flourishes, his signature as the last witness on the same charter. His versatility is demonstrated from this early date. He was then a workhorse in the scriptorium over the next twenty-five to thirty years; the appearance of his hand in Monte Cassino, MS 333, dated to Oderisius's abbacy (1087–1105) before the Hague manuscript was identified.[25] Table 1.1 organizes the surviving manuscripts containing Geraldus's hand chronologically, thus demonstrating the position of the *Pantegni* manuscript in his known scribal career.

The extraordinary textual importance of the array of manuscripts in which his hand is found will be discussed later; but we may state here that based on both the early and late evidence, Geraldus remained a trusted, faithful servant of the abbot of Monte Cassino. It is therefore unsurprising that he was entrusted with the task of preparing, in the course of its production, a 'fair copy' of the masterpiece of the resident foreign scholar Constantine the African; a masterpiece dedicated to Constantine and Geraldus's father in God, Desiderius.

[25] This important manuscript would have been named in the Desiderian book list if it had been completed under that abbot. The fact that it was not, and the palaeographical evidence within the manuscript itself, makes it a product of Oderisius's time (Newton, *Scriptorium and Library*, pp. 255–59; 374). As is demonstrated in this monograph, the Hague manuscript represents a stage in the development of the text of Constantine's translation which continued at Monte Cassino; since the dedicatory words do not address Desiderius by his papal name (Victor III), the book must date from before May 1086.

Caroline Minuscule Script in the Beneventan Zone

When Desiderius of Monte Cassino (abbot from 1058–87) generously welcomed Constantine the African to his monastery in the 1070s, it was enjoying a 'golden age'. It was also, in many ways, the golden age of Beneventan script. In the previous decade, the abbey had achieved a new and handsome form of the revered, traditional hand (fig. 1.2).[26] On the other side of the peninsula, in the region of Bari, a very different, yet equally calligraphic, form of Beneventan was dominant.[27] Other houses or regions (as manuscripts not yet localized show) were producing beautiful books with their own variations on the style. *Beneventana* held sway as the dominant script from just below the Alban Hills of Rome southwards. In fact, in Abruzzi and the Marche, it had strongly penetrated far northwards, and from Apulia had spread across the Adriatic to hold a principal position in the Dalmatian coastal regions. From Teramo in Central Italy to Brindisi and Montescaglioso in the south, and eastwards at least as far as Split, the script had extended its domain.

Still, this hegemony was challenged by non-Beneventan script types, especially by Caroline minuscule.[28] This did not happen only at the fringes and borders of the Beneventan zone; anyone who closely examines Beneventan manuscripts from the heart of the territory will encounter this phenomenon. At Naples a beautiful tenth-century Virgil manuscript in the Beneventan style of that city (Naples, Biblioteca Nazionale, Vindob. lat. 5) contains an added line in almost contemporary Caroline minuscule (fig. 1.11). At Benevento a locally made liturgical roll, a Pontifical, of the same century (now Rome, Biblioteca Casanatense, MS 724 [B I 13], part I, has rubrics added not much later in fine Caroline minuscule (fig. 1.12). More examples are found at Monte Cassino: that prince of early Desiderian scribes, Grimoald, corrects his own handsome Beneventan text with marginal suppletions in stately Caroline minuscule in Monte Cassino, MSS 104, 109, and 434.[29]

[26] Newton, *Scriptorium and Library*, pp. 52–74.

[27] Lowe, *Beneventan Script*, pp. 150–51 and pl. 6,8; and especially Magistrale, *Cultura grafica e circolazione libraria*.

[28] For some of the contributions to discussion of this subject, see Lowe's chapter, 'Ordinary Minuscule in the Beneventan Zone', in *Beneventan Script*, pp. 84–92; Tristano, 'Scrittura beneventana e scrittura carolina'; Newton, 'One Scriptorium, Two Scripts'; and his *Scriptorium and Library*, pp. 87–95, 113–14.

[29] Newton, 'Fifty Years of Beneventan Studies'.

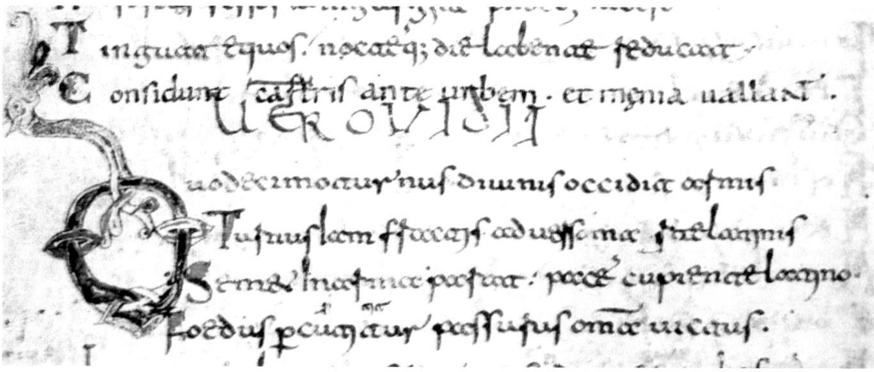

Figure 1.11. Omitted line in contemporary Caroline minuscule (here line 2) added to a Virgil manuscript copied in Beneventan script, Naples, Biblioteca Nazionale, Vindob. Lat. 5, fol. 168v. Tenth century.

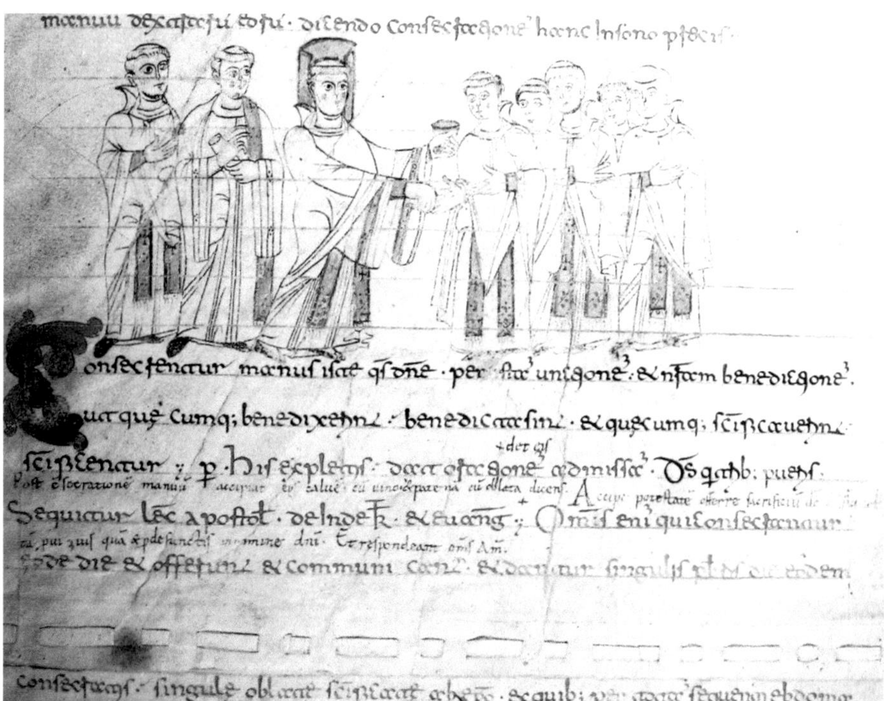

Figure 1.12. Contemporary interlinear additions in Caroline minuscule added to a liturgical roll copied in Beneventan, Rome, Biblioteca Casanatense, MS 724 [B I 13]. Tenth century.

In these examples from the great centres of Naples, Benevento, and Monte Cassino, the Caroline minuscule parts have something in common: they are all marginal. In Grimoald's manuscripts Caroline minuscule additions are literally in the margin: they are words, phrases, or clauses that Grimoald happened to omit when copying, and proofreading had revealed the need for correction. It is striking that Grimoald, who himself entered these suppletions, chose to do so not in the text's Beneventan, but also in a large, formal Caroline minuscule. In other words, Grimoald thought in terms of a hierarchy of scripts. In his mind, in display manuscripts such as these, the text hand must be Beneventan, but the textual additions *in margine* could be entered in a different script, one that Grimoald and his contemporaries perhaps regarded as more suitable for such things as glosses, suppletions, and other additions. Indeed Caroline minuscule, *in its place*, was not thought to disfigure the look of the page or opening.

The homiliaries of Grimoald (Monte Cassino, MSS 104 and 109) are display manuscripts, very carefully written, with splendid initials and even, in an initial **O** in Monte Cassino, MS 109, a miniature (fig. 1.13 and pl. V). There, the enthroned Christ is flanked by the Virgin and St Benedict, and the scribe, guided by Benedict, presents the volume and gives his own name: 'Grimoaldus diaconus et monachus scriptor'.[30] Grimoald's volumes, then, are on the same level as the Benevento Pontifical (if not quite so grand); they are meant for ceremonial use. In both, Caroline minuscule appears in a subordinate position, for textual additions or suppletions in the homiliaries, and for additional rubrics in the Pontifical. The relationship may be summed up in a quasi-mathematical diagram:

littera Beneventana: *littera Carolina*:: *domina*: *ancilla*.

In other words, Beneventan is to Caroline minuscule as mistress to maid (that is, of course, only in the Beneventan zone).

Now, but a little lower than these radiant creations, stands our other non-Cassinese example, the Naples Virgil. The script of this volume is the spidery Neapolitan type of the tenth century: one of the crowning calligraphic achievements in the history of Beneventan script. The initials of the Virgil have no gold, but they are large and dramatic evocations of the text. This manuscript also features corrections in Caroline minuscule, but here in a most inconspicuous fashion. It also illustrates a tendency in handwritten books in general: it is

[30] The abbreviation 'scrip' is expanded here as the noun (parallel to the titles of the Virgin and St Benedict), rather than as the verb 'scripsit'.

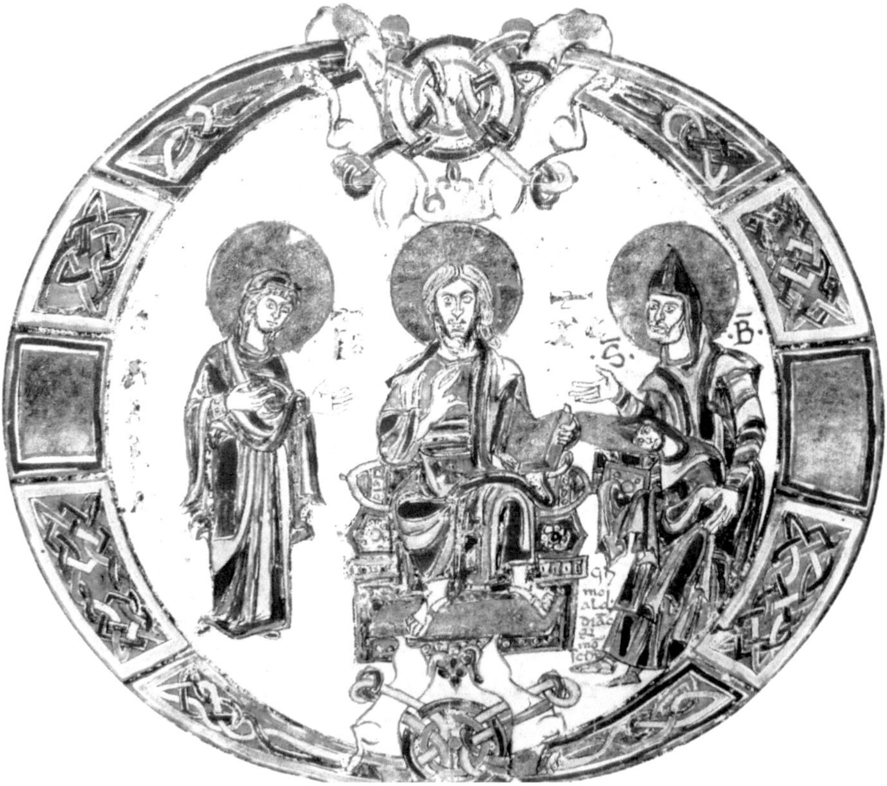

Figure 1.13. Decorated initial **O** showing the enthroned Christ. Grimoald the scribe, with his golden shoes, shelters beneath the arm of St Benedict on the right. He self-identifies in the inscription, 'Grimoald, deacon and monk, the scribe'. Monte Cassino, Archivio della Badia, MS 109, p. 295. *c.* 1058–75.

the final line of book XI (the penultimate book) of the *Aeneid* that the scribe omitted. For even highly skilled scribes, as one approaches the end of a work or of a section, attention wanders and vigilance flags.

Other manuscripts of the classics are not of such high quality as the Virgil. In fact, most classical texts, and most patristic texts as well, are copied in manuscripts that fall in the category of common books (*libri plebeii*).[31] In such cases a number of scribes may work in a single manuscript, and there may be a wide range of skill among them. Experienced students of medieval Latin manuscripts know where to look for the very best script a house could show; it is precisely in the class of display manuscripts, or *libri nobiles*. Conversely, the scribes of least

[31] Newton, 'One Scriptorium, Two Scripts'.

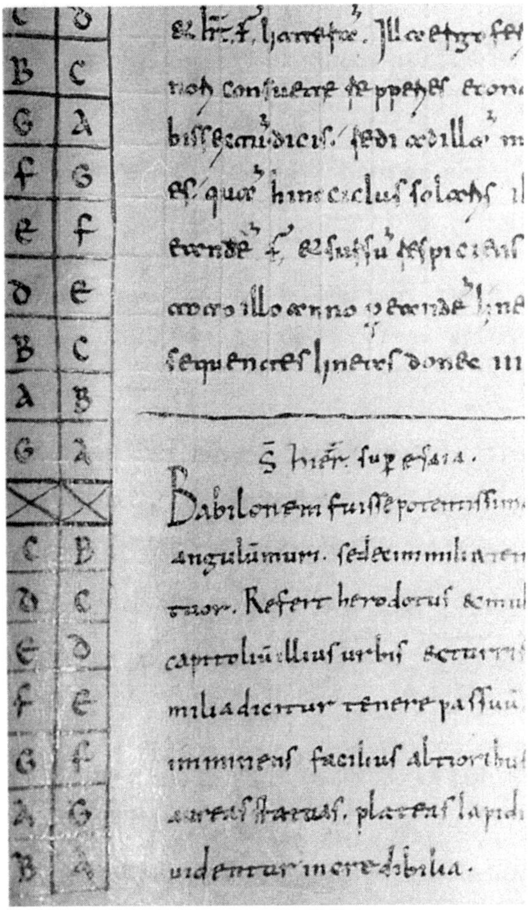

Figure 1.14.
Computus manuscript copied by Grimoald. The lower half of this passage (Jerome on Isaiah) is copied in Caroline minuscule by Grimoald due to tight space. The upper half shows his Beneventan hand. Monte Cassino, Archivio della Badia, MS 230, p. 34. Early Desiderian period.

ability are visible in *libri plebeii*. Scholars also know that within manuscripts, the poorest scribes were pressed into service towards the end of a given book. As shown elsewhere, an example of such an incompetent at work is found in the last quires of an Augustine manuscript preserved at Monte Cassino (Monte Cassino, MS 13).[32] Medieval scribes liked to compare themselves, as they guided the pen over the virgin parchment, to farmers ('aratores') ploughing the untouched fields. In this respect (the quality of writing/ploughing), the two shared a pride that survives in agriculture even today. Farmers in the Old World and the New tend to devote more care to fields that are seen by neighbours and travellers passing by than they do to fields remote from the road or highway.

[32] Newton, *Scriptorium and Library*, p. 82.

There is a further aspect to marginality. In this hierarchical world, some books were considered by their very nature, so to speak, marginal. In this category fall works that Bernhard Bischoff sometimes referred to as 'Fachliteratur': the technical texts essential to a monastic community. The practised palaeographical eye (and perhaps the codicological one as well) can often discern the differences. These books were not intended for display in the liturgy of the community (*libri nobiles*), nor were they designed for the individual, extended, profound, contemplative, scholarly reading of patristic or even classical texts (a type of *libri plebeii*, or what the French call 'livres d'étude'). This third type, also plebeian, was restricted to practical consultation or teaching. Many medical books fall into this category, as do grammatical and rhetorical works. For example, among the technical books that every monastery needed was the *computus*. Here again, perhaps surprisingly, the scribe Grimoald makes an appearance. The *computus* manuscript Monte Cassino, MS 230 (fig. 1.14) was produced almost entirely by this master. The book was certainly partly copied from a manuscript produced in the years 969–87, as the Paschal Tables suggest, and the manuscript has been misdated through a reliance on this sole criterion.[33] In reality, it is a product of the Desiderian period almost a century later.[34] A curious feature of the book, which has also caused confusion, is the presence of both Beneventan and Caroline minuscule. As has been set out elsewhere *in extenso*, it seems that in copying a fixed text (in the *computus*) with 'tight' layout, Grimoald found it convenient to use Beneventan where space was restricted because of the 'knitted' quality of that script, and Caroline minuscule where more flexibility and space was possible.[35] In this book Grimoald was seemingly unconcerned about consistency.

If this analysis is correct, Grimoald's script alternation in Monte Cassino, MS 230 was quite deliberate, but in common, plebeian manuscripts there are occasions when the scribe's alternation in scripts is not due to any intention on his part. It is an accident. The problem arises from a particular circumstance, with scribes whose original training had been in Caroline minuscule. Those who came to the Beneventan zone and there learned to write a Beneventan of passable or even good quality (and there seem to have been a fair number of them) were liable, when weary or distracted for whatever reason, to fall back into their native Caroline minuscule for a few words, or even for some clauses.

33 Lowe, *Scriptura Beneventana*, pl. 51.

34 Newton, *Scriptorium and Library*, pp. 43–47.

35 Newton, *Scriptorium and Library*, pp. 43–47.

Inattention at the foot of a page probably explains why the last two lines of text in the famous unique copy of Hilary's *Hymni* (Arezzo, Biblioteca della Città, MS 405, p. 29) are in Caroline minuscule, but by the same early-Desiderian scribe who wrote the rest. Another manuscript of great textual interest is that containing the works of Peter Damian (Monte Cassino, MS 359), copied by a team of Monte Cassino monks from the exemplar(s) held at Fonte Avellana shortly after the death of Peter, and hence in the early 1070s. One member of the team, as has been demonstrated,[36] perhaps because of pressure to complete the work or out of weariness, lapsed from his quite serviceable Beneventan into his native Caroline minuscule.

Geraldus and the Scriptorium at Monte Cassino

It is clear that the script of Geraldus represented the unorthodox in the context of the scriptorium of eleventh-century Monte Cassino. In a house, and indeed in a region, where the favoured hand was *littera Beneventana*, Geraldus's Caroline minuscule was somewhat alien. Caroline minuscule was, however, far from unknown in South Italy, as the present discussion has shown. Caroline minuscule appears, in fact, in some of the finest manuscripts produced at Naples and Benevento. Moreover, at Monte Cassino itself a master scribe of the early Desiderian years, the superb Grimoald, used it alongside his stately Beneventan for two purposes: in the margins of his great homiliaries (Monte Cassino, MSS 104 and 109) and his psalter (Monte Cassino, MS 434) for portions of the text that had been omitted in his original copying, or suppletions; and for sections of the *computus* (Monte Cassino, MS 230), a species of technical treatise, or 'Fachliteratur'. In both these instances, Grimoald's work makes a fine distinction: Caroline minuscule is deployed by the master scribe in a subordinate or ancillary position, whether in a certain place in a book (the marginal additions in fine manuscripts), or type of book (the lowly handbook that is the *computus*).

It is important to underscore that both these functions are paralleled in the *oeuvre* of Geraldus. The former type (a technical work) is seen in Geraldus's Hague manuscript of the *Pantegni*.[37] A precise parallel to the latter type is

[36] Newton, *Scriptorium and Library*, pp. 86–88, and especially fig. 4.

[37] The Hague manuscript is written entirely in Caroline minuscule. Perhaps a more precise parallel to Grimoald's Monte Cassino, MS 230 is found in Monte Cassino, MS 580, the *Lexicon prosodiacum*, which is partly in Beneventan and partly in Caroline minuscule.

seen in Paris, BnF, NAL 1628, fols 19–26, where the main text is written in Beneventan and marginal suppletions are added in Geraldus's Caroline minuscule, or in Monte Cassino, MS 333, containing works of Maximus Confessor, with main text in Beneventan and marginal *scholia* in Geraldus's Caroline minuscule. Of course, in the Cassinese scriptorium, as in any monastic scriptorium, the most beautiful manuscripts were for liturgical use. They did honour to Holy Writ, and to the ritual that centred around the altar. The scribes who produced those glorious books were at the cutting edge of their handsome script.[38] In the division of labour they were favoured, it appears, to execute these books, as the examples in table 1.2 show (Section A).[39] Yet there was another group of favoured scribes within the scriptorium, with a different focus, who worked at the cutting edge as well, but who stand almost at the opposite pole. Their attention was directed toward the recovery of old learning or the creation of new learning (table 1.2, Section B).

Notably, in Section B we encounter the works of 'house authors' such as Alberic, with his revolutionary new treatises on prosody and instruction in that art, and Constantine the African, with a long series of medical texts unknown before in Western Europe, now translated out of Arabic. These books are a stunning enough achievement in themselves, but their scribes were very closely associated with, or identical to, the scribes of some of the rarest classical texts to come down to us.[40] As was noted above, the Copenhagen manuscript of rare gynaecological texts (Copenhagen, KB, GKS 1653 4°) shows Geraldus entering passages in a volume copied in part by the same scribe whose work is seen in the Florence Apuleius (Florence, Laurenziana, MS Plut. 68.2, part II); it was Monte Cassino, and this manuscript, that preserved the famous novel filled with magic and the occult, and lesser works of the second-century Latin sophist. In the case of Geraldus's suppletions in the Paris *Isagoge* (fig. 1.4), the main text was produced by the same scribe who wrote the Bodleian Juvenal (Oxford, Bodleian, MS Canon. Class. Lat. 41), which preserves, uniquely, the thirty-four verses discovered by E. O. Winstedt (fig. 1.15), and so properly called the 'Winstedt

[38] For this reason, these dated or datable manuscripts of the eras of Abbot Desiderius and Abbot Oderisius form the framework of Newton's study of the Cassinese scriptorium in that period. See Newton, *Scriptorium and Library*, pls 1–47, and Irving, '(Not) Identifying a Desiderian Evangelistary Fragment'.

[39] The identifications in this table are new, except for the Geraldus manuscripts, which are introduced above.

[40] For the role of the classics in the education of monks at Monte Cassino in the eleventh century, see Newton, '"Expolitio" per l'Umanesimo'.

Table 1.2. Two elites of the Monte Cassino scriptorium (late eleventh century).

Section A: Liturgical Use		
Manuscripts	**Content**	**Scribe**
Monte Cassino, MSS 104 and 109[41]	*Homiliaria*	Grimoald
Monte Cassino, MS 434[42]	*Psalterium*	Grimoald
BAV, Vat. lat. 3784[43]	Exultet	Grimoald
Monte Cassino, MS 99	*Homiliarium*	Leo
Pisa, Museo Nazionale di San Matteo, Exultet Roll 2[44]	Exultet	*Dialectica* Scribe
Monte Cassino, Exultet Roll 1[45]	Exultet	*Dialectica* Scribe
Section B: Scholarly Use		
The Hague, KB, MS 73 J 6	*Pantegni*	Geraldus
Paris, BnF, NAL 1628, fols 19–26	*Isagoge*	Bodleian Juvenal Scribe + Geraldus
Oxford, Bodleian, MS Canon. Class. Lat. 41	Juvenal	Bodleian Juvenal Scribe
Copenhagen, KB, GKS 1653 4°	Oribasius	Apuleius Rubricator + Geraldus
Florence, Laurenziana, MS Plut. 68.2, part II (fols 104r–191r)	Apuleius	Apuleius Rubricator
Monte Cassino, MS 580	*Lexicon prosodiacum*	Geraldus
BAV, Ottob. lat. 1406[46]	Aristotle, *Categories* and other works	*Dialectica* Scribe

41 Newton, *Scriptorium and Library*, pp. 328–29; pls 1 and 2.

42 Newton, *Scriptorium and Library*, p. 379; pl. 176.

43 Newton, *Scriptorium and Library*, p. 335; pl. 22.

44 Newton, *Scriptorium and Library*, p. 332; pl. 14.

45 Newton, 'Un *codex Casinensis nobilissimus* di testi classici'. This Monte Cassino roll, now identified as being copied by the *Dialectica* Scribe, is of particular interest as it gives us, for the first time, two Exultet rolls (this and the Pisa roll also listed) that are the work of the same scribe.

46 Newton, 'Un *codex Casinensis nobilissumus* di testi classici'. This manuscript demonstrates that scribes of this calibre (copyists of liturgical books) might stray into the field of the other group (copyists of school texts). Grimoald apparently did so in the case of Monte Cassino, MS 230, *computus* (see above), and in the case of this *Dialectica* volume; the latter was produced for quite extraordinary reasons, discussed in this 2013 article. The reverse, of scribes of school books straying into the production of luxury liturgical manuscripts did not occur, as the article notes.

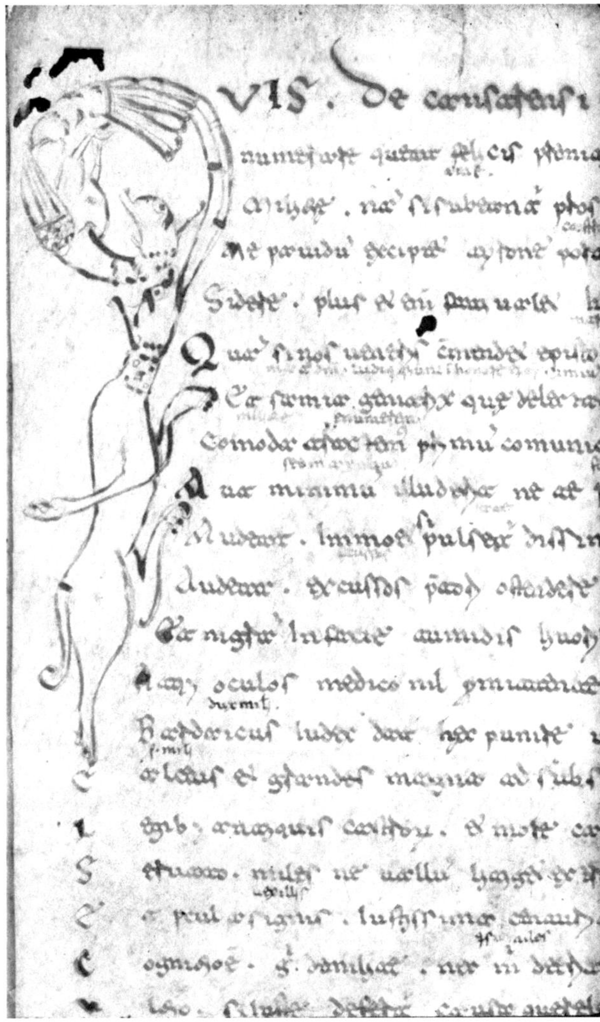

Figure 1.15.
The Bodleian Juvenal Scribe, Oxford, Bodleian Library, MS Canon. Class. Lat. 41, fol. 23r. *c.* 1075–*c.* 1100.

lines', in the satire directed against women (Satire 6). When it comes to Greek works, the text of John Scotus Eriugena's translation of Maximus Confessor must have been rare in the West: Geraldus's hand is responsible for the *scholia* in Monte Cassino, MS 333 (see fig. 1.5 and pl. II).

In fact, it is certainly true, as Jacquart and Micheau have pointed out in regard to medicine, that the Cassinese monks of the late eleventh century were interested in recovering the Greek texts of antiquity.[47] The monks would have been

[47] Jacquart and Micheau, *La médicine arabe et l' occident medieval.*

thrilled to read, in the Prologue to Constantine's translation of the *Pantegni*, al-Mağūsī's stately survey of great Greek medical writers: Hippocrates, Galen, Alexander of Tralles, Paul of Aegina, and Oribasius. Of course, the list begins with classical works, but it includes Byzantine authors (*novi*) as well. Moreover, we have noted in the list of manuscripts works of Maximus Confessor and Oribasius, of the Byzantine era. Monte Cassino still possesses a manuscript of Paul of Aegina's work (Monte Cassino, MS 351) that is contemporary with Constantine's residence there. Alfanus of Salerno translated what he called the *Premnon physicon* (originally *Peri tou anthropou physeos*) of Nemesius of Emesa, with its great roll-call of classical thinkers and their conceptions of the human soul.

Yet it must be remembered that, in terms of script, these scribes were poles apart from the other cutting-edge scribes who worked *in usum liturgicum*. The scribe of the Bodleian Juvenal, for example, practised a style of Beneventan that was so unlike the Monte Cassino script that he, and the Juvenal manuscript, have been assigned by modern scholars to a wholly different section of South Italy.[48] It is only by understanding the unorthodox and the un-Cassinese as having been an acceptable part of this textually innovative group that we can see how he and his unique manuscript fit into the picture of the same scriptorium. Furthermore, as for Geraldus, his Hague manuscript is written not in unorthodox Beneventan but in non-Beneventan altogether, being from start to finish in Caroline minuscule. And his script, as described here, is not even calligraphic Caroline minuscule. It was, in sum, an ill-assorted crew. Yet, from the standpoint of transmission of important texts, Geraldus was rubbing scapulars with, and part of, the scriptorium's elite.

[48] Cavallo, 'La trasmissione dei testi nell'area beneventano-cassinese', pp. 357, 406–07. The present discussion is part of a planned study of the manuscripts of the Scribe of the Bodleian Juvenal.

Chapter 2

Producing the Manuscript

The Beginnings: Monte Cassino, c. 1050–c. 1100

The story of The Hague, KB, MS 73 J 6 begins at Monte Cassino. Like any Benedictine abbey, Monte Cassino had an active scriptorium, which in the eleventh century produced a significant number of books.[1] The monastery is well known for its high-end illuminated books written in Beneventan script. MS 73 J 6, however, is not such a book: its appearance is notably plain (see the manuscript description in Appendix A).[2] For example, it contains only a single coloured initial, at fol. 1^{r}, and its parchment is mediocre. Moreover, it is written in Caroline minuscule, which represented a lower register of book production in Monte Cassino.

In a study of the coexistence of Caroline minuscule and Beneventan script in South Italian scriptoria like Monte Cassino, three grades of books are distinguished which form a hierarchy of quality, as discussed in Chapter 1.[3] The Hague manuscript can be placed on the lowest tier of this ladder in that it represents a book with 'every-day, utilitarian texts, many of them for school use it would seem, or for the pursuits of scholars'.[4] The books in this category pertain to dialectic, law, medicine, and grammar and are partly written in Beneventan and partly in Caroline minuscule. In physical respects as well, both palaeographically and codicologically speaking, the Hague manuscript sits on a lower tier.

[1] For the scriptorium and its output during the time of the Hague manuscript's production, see Newton, *Scriptorium and Library*.

[2] All material details explored in this chapter are summarized in Appendix A.

[3] Newton, 'One Scriptorium, Two Scripts', p. 120.

[4] Newton, 'One Scriptorium, Two Scripts', p. 122.

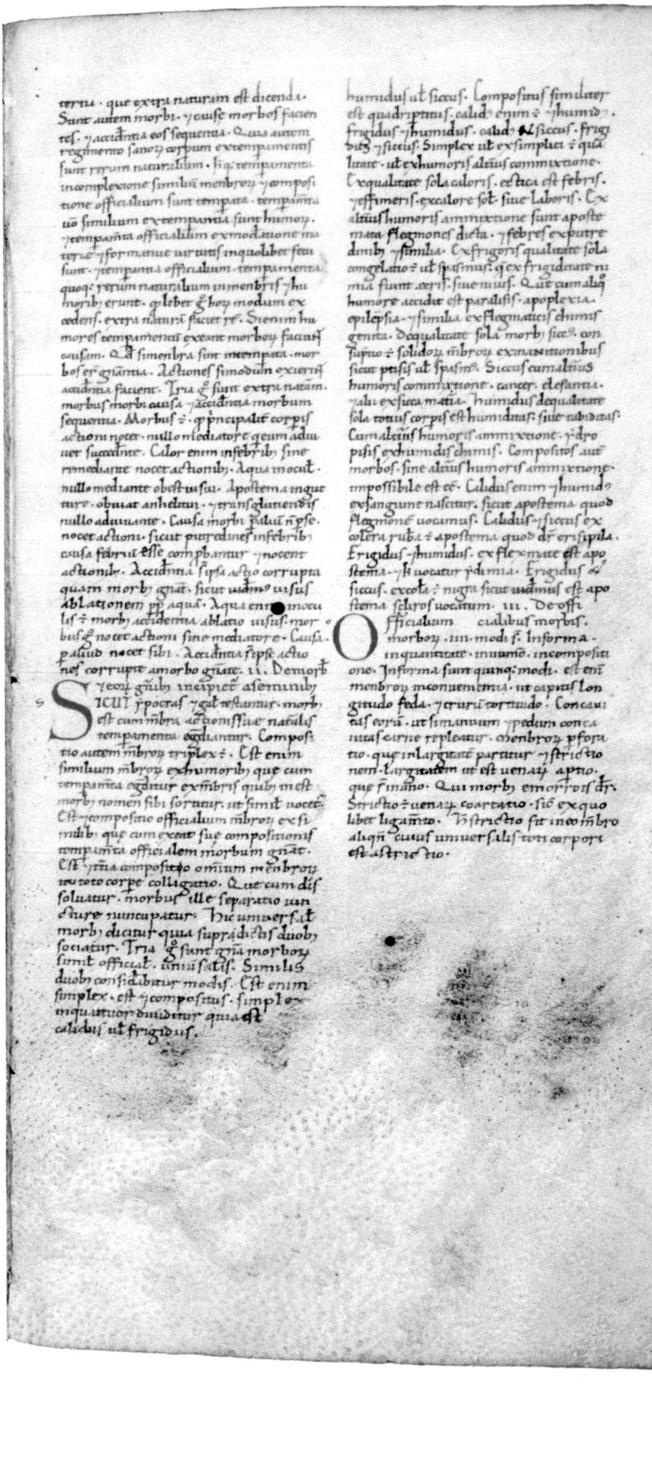

Figure 2.1.
Section of very thin parchment (lower end of col. B), skipped by the scribe. Indeed, the parchment is so thin that the writing on the verso shows through. The Hague, Koninklijke Bibliotheek, MS 73 J 6, fol. 37[r]. Late 1070s–early 1080s.

While MS 73 J 6 does not contain pages fully copied in Beneventan and others in Caroline minuscule, like some of the other lower-quality books, the individual who designed the pages and copied much of the *Pantegni* does employ Beneventan features in his predominantly Caroline minuscule script, the most prominent of which is the **ri** ligature.[5] Thus MS 73 J 6 represents a palaeographical mix. As discussed in Chapter 1, this individual, also identified here as Scribe A, is actually known by name: Geraldus.

Geraldus prepared eleven quaternions for the Hague copy of the *Theorica*. At some point a singleton was added to the end of the manuscript (fol. 89) to serve as a pastedown (now lifted).[6] The parchment used for these quires has some striking features that show that the scribe aimed to economize: a great many leaves contain translucent patches, a pronounced follicle pattern, discolouration (dark and yellow streaks or patches), or gaps at the edge of the page.[7] Moreover, the surface of the sheets was such that the ink often adhered poorly to it. Evidently, it was deemed unnecessary to present this copy of the *Pantegni* on better quality parchment.

The features noted here are typical for the outer edge of pre-cut skins, and were normally removed by scribes when cutting parchment into usable sheets. The scribe decided to include this outer edge (with its imperfections) because it meant that more surface would be retained for writing, even if that surface was indeed poor.[8] This enabled the scriptorium to use its available parchment more efficiently, which must have been particularly important in especially prolific copying periods. While Geraldus seems to have taken the imperfections in stride, at one point he does encounter problems because of them, which shows just how mediocre the writing support is: fol. 37^{r} contains a large section of parchment that is so poor that the scribe had to avoid it altogether, 'draping'

[5] A detailed palaeographical analysis of this hand is provided in Chapter 1.

[6] Some dark patches of the glue which adhered fol. 89 to the binding are still visible on the verso, which is otherwise blank. The recto contains medical excerpts, as discussed in this chapter and in Appendix A.

[7] Leaves with a pronounced follicle pattern and/or discolouration include fols 13^{r}, 14^{r}, 22^{v}, 25^{r}, 27^{r}, 28^{v}, 59^{r}, 60^{v}, 62^{v}, 66^{r}, 66^{v}, 68^{r}, 73^{r}, and 87^{r}. Translucencies are visible at fols 17, 18, 57, 58, 63, 64, 75, 76, and 80. Gaps occur at the edges of fols 36, 49, 52, and 55. A small tear or pebble-hole is found on fol. 50. Furthermore, some holes from the parchmenter's knife are present, for example at fols 15 and 25.

[8] About this procedure and its economical upside, see Kwakkel, 'Discarded Parchment as Writing Support'. In a commercial setting, the cost of labour was most expensive, followed by the cost of the writing support. In the case discussed here there were of course no writing costs, making the parchment the most expensive resource in book production.

the text around it, thus avoiding the lower five lines of column A and lower sixteen lines of column B (fig. 2.1).

Geraldus's book measures 235 × 128 mm. Once the sheets were cut he prepared them by pricking and ruling them according to the two-column *mise en page* he had designed. The ruling is dry-point, as per eleventh-century custom, and the pricking is still visible along the outer edge of most pages, which suggests that the bookbinder trimmed modestly. The textblock that Geraldus defined for himself offers 189 × 98 mm of written space (including the space between the two columns). This layout is unusual for several reasons. First, scribes in the late eleventh century were not in the habit of dividing such a narrow textblock into two columns. Codices in the *Catalogues des manuscrits datés* from 1075–99 show that the width of the textblock in two-column manuscripts ranges between 160 and 260 mm (including the space between the columns). A width over 190 mm was most common.[9] Evidently, the space reserved for the textblock of the Hague manuscript was unusually narrow: one would expect one column here, not two. A second feature worth noting is the remarkably small script used by Geraldus: each column holds sixty-two lines. Considering the column is 189 mm high, only 3 mm of space is available per line. Such compressed lines are uncommon in medieval books. The line height of MS 73 J 6 is equivalent to the very smallest of the famous thirteenth-century pocket bibles, which may well feature the tiniest handwriting of the Middle Ages.[10]

There is a third notable observation regarding the layout: Geraldus planned very little marginal space around the two text columns. The amount of unwritten space on the page, combined from all four margins, is only 38 per cent; as noted, surviving pricking suggests limited trimming by the binder. Considering margins as they survive today, about 50 per cent of the page is reserved for margins in codices written in 1075–99 which is also consistent with the twelfth-century average.[11] That the scribe used a tiny script and kept the mar-

[9] This information was retrieved from Kwakkel's unpublished Database of Dated Manuscripts, 1075–1225. Ten manuscripts with two columns are included from 1075–1100, the textblocks of which have a width of 160, 170, 170, 192, 195, 192, 203, 230, 250, and 260 mm. Dated codices in two columns written between 1101 and 1200 show roughly the same pattern.

[10] Large 'Paris Bibles' with a height of 380–420 mm may have a line height of 6–7 mm, while in pocket versions of some 150 mm in height the lines measure only 3–5 mm. For these measurements see Kwakkel, 'The Cultural Dynamics of Medieval Book Production', p. 247 n. 12. A smaller script is sometimes encountered in glosses, especially scholastic ones, but generally not in the main text.

[11] Kwakkel, 'The Margin as Editorial Space', p. 323 n. 1. These books may be trimmed,

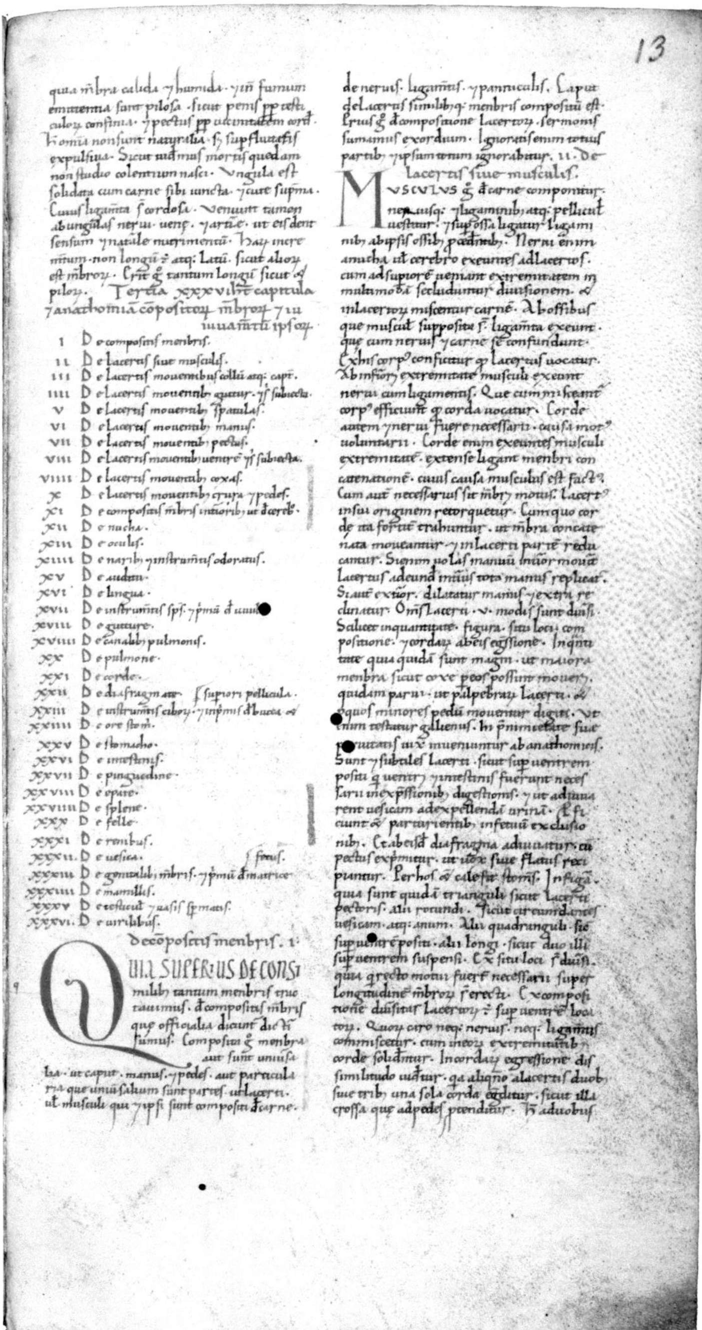

Figure 2.2.
Page with different types of rubrication in col. A (numbers in the *capitula* list, rubrics, initials), The Hague, Koninklijke Bibliotheek, MS 73 J 6, fol. 13r (*Theorica Pantegni*, beginning of book III). Late 1070s–early 1080s (before 1086).

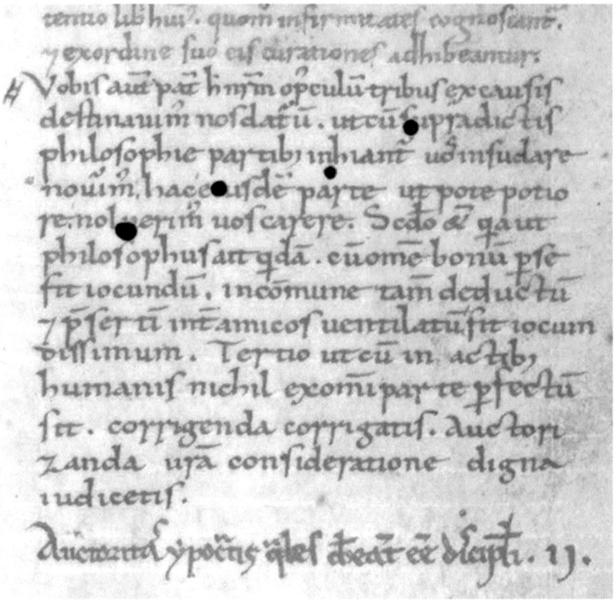

Figure 2.3.
Script of the Hague Rubricator, a.k.a. Scribe B, writing Prologue Part C. Late 1070s–1080s (before 1086). In the lowest line, Scribe C gives the rubric to chapter 2, the authority of Hippocrates on what type of persons medical students should be (*c.* 1150). The Hague, Koninklijke Bibliotheek, MS 73 J 6, fol. 1^r (detail).

gins particularly small suggests that he attempted to fit as much text per page as possible. This, subsequently, limited the number of sheets needed for the manuscript, which was apparently the scribe's ultimate goal. As discussed in Chapter 4, he tried to create a manuscript that was both lightweight and able to be held in one hand for consulting.

Once his folia were prepared, Geraldus began to copy out the *Pantegni*. At the opening of each of the ten books he wrote a *capitula* list (a table of contents without references to specific folia, which were not numbered). These tables are written in a slightly smaller script so as to set them apart clearly from the main text that followed. A second scribe rubricated much of the manuscript (fig. 2.2 and pl. VI). Scribe B, the 'Hague Rubricator', as we call this anonymous individual for convenience (for we encounter him in other manuscripts), is most likely a peer of Geraldus; note for example that his script still includes a long **r** that descends below the line, and a long-stemmed **s** with a broad headstroke, both of which are eleventh-century features (fig. 2.3 and pl. XI). In contrast to Geraldus's hand, however, his minims move in the same direction, and their feet are fully formed. This is not an eleventh-century feature, but

of course, but this would increase the percentage of text on the page. The fact that the Hague manuscript contains substantially more text on the page than average is therefore significant.

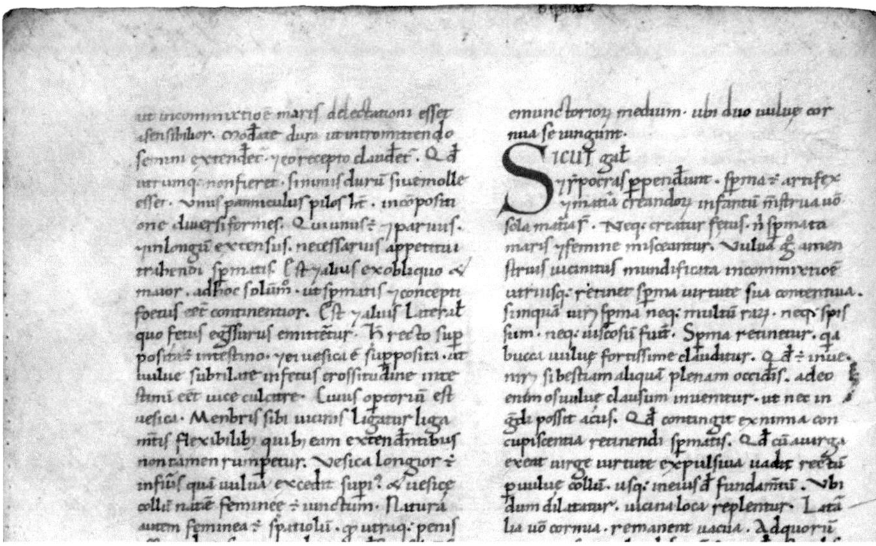

Figure 2.4. Rubric skipped by Scribe B. In later manuscripts the rubric is 'De spermate'. The Hague, Koninklijke Bibliotheek, MS 73 J 6, fol. 19^{v} (detail). Late 1070s–early 1080s (before 1086).

rather belongs to *littera praegothica*, the transitional script that came to replace Caroline minuscule. Additionally, the head-stroke of **r**, and occasionally the right limb of **h**, are angular rather than round. This angularity is another feature of the developing transitional script.[12] The inclusion of these 'new' features shows the scribe was in touch with current developments in handwriting. This may be reason to suppose that while the two likely worked as a team, the Hague Rubricator may have been the younger.

Whatever their age difference, the duo's collaboration was carefully planned and executed. The main scribe, Geraldus, calculated how much space each rubric required and left just enough room; the rubrics fit remarkably well into the space reserved for them. While they show experience in both their script and the execution of their tasks, the two individuals are jointly responsible for an intriguing irregularity in the manuscript: a rubric that was planned at fol. 19^{v} but which was never completed. At the folium in question, Geraldus, as usual, leaves blank space for the rubric (a long one, apparently, for one full line is left blank as well as two-thirds of a second line) and for a majuscule

[12] For the features of the *littera praegothica*, see Derolez, *The Palaeography of Gothic Manuscript Books*, pp. 56–71. For the term 'transitional script' and some of its features, see Kwakkel, 'Biting, Kissing and the Treatment of Feet'.

S three lines tall, the customary height for an initial at the outset of a chapter. He then writes the first word in majuscule before continuing in minuscule ('SICUT Galienus et Ypocras perpenderunt'), which is also typical for the start of a chapter.[13] While the rubricator did fill in the **s** initial, he did not add a rubric (fig. 2.4).[14]

The text segment marked with the enlarged **S** is part of an independent tract on the anatomy of the sex organs called *De genitalibus membris*, translated by Constantine. The tract is included in the *Theorica*, where it makes up the last four chapters of book III (chapters 33–36).[15] The full title of this tract, *De genitalibus membris et primum de matrice*, is the same as the rubric of chapter 33 (see fol. 19r). In the independent tract our would-be chapter starts in line 49, according to the edition of Monica Green.[16] However, no rubric accompanies the text here and so Geraldus's preparations seem out of place. Still, he is clearly under the impression that a new chapter is about to start. Indeed, he reserved a calculated amount of blank space, custom-tailored to this particular instance, which may suggest that his exemplar did indeed have a rubric at that point. This is an important observation given that the exemplar used for MS 73 J 6 likely originated from Constantine's milieu, and moreover was possibly provided by the translator himself. Curiously, the 1539 *Pantegni* edition also has an enlarged majuscule **S** at the start of the text segment beginning with 'Sicut Galenus' (executed in the fashion of a chapter start), but a rubric or a chapter number is not found here either; thus the Basel edition shares a striking resemblance in physical presentation to MS 73 J 6.[17]

[13] The full incipit of the text segment is 'SICUT Galienus et Ypocras perpenderunt, sperma est artifex et materia creandorum infantum, menstrua vero sola materia sunt' (fol. 19v, col. B, lines 3–5).

[14] The ink colour suggests that the rubricator executed both the rubrics and the capitals.

[15] For the text and its authorship, see Green, 'The *De genecia* Attributed to Constantine the African', p. 308.

[16] Green, 'The *De genecia* Attributed to Constantine the African', p. 315.

[17] Constantine the African, *Summi in omni philosophia viri Constantini Africani medici*, ed. by Petrus, p. 74. Mark Jordan argues that, aside from a missing Prologue, this Basel edition of the *Pantegni* is closer to the older, and larger number, of manuscripts of the text. It does not, however, include the *Practica*. Consequently, scholars working on the *Practica* and its reconstruction customarily rely on Trot's Lyon edition of 1515 (*Omnia opera Ysaac*), and on the earliest manuscripts available. See Jordan, 'The Fortune of Constantine's *Pantegni*', pp. 286–302, and Green, 'The Re-Creation of *Pantegni*, *Practica*, Book VIII', p. 121 n. 1.

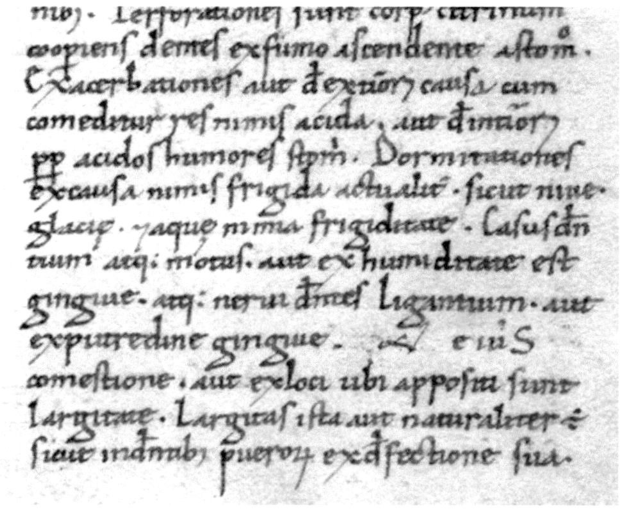

Figure 2.5.
Erased text in the fourth line from the bottom is modified by Scribe A, with 'et eiuS' inserted over the erasure. The Hague, Koninklijke Bibliotheek, MS 73 J 6, fol. 67^{r} (detail). Late 1070s–early 1080s (before 1086).

In several instances Geraldus made corrections to the text. These corrections range from very superficial to more elaborate interventions and occur throughout the manuscript. For example, he frequently inserts text. Sometimes it is limited to a few words (fol. 1^{v}, col. B, above line 21), but at other times the suppletions are much longer and extend to a full line (for example, those on fol. 1^{v}, col. B, above line 54, and fol. 2^{v}, col. B, above line 25). These insertions are all in a slightly different ink (which is a bit darker), suggesting that these were perhaps added later while he was checking the text to verify the accuracy of his copying from the exemplar. There are also instances where text was erased and replaced by a new reading. At fol. 67^{r}, col. B, fourth line from the bottom, an earlier text of substantial length was erased (about half a line) and replaced with only two words — 'et eiuS' — which is the reading found in the printed edition as well as other manuscripts.[18] The majuscule **S** that is used for 'eiuS' is likely a carryover from this older reading, which shows just how adaptive the scribe is (fig. 2.5). This is also shown by cases where a word was changed by erasing parts of its letters: in the bottom line of fol. 5^{v}, col. A, we see how the word *ultima* is created out of the word *humida* by erasure of **h**, extension of the first minim of **m**, and erasure of the ascender at **d**.[19] In this case the main hand also placed the word in the far left side of the margin, perhaps to clarify the mess he had made. Some marginal additions are found in the manuscript as well (for

[18] Compare Helsinki, Yliopiston kirjasto, MS EÖ II 14, fol. 158^{v} (*c.* 1150).

[19] Another such revamp through erasure is found at fol. 7^{r}, col. B, line 32.

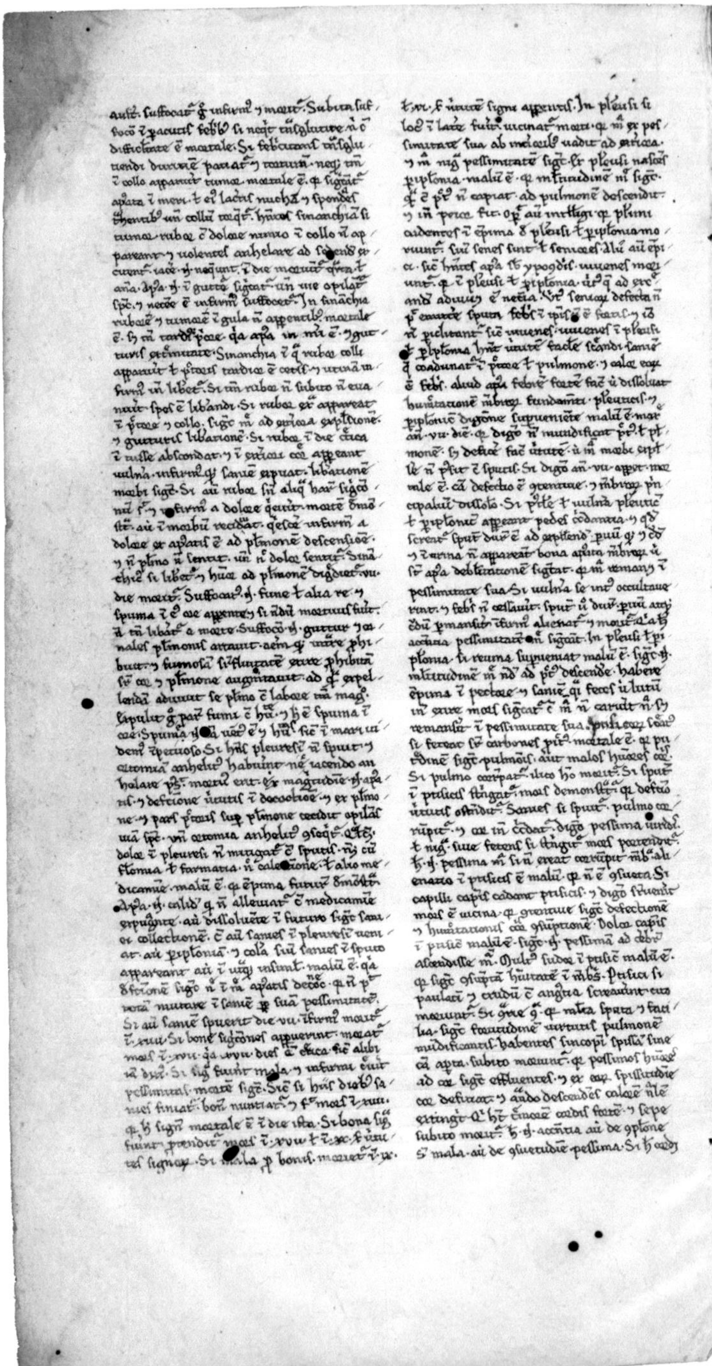

Figure 2.6.
First page of Scribe C, who completed this abandoned manuscript of the *Pantegni*. The Hague, Koninklijke Bibliotheek, MS 73 J 6, fol. 85ᵛ. *c.* 1150.

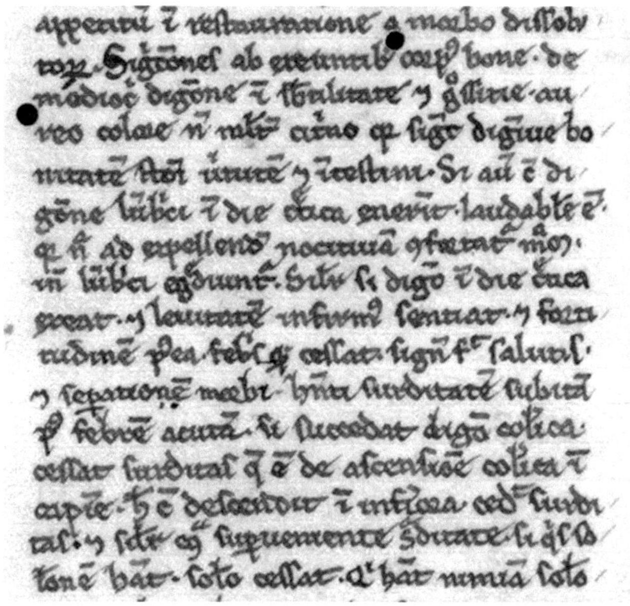

Figure 2.7.
The script of Scribe C, with **pp** biting in line 1, an important characteristic for dating his hand. The Hague, Koninklijke Bibliotheek, MS 73 J 6, fol. 87ʳ (detail). *c.* 1150.

example, at fol. 1ᵛ in the inner margin next to lines 7–11).[20] The most invasive correction, however, is the practice of leaving blank space where an improved reading was planned. This intervention will be discussed later in this chapter.

The End: Completing and Expanding the Codex (c. 1150–c. 1200)

While Geraldus copied most of the *Theorica*, he did not finish the task. He wrote from the beginning of the first quire until almost the end of the last (fols 1ʳ–85ʳ). However, at the very beginning of fol. 85ᵛ, from the very first line in column A, we encounter yet another copyist, who will be addressed as Scribe C (fig. 2.6 and pl. VII). His hand can be dated to the middle of the twelfth century. Features that point in this direction are the use of angular strokes, feet formed on minims, and that these feet all veer to the right, as is typical for developed Pregothic script.[21] His script shows fusion in **pp** (the letter forms 'bite' one another), which is a feature encountered from *c.* 1150 onwards (fig. 2.7).[22] Scribe C was evidently not part of the late eleventh-century Team

20 See also fol. 19ᵛ, col. A, line 8 (with insertion mark).

21 Kwakkel, 'Biting, Kissing and the Treatment of Feet', p. 90.

22 Kwakkel, 'Biting, Kissing and the Treatment of Feet', p. 97.

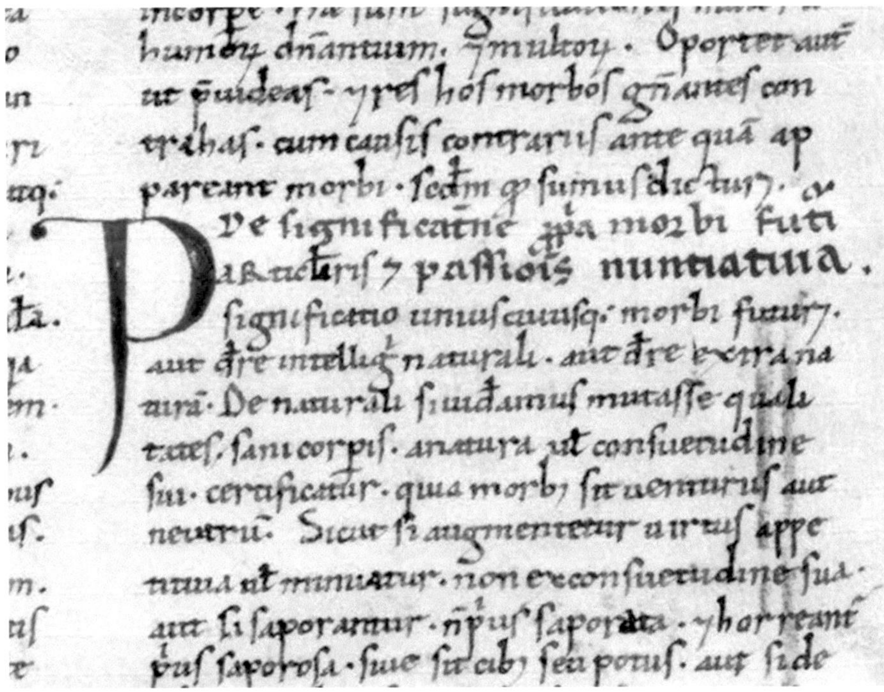

Figure 2.8. Rubric executed by Scribe C in space left blank by Scribe B, the usual rubricator. The text itself is copied by Geraldus. The Hague, Koninklijke Bibliotheek, MS 73 J 6, fol. 78ᵛ, col. B (detail). *c.* 1150.

Constantine. Even so, his Pregothic script contains Beneventan traits, which puts him in the Beneventan zone, perhaps even in Monte Cassino, although this cannot be certain.[23]

It is thus noteworthy how this copy of the *Pantegni*, in a composite manner, came to be. Most remarkable, of course, is that Geraldus halted his work so close to the finish line. Having filled 169 pages with carefully written and corrected text, he stopped just four pages short of completing the job. To put this in perspective: it would probably have taken him only a day or so to finish.[24] Did he run out of text to copy? We will return to this matter shortly. The

[23] Note the Beneventan abbreviation for *autem* ('au' with macron) at, for example, fol. 86ᵛ, col. A, line 22 and at fol. 87ʳ, col. B, line 53.

[24] In a medium-quality script, a scribe could copy an average of two or three folia per day (four to six pages), while a scribe writing high-grade script averaged a little over one folium per day (two pages). See Gumbert, 'The Speed of Scribes', especially pp. 62–63, 68–69; Bozzolo and Ornato, *Pour une histoire du livre manuscrit au moyen-âge*, pp. 46–48.

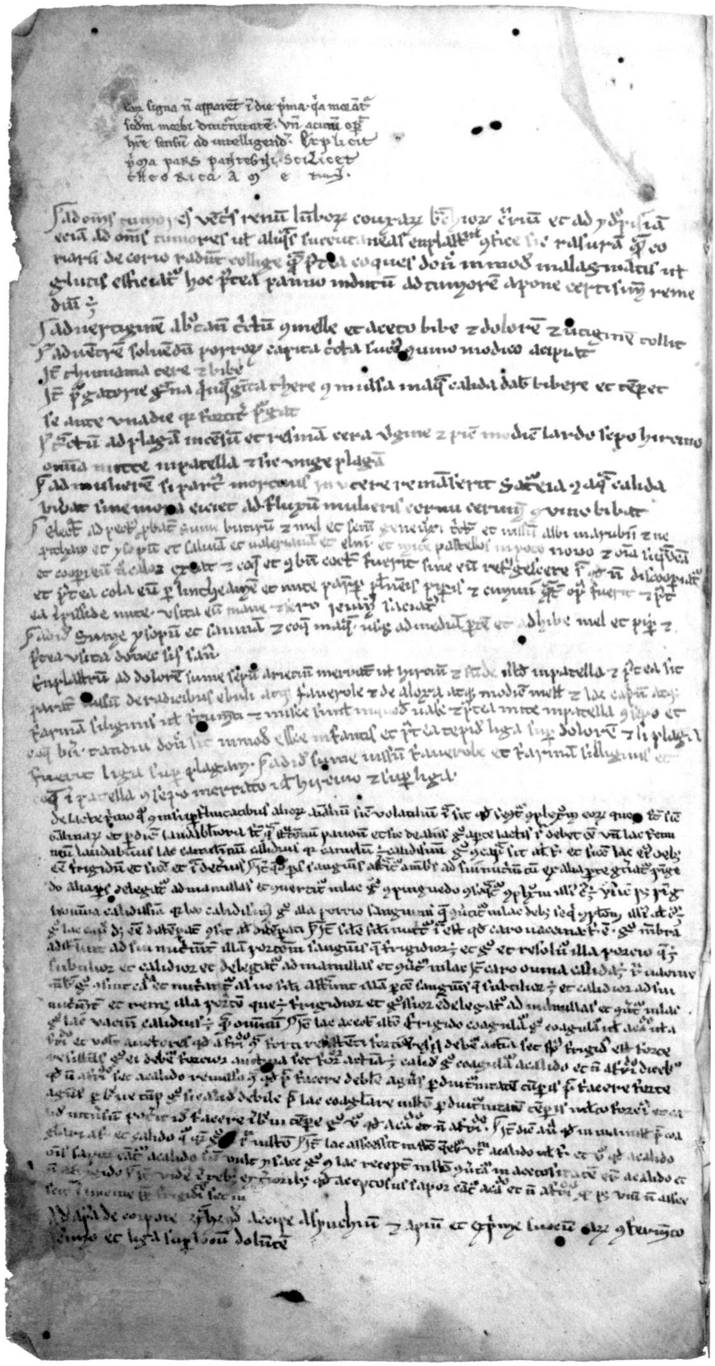

Figure 2.9.
Following the *explicit* of the *Theorica* by Scribe C (top five lines), the rest of the page is filled with excerpts by Scribe D. The Hague, Koninklijke Bibliotheek, MS 73 J 6, fol. 87v. Excerpts, *c.* 1150–*c.* 1200.

individual who completed this abandoned early manuscript of the *Theorica* did so by copying the remainder of the text on fols 85^{v}–87^{r} and adding the translator's colophon on fol. 87^{v}. It is possible that Scribe C used a different *Pantegni* copy as exemplar (potentially from a different branch of the textual tradition), given that so much time had passed since Geraldus first started copying the text. Scribe C also added three omitted lines (at fol. 21^{r}, inner margin; fol. 26^{r}, inner and lower margin; and fol. 68^{r}, inner margin), which may indicate that he checked the manuscript or portions of it against his exemplar. Scribe C also completed nine remaining rubrics in the portion by Geraldus, starting at fol. 78^{v} (fig. 2.8) because the Hague Rubricator, Scribe B, had stopped executing these at fol. 78^{r}. The slightly dull red ink of Scribe C can be easily distinguished from that of the main rubricator, whose red ink is particularly bright. Scribe C also noticed that the rubric at fol. 19^{v} was unexecuted, and preparing to do so, he wrote 'De spermate' just below the upper edge of the leaf, now partly cut away (fig. 2.4). These words form a rubric that was to be placed in the vacant space in red ink, but it never was, adding to the mystery of this would-be chapter.[25]

In the second half of the twelfth century a number of recipes and excerpts from other medical texts were added to the manuscript. It is surely noteworthy that these additions were of a purely practical nature, and thus augmented in useful fashion the older *Theorica Pantegni*, which had no therapeutic utility. The individual who copied these is here called Scribe D.[26] His first batch is found in the space that was left blank after Scribe C had finished copying the *Theorica* (most of fol. 87^{v} and all of fol. 88^{r}). But for one large excerpt at the bottom of fol. 87^{v} (fig. 2.9 and pl. VIII), Scribe D marked the beginning of each excerpt with a paragraph mark, eleven of which are found at fols 87^{v}–88^{r}. The excerpts added to these blank pages were written down intermittently, as is shown by their differences in ink colour, duct, and thickness of the nib. It is probable that Scribe D was a user of the book who added relevant material over time.

A smaller batch of recipes and excerpts, copied by the same hand, is found on the recto of the pastedown in the back of the manuscript (fig. 2.10). This

[25] A similar occurrence is encountered at fol. 87^{r}, where Scribe C wrote the text of the rubric just below the top edge of the page as well. In this case, the text was actually turned into a rubric by Scribe C himself. The identification of Scribe C as the writer of the rubric at the top of fol. 19^{v} is based on the distinctive slightly tilted **e** in the last letter of *De spermate*.

[26] Distinctive palaeographical features of this hand include the occasional extension of the third minim of **m** below the line, lower compartment of **g** with a flat bottom, and frequent extension of **r** below the line.

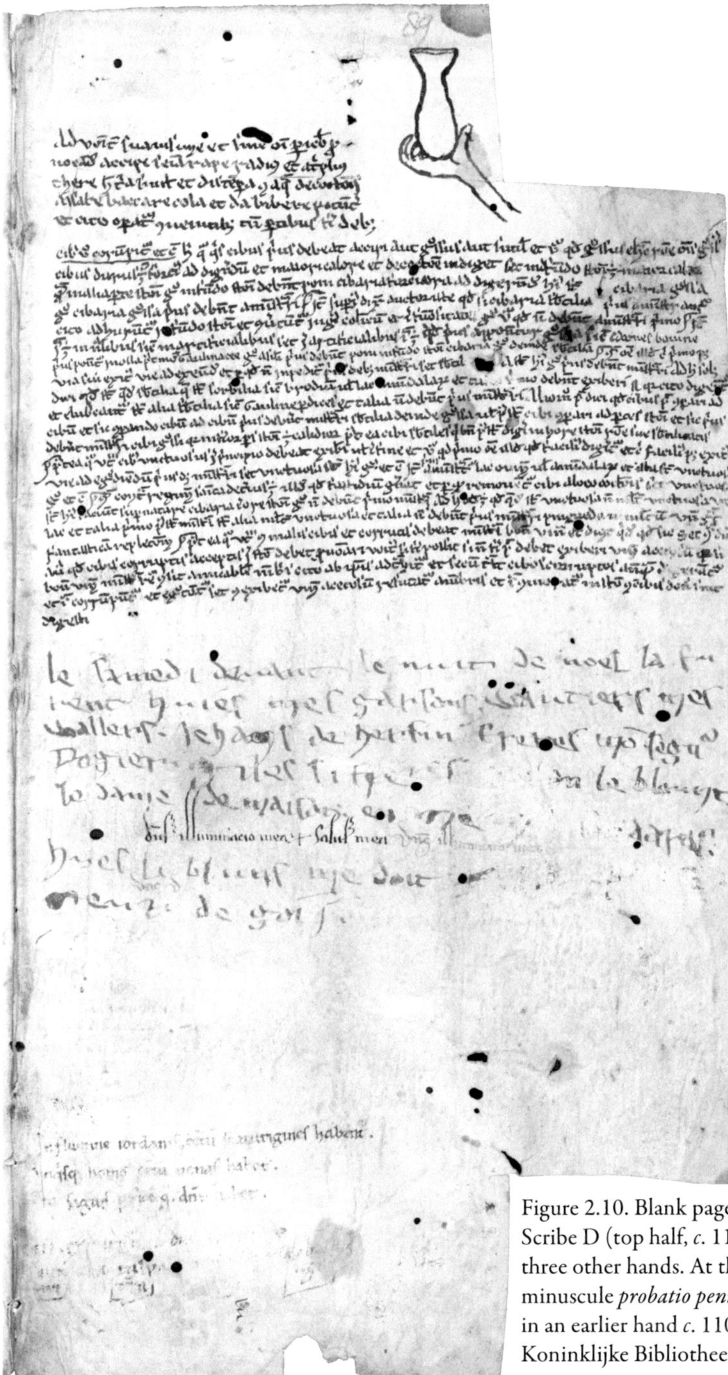

Figure 2.10. Blank page filled with excerpts by Scribe D (top half, *c.* 1150–*c.* 1200) and at least three other hands. At the bottom is the Caroline minuscule *probatio pennae* on the River Jordan in an earlier hand *c.* 1100– *c.* 1125. The Hague, Koninklijke Bibliotheek, MS 73 J 6, fol. 89[r].

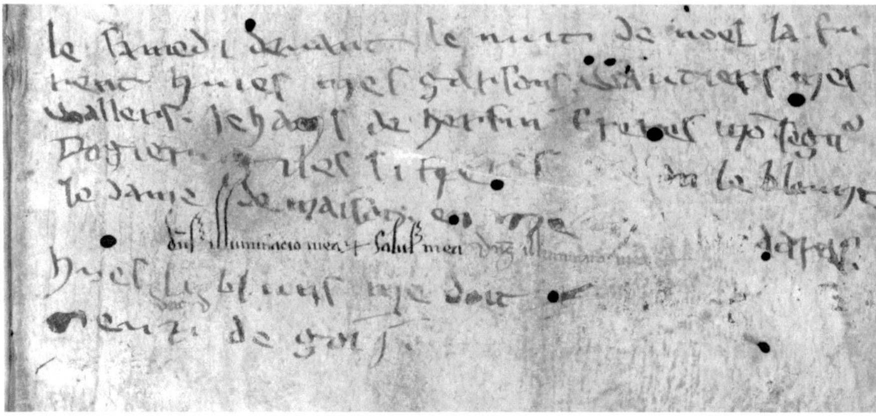

Figure 2.11. French note, The Hague, Koninklijke Bibliotheek, MS 73 J 6, fol. 89^{r}. *c.* 1200–*c.* 1300.

leaf was already part of the manuscript in the early twelfth century, as shown by a *probatio pennae* from *c.* 1100–*c.* 1125 near the bottom of fol. 89^{r} which reads 'In flumine Jordanis centum scaturigines habentur. | Unus quisque homo centum venas habet. | ita sanguis perficere quod dominus iubet' (In the River Jordan are a hundred channels | Each single man has a hundred veins | So blood can accomplish what things the Lord commands). In addition to the excerpts added to fol. 89^{r}, Scribe D drew a picture of a hand holding a urine flask, as if to demonstrate how to hold such an object. In the thirteenth century a long note was added between the two twelfth-century additions at fol. 89^{r}. The note holds references to one John of Hersin and the city of Arras in northern France: 'le samedi deuant le nuit de noel la furent huies mes garsons, wautiers mes wallers. jehans de hersin freres mon segneur Rogier. miles li freres [...]n le blannc le dame de maison. en m[...] aaras. Hues li blains me doit [...] men doit i de goi[s..]' (The Saturday before Christmas night were present: Huies, my servant; Wautier, my friend; John of Hersin, the brother of my lord Rogier; Miles, the brother of [...] le Blanc, the lady of the house; and [...]. Hues le Blanc owes me [...], [...] owes me a [...].) (fig. 2.11).[27] The pastedown thus provides various snapshots of later users of the manuscript.

While these additions were all placed in vacant space, another expansion took place through codicological intervention. At some point early in the second half of the twelfth century a bifolium and a singleton were placed in

[27] Transcription by Ed van der Vlist (The Hague, Koninklijke Bibliotheek), translation by Julia Szirmai (Leiden).

front of the eleven quires that were originally prepared and filled with text by Geraldus (the bifolium entails fols i–ii, the singleton fol. iii). These added leaves are now filled with excerpts, which were copied there by four different individuals. One of these, Scribe E, wrote the majority of the excerpts. Working in the second half of the twelfth century, most likely in *c.* 1150–*c.* 1175, judging from his script, Scribe E started writing at the top of fol. i^{v} and continued until near the bottom of fol. ii^{v}. First, he copied the full and extensive chapter 6 of *Viaticum*, book III, 'De tussi', followed, in its entirety, by 'De fastidio', chapter 9 of the *Viaticum*'s book IV (figs 2.12–2.14 and pl. IX).[28]

The first of these chapters features dozens of complex recipes containing exotic ingredients and preparations: syrups of jujube, hyssop, horehound, and poppy; *diapapaveris*; *tiriaca maiore* (the great theriac); and various electuaries. It is clear that the scribe was particularly interested in these remedies, as he noted them by name in the marginal spaces, twice surrounding them in an informal cartouche. These are precisely the types of therapeutic preparations that were entirely lacking from the *Theorica Pantegni*, but which would have been of great use to any practitioner.[29]

The textblock dimensions of these two *Viaticum* excerpts are the same as the *Theorica*, the main component of the manuscript, suggesting that Scribe E intended them as additions to this copy of the *Pantegni*; after all, the folia of the eleven quires prepared by Geraldus have unusual relative proportions — the pages are quite tall — and the leaves prepared by Scribe E match this rare design. The parchment of the added leaves may have been discarded during an earlier book project: the bifolium contains two long horizontal cuts that reach across both sides. As the singleton features the same flaw, we can assume it was added at the same time, by the same person, as the opening bifolium. At fol. ii the cut was so deep that Scribe E had to write his text around it on both sides of the leaf.

When Scribe E started copying down selections of the *Viaticum*, the other side of the leaf, fol. i^{r}, was still empty. Medieval scribes would often refrain from writing on recto when it concerned an opening leaf, so that the first (blank) page could be pasted against the inside of the wooden board of the binding. In the second half of the twelfth century, probably contemporary to the writing

[28] Book III, chap. 6, 'De tussi', and book IV, chap. 9, 'De fastidio' correspond with only minor variation to Basel 1536, pp. 48–51 and 73–74, respectively. Identifications by Eliza Glaze.

[29] We owe this information to Eliza Glaze.

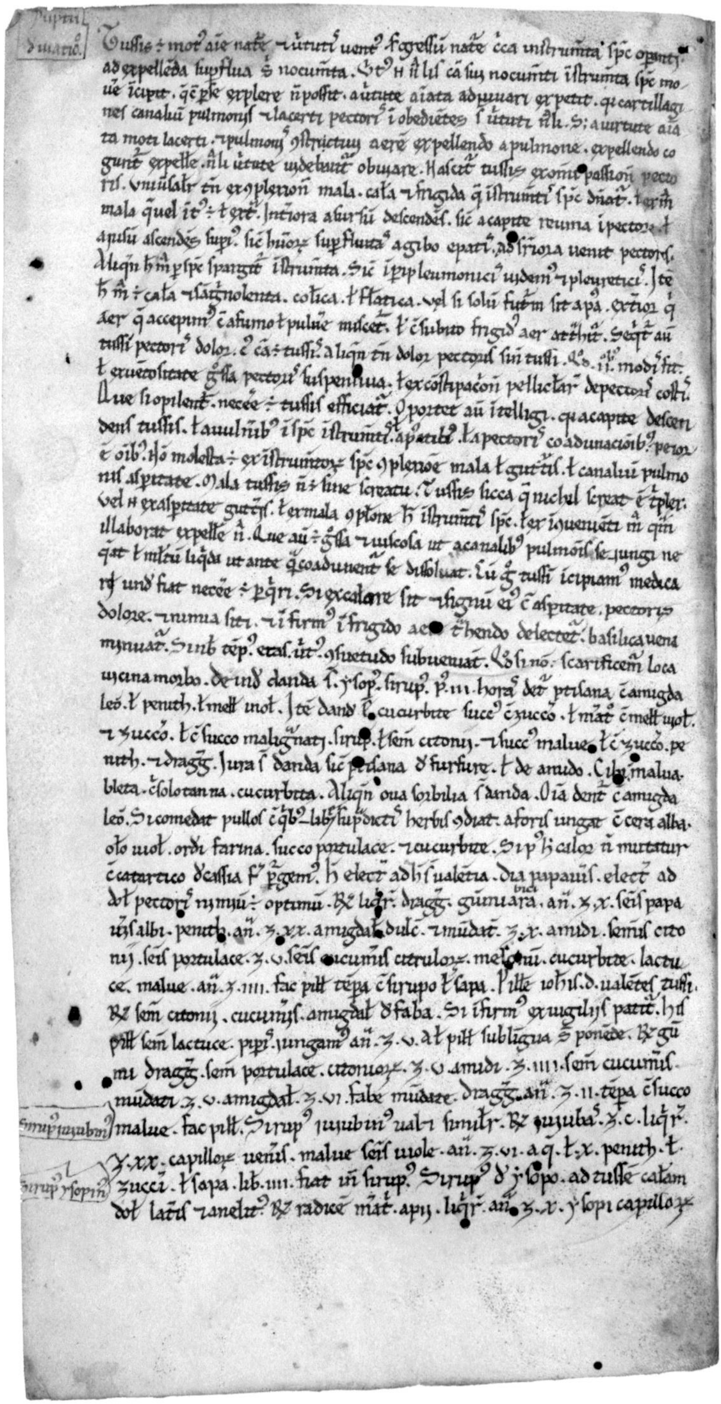

Figure 2.12. Second page of medieval excerpts copied by Scribe E, containing the first part of *Viaticum* book III, chapter 6, 'De tussi'. The Hague, Koninklijke Bibliotheek, MS 73 J 6, fol. i^{v}. *c.* 1150–*c.* 1175.

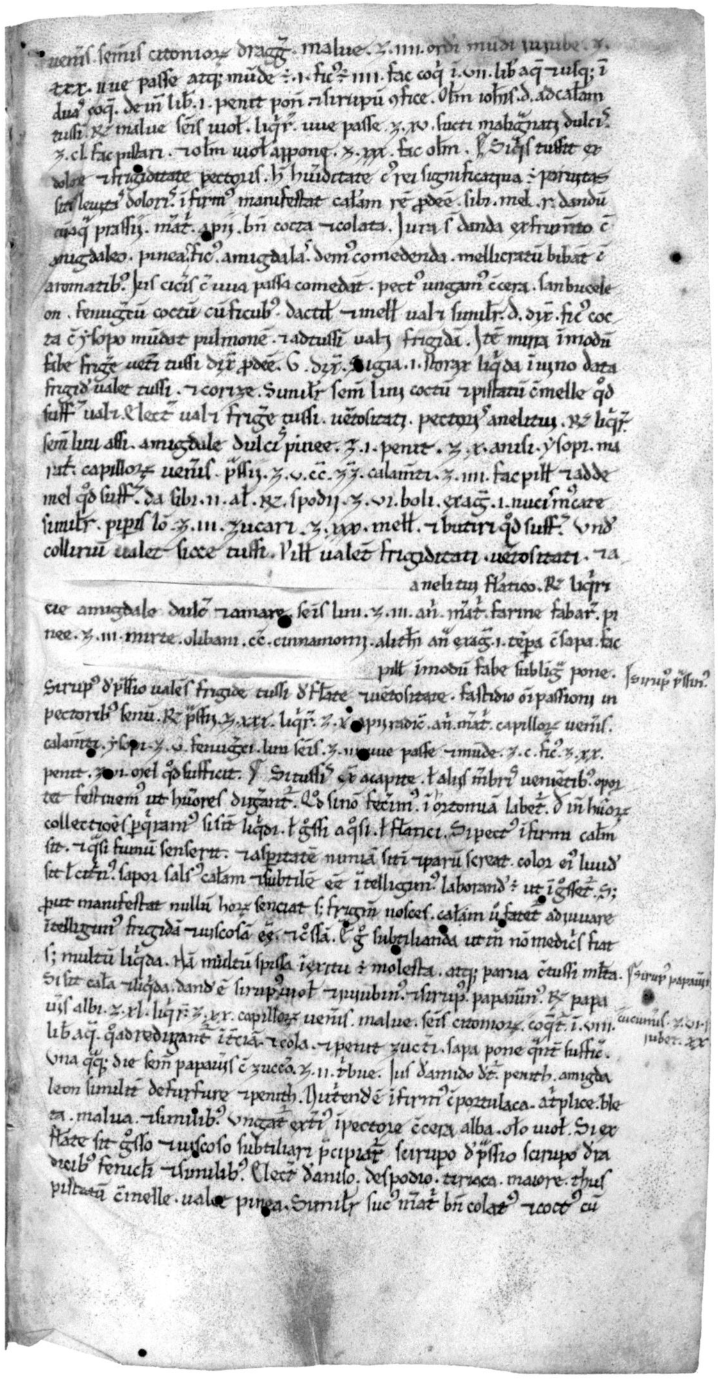

Figure 2.13.
Third page of medieval excerpts copied by Scribe E, containing the second part of *Viaticum* book III, chapter 6, 'De tussi'. The Hague, Koninklijke Bibliotheek, MS 73 J 6, fol. ii[r]. *c.* 1150–*c.* 1175.

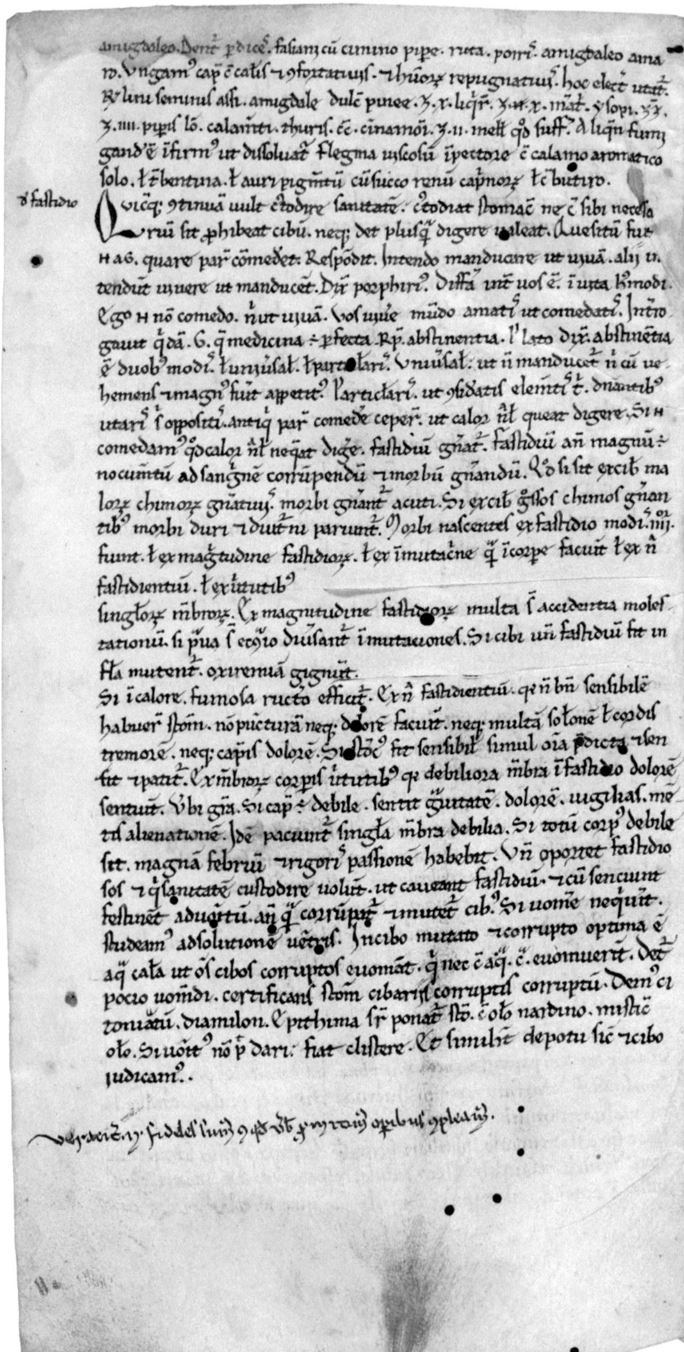

Figure 2.14.
Fourth page of medieval excerpts copied by Scribe E, containing the final part of *Viaticum* book III, chapter 6, 'De tussi', and book IV, chapter 9, 'De fastidio'. The Hague, Koninklijke Bibliotheek, MS 73 J 6, fol. ii^{v}. *c.* 1150–*c.* 1175.

stint of Scribe E (so *c.* 1150–*c.* 1175), this blank page was filled with various medical excerpts, which were added by three different hands (fig. 2.15).

The first of these, Scribe F, copied lines 1–10 of fol. i^{r}: an excerpt from chapter 21 of *Viaticum*, book VII, 'De carbunculis'.[30] In line 10 we see a switch to a different hand, Scribe G, who copied additional short extracts of simple cures from the *Viaticum*, book II, chapter 22, 'De gingivis', and, starting in line 12, from chapter 23, 'De fetore oris'.[31] These are followed, starting in line 22, by extracts on laxative food and drink, still by Scribe G. The last section of these extracts on laxative food and drink, however, were done by a third individual, Scribe H, who used a much larger script.

In addition to the excerpts penned by Scribes E–H on the bifolium fol. i–ii, the singleton fol. iii also holds text. It contains notes written down in lead point (fig. 2.16). The individual who wrote down these notes, Scribe I, filled both sides of fol. iii. Based on the style of his handwriting, his additions can likely be dated to *c.* 1200, or perhaps very early in the thirteenth century. At the top of fol. iii^{r} the handwriting of Scribe I is still somewhat legible, but the legibility decreases rapidly until, at the bottom of the page, the script even starts to include cursive features, most notably in tall **s**, which extends below the line, making his hand very difficult to read and identify (fig. 2.16).[32]

Judging from what can be read, the text at fol. iii^{r} appears to be medical, as suggested by words such as 'mala', 'toto corpore', 'figura', and 'corrumpitur'. The text on the verso is, however, completely illegible. Scribe I also added a short tract in plummet on a blank page at the very back of the codex (fol. 88^{v}). Moreover, throughout the volume he is encountered in the margins (for example, at fol. 65^{v} in the top margin) and at one point in the space between the columns ('malum' at fol. 83^{v}). It is quite possible that the *nota* signs in plummet throughout the manuscript are also his.[33]

[30] The incipit reads: 'Carbunculi de sanguine crosso nascuntur et corrupto. Vnde deforis est super ponen[-]'. Transcription and identification by Ed van der Vlist (The Hague, Koninklijke Bibliotheek). This excerpt corresponds, with minor word order modifications, to Petrus's 1536 printing of the *Viaticum*, in *Summi in omni philosophia viri Constantini Africani medici*, p. 163.

[31] These very spare extracts, with heavily abbreviated recipes, correspond to Petrus's Basel 1536 printing of the *Viaticum*, pp. 40–41. Identifications by Eliza Glaze.

[32] Unfortunately, writing in plummet cannot be enhanced with ultraviolet light.

[33] We find *notae* at fols 4^{r} (inner margin), 16^{r} (outer margin), 21^{r} (inner margin), 55^{r} (inner margin), 62^{r} (inner margin), 64^{r} (inner margin), 65^{v} (inner margin), 66^{v} (inner margin), 75^{r} (inner margin), and 78^{r} (outer margin). A particularly high volume is encountered at fols 58^{v}–59^{r}.

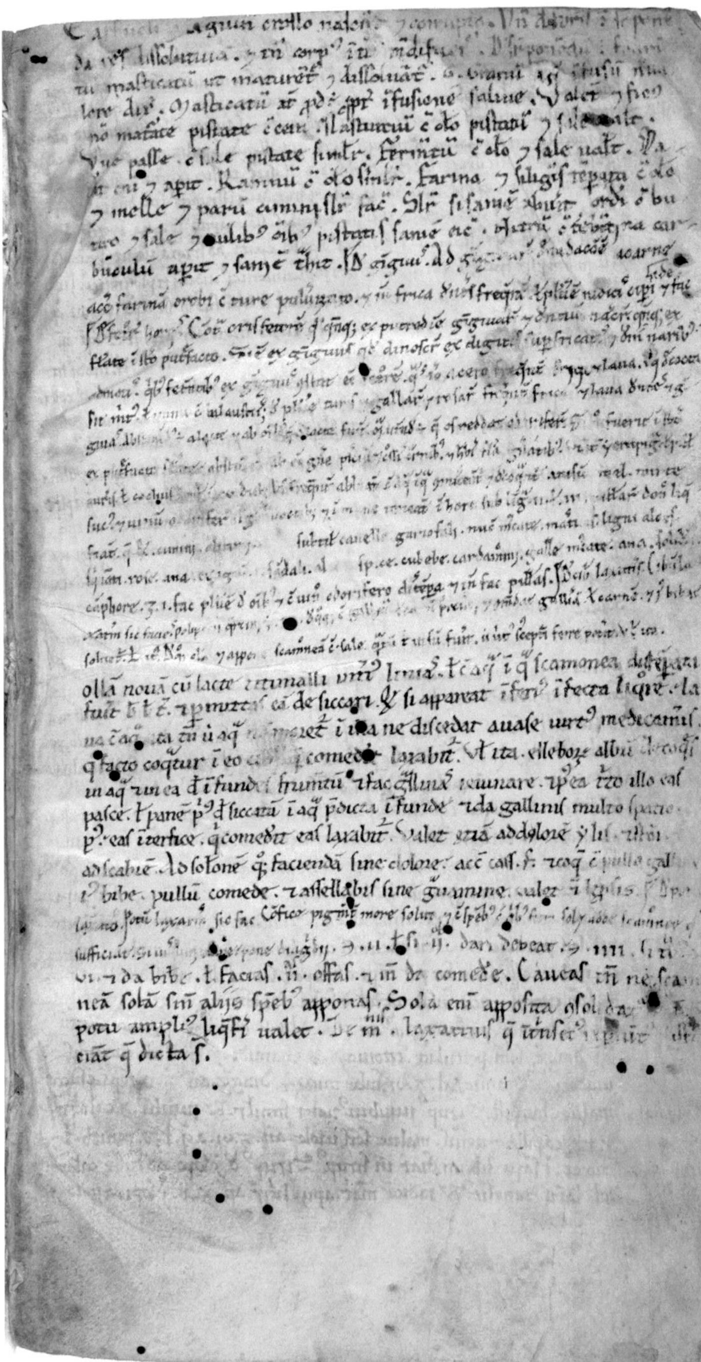

Figure 2.15.
First page of medieval excerpts copied by Scribes F–H. The Hague, Koninklijke Bibliotheek, MS 73 J 6, fol. i[r]. *c.* 1150–*c.* 1175.

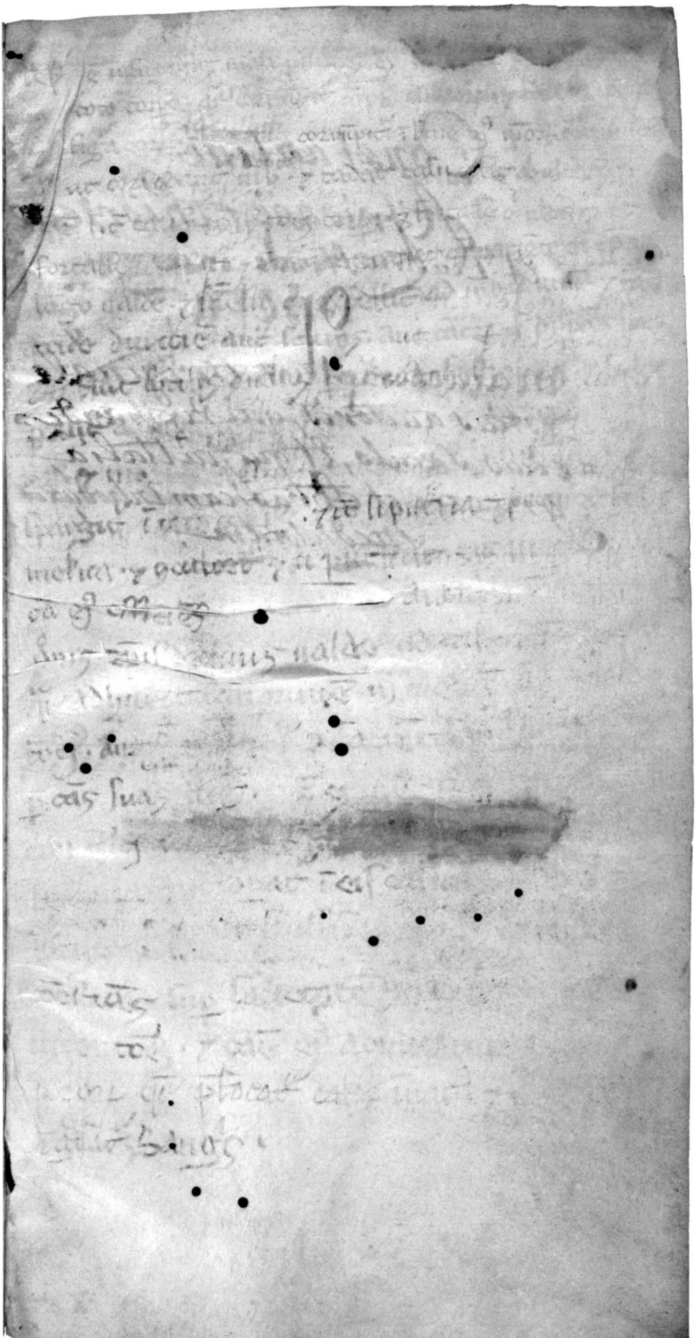

Figure 2.16. Blank page filled with notes in lead by Scribe I, The Hague, Koninklijke Bibliotheek, MS 73 J 6, fol. iii[r]. *c.* 1200–*c.* 1225.

The added leaves thus provide us with clues related to the later users of the oldest *Pantegni* copy: they were evidently individuals interested in practical medical knowledge. In fact, one of them appears to have been so involved in this subject that he even used some blank pages for putting down notes. They may provide us with even more important information about the manuscript as a whole: the whereabouts of the oldest *Pantegni* copy in the century after its production. Fortunately, two of the hands found on the added leaves can be localized with some certainty. Scribe E uses a 7-shaped Tironian note for *et* in the distinct style of Southern France: it has a notably upright vertical stroke and a particularly long horizontal top bar which gives it a top-heavy appearance. Moreover, the *con* symbol is formed as a figure 9 placed on the baseline, which is also a feature of Southern France (fol. ii^v^, line 2, 'confortatiuis').[34] Additionally, the style of long **s**, which is rather narrow and upright, also points to Southern France, as does the positioning of round **s**, which tilts slightly backwards (fol. ii^v^, line 4, 'obedientes', and line 5, 'tussis').

It appears, then, that one of the hands found on the added leaves had learned to write in Southern France. While this is not evidence that the manuscript itself was in Southern France during the second half of the twelfth century (scribes, after all, did travel), the combination with the discussed thirteenth-century note related to Arras in northern France demonstrates that the book had made its way to France. Moreover, Scribe H shows some palaeographical features of Southern France as well: the 7-shaped Tironian note for *et*, the figure 9 for *con* (fol. i^r^, line 3 from below, consolidatur), and the tilted **s** (fol. i^r^, line 3 from bottom, *sola*). The combination of these features (a later French provenance and two occurrences of scribes trained in Southern France) strongly suggests that the manuscript had reached Southern France by the early years of the second half of the twelfth century, when Scribes E and H added their excerpts.

Lacunae

It is striking that the ending of the text of the *Theorica* on the last five folia (fols 85^v^–87^v^) in MS 73 J 6 was added almost one hundred years after Geraldus completed his work. Remarkably, the missing end of the text is not the only way in which the late eleventh-century copying process remained unfinished. As Geraldus copied the *Theorica*, he occasionally left blank spots within the text.

[34] For the localization of these features, see Derolez, *The Palaeography of Gothic Manuscript Books*, pp. 116–17.

Table 2.1. Lacunae in The Hague, Koninklijke Bibliotheek, MS 73 J 6.

	Fol., col., line	Text (book, chapter in *Theorica*)
1	11^{r}, A, 12	Quod inde remanet [lacuna] ascendit, quam graeco lauda assimilatur, ibique dividitur (book II, chap. 12)
2	12^{v}, B, 36	Sunt et [lacuna, with strike-out line] onestantia [honestantia *by later hand*] quia homo non decoratur eorum carentia (book II, chap. 16)
3	33^{v}, B, 28–29	Mel vel zuccarum [lacuna, with strike-out line] cum farina cocta, sunt indigestiva (book V, chap. 27)
4	42^{r}, B, 45	Defectio vel ex dolore est nimio, cum in interiora corporis calor fugiat naturalis, vel ex defectione virtutis spiritualis, cum arterias dilatare in omnes suas extremitates non possit sicut [lacuna, with strike-out line] videmus (book VI, chap. 26)
5	57^{v}, A, 8–9	Si de flegmate crosso est et viscoso, [lacuna] vocatur et glans, scrofula, et verruca, et nodi similes glandi (book VIII, chap. 11)
6	65^{r}, B, 24	Quae autem nascuntur in cornea, cancer sunt, & uulnera, [lacuna, with strike-out line] pustula, & pustulae albedo (book IX, chap. 15)
7	70^{v}, B, 47–48	Aut in substantia cibi crossi sicut caro est uaccina, & panis azymus, quae [lacuna, with strike-out line] aut in ordinatione cibi, sicut cum quis crossum aut stipticum manducaverit cibum, postea subtilem apponat, qui antea corrumpitur quam crossus, a stomacho egrediatur, aut cum cibum accipiat quem antequam digerat alium rursum suscipiat (book IX, chap. 27)
8	71^{r}, B, 12	Si aut dieta [lacuna] aliquando hoc in tertiana est febri cum colericos humores natura expellit in die accessionis (book IX, chap. 27)
9	83^{v}, A, 20	Cum autem malum [lacuna] dixerit possibile est infirmum sanari si bona signa apparuerint (book X, chap. 10)

These blanks or 'lacunae' vary from the space equivalent to a single word up to two full lines. While only nine of them are found in the manuscript (table 2.1), they significantly benefit our understanding of Geraldus's intentions when he copied the book. Moreover, the blanks provide insight into some of the problems Constantine experienced when he translated al-Mağūsī's text from Arabic into Latin. Overall, these lacunae warrant closer inspection, beyond what is observed below. The following, however, is a first attempt to map these gaps and deduce what Geraldus may have planned to write in them.

Although few manuscripts with such lacunae have been identified, the practice is clearly connected to manuscripts for which the final text was still in flux, perhaps because some passages still needed to be translated or revised.[35] A four-

[35] For the technique, see Kwakkel, 'Behind the Scenes of a Revision', pp. 121–25.

teenth-century example illustrates how the correction technique worked. Brussels, KBR, MS 2849–51, produced at Herne Charterhouse near the end of the fourteenth century, is a Middle Dutch epistolary.[36] This manuscript's scribe copied the texts while comparing the Middle Dutch translation to the Latin Vulgate reading. When he encountered a passage that was poorly translated, he left blank space and wrote the Latin equivalent for the skipped Middle Dutch passage in the margins. The length of the blank space depended on the length of the skipped passage. A fellow Carthusian monk subsequently translated these Latin passages in the margins, placing the improved reading right below it, and then returned the quires to the first scribe. This scribe then placed the newly translated passages into the lacunae he had originally left throughout the manuscript. When the translator thought a Middle Dutch translation marked for improving was in fact fine, he wrote 'This is fine' (*Dits wel*) next to the Latin, to explain why he had not retranslated it.

As Brussels, KBR, MS 2849–51 shows, the lacunae technique is unusual in that an identified flaw was not corrected immediately, but after the copying of the entire main text was completed. This was done because the scribe needed input from a fellow brother to correct the skipped text. The technique thus divides two tasks that are otherwise entwined: copying and correcting text. It also raises the status of the latter from the relatively quick and 'automated' task done during or right after copying the text, to something that was done with care by an 'outside' party, perhaps even a specialist. The very use of the lacunae technique suggests, in other words, that the pair of artisans set out not only to copy the text but also to improve it, in this case by upgrading the quality of the translation. The hundreds of substantial interventions on the pages of MS 2849–51 demonstrate just how much improvement was necessary in this old, rusty translation dating from the late thirteenth century.[37]

To make their collaboration easier, the scribe and translator of the Brussels manuscript divided the text across seven booklets, which enabled the corrector to begin his share of the work while the scribe continued his own, allowing the copying and correcting to be undertaken as two independent, but concurrent, activities.[38] It meant that the translator did not have to sit next to the scribe for

[36] See de Bruin, '"Retractationes"' and Kwakkel, 'Behind the Scenes of a Revision', pp. 113–14. A deeper analysis is found in Kwakkel, *Dit sijn die Dietsche boeke die ons toebehoeren*, pp. 122–24.

[37] For more on this translation, see de Bruin, '"Retractationes"'.

[38] The collation of Brussels, KBR, MS 2849–51 is described in Kwakkel, *Dit sijn die Dietsche boeke die ons toebehoeren*, pp. 210–14.

the duration of the copying process, waiting until his input was needed, and also that there was no time pressure for him. In fact, because the correction of translation errors was undertaken separately from the main activity of copying, the translator was able to read through the entire text himself, which is evident from the occasional unprompted corrections where he crossed out the Middle Dutch (there were no blanks, after all) and wrote his improved text above it interlineally: 'Dus soudic dat dietschen' (This is how I would translate it into Dutch) he wrote in the margins to the scribe, to whom he returned the corrected quires, as explanation.[39]

An example perhaps closer to the scenario in the Hague manuscript, where the lacuna technique was used to improve an Arabic–Latin scientific translation, is witnessed in the oldest copy of Michael Scot's *Abbreviatio Avicennae*, his Arabic–Latin translation of Avicenna's commentary to Aristotle's *De animalibus* (BAV, Chisianus E VIII 251). This codex was made in close proximity to the translator himself at the court of Frederick II, and it is likely that Michael personally oversaw the textual revision.[40] While copying the text, the scribes carefully examined the reading of their exemplar, which was probably supplied by Michael himself, and used a variety of correction methods. One of the scribes used the lacuna technique when he encountered readings in the exemplar that he thought needed amendment. A consultant behind the scenes of this operation, most likely Michael Scot himself, subsequently went through these proposals for improvement. He gave his approval where appropriate, after which the scribe inserted the improved text in the blank spaces. These later insertions by the same scribe can be recognized as such because they were written in a slightly different duct and ink colour. Sometimes the scribe had miscalculated how much blank space was needed; space that was left blank after the corrected text was inserted was filled with a thin line. At other such occasions the scribe resorted to using abbreviations, including those that did not formally exist, such as 'ap'ema' for 'apostema'.[41]

The use of lacunae in the Vatican manuscript is surprisingly similar to that of the Brussels manuscript discussed above: there is a clear division between the stages of copying and correcting the text, and there is an individual other than the scribe assigned or available to improve it. There is however another, more

[39] Kwakkel, *Dit sijn die Dietsche boeke die ons toebehoeren*, p. 124.

[40] Kwakkel, 'Behind the Scenes of a Revision'.

[41] Kwakkel, 'Behind the Scenes of a Revision', pp. 121–25; see p. 132, fig. 2 for the line used as filler. The case of 'apostema' is found at fol. 157v, col. B, line 11.

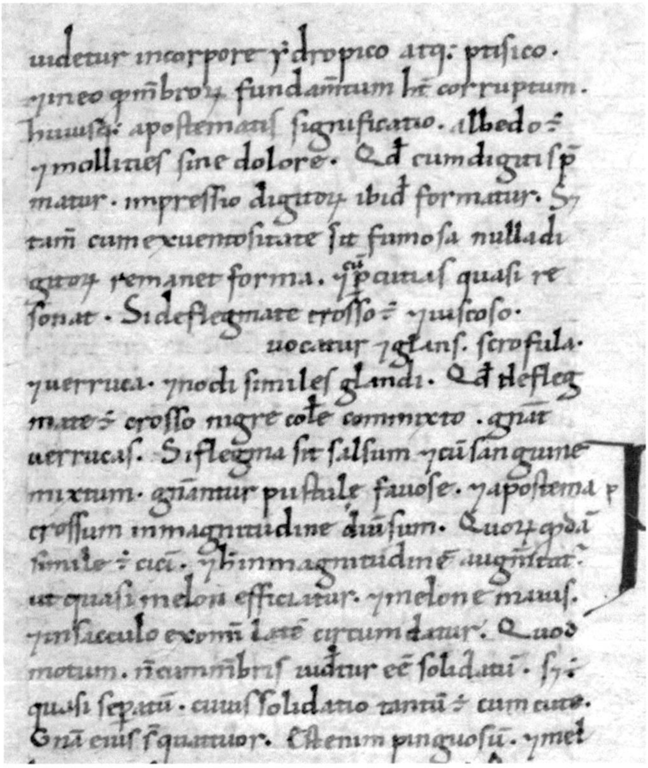

Figure 2.17. Lacuna left by Geraldus (lines 8–9, no. 5 in table 2.1), The Hague, Koninklijke Bibliotheek, MS 73 J 6, fol. 57[v], col. A (detail). Late 1070s–early 1080s (before 1086).

pertinent similarity between the two manuscripts: in both cases the copyist goes well beyond the normal tasks of a scribe. After all, in both cases he critically judges whether the text in the exemplar is of sufficient quality. The scribes do not simply reproduce the words before them, but they influence, potentially, the ultimate text. In the Vatican manuscript the scribe at first skipped the reading of some technical terms — such as *furcula* (the wishbone in birds), *culcitra* (a mattress), and *apostema* (an abscess) — which are all subsequently copied into the spaces he had previously left blank.[42] We may assume, then, that these filled-in lacunae resulted from an intervention whereby the scribe decided not to copy these words from his exemplar until he had them checked by the translator.

The cases presented thus far show how manuscripts with lacunae could be produced with a certain agenda in mind. The goal does not appear to have been only to copy an exemplar, but also to improve the text found in that exemplar.

[42] Kwakkel, 'Behind the Scenes of a Revision', p. 124.

The varying length of the gaps in MS 73 J 6 shows that Geraldus attempted to calculate precisely how much space was needed: the gaps are dynamic and designed to contain certain words, phrases, and sentences. It is tempting to infer that a similar practice takes place in this codex, that the lacunae were meant to upgrade Constantine's translation, perhaps even with the translator's own involvement. Before further addressing this possibility, it must be confirmed that the lacunae in MS 73 J 6 indeed represent readings that were skipped so they could be improved. While the analysis here presents such evidence, it must be emphasized that the case of MS 73 J 6 is harder to make because improved readings were not actually written into the gaps. Because of the absence of actual revisions, the only tool we have at our disposal to reconstruct Geraldus's intentions is a comparison to the original Arabic text. Such a comparison does in fact suggest that Geraldus attempted to revise the text in his exemplar.

A straightforward case is encountered in book VIII, chapter 11, where the Hague *Theorica* reads: 'Si de flegmate crosso est et viscoso, [lacuna] vocatur et glans, scrofula, et verruca, et nodi similes glandi' (table 2.1, no. 5, and fig. 2.17). This passage describes how a certain abscess, 'if it arises from a heavy thick phlegm, [lacuna] *it is called* also an "acorn" [a cancerous tumour], scrofula, wart, and knots similar to an acorn'. The Arabic text translates to: 'This abscess comes from thick phlegm, *which causes* ulcer, scrofula, indigestion'.[43] The translator, it seems, had picked the Latin verb 'to call' instead of the proper 'to cause': while something *caused* a cancerous growth, Constantine's translation refers to something that is *called* a cancerous growth.[44] This, of course, would lead to some confusion later on in the sentence, as it now seemed as if a technical term was missing. Geraldus likely planned to fill in that term to remedy this confusion.

A second example of a revision also involves a missing technical term:

> [no. 6, Arabic] And the diseases concerned which originate in the [lacuna] of the cornea, these are cancer, abscesses, pus, pustules, growths, and glaucoma.[45]
>
> [no. 6, Latin] Quae autem nascuntur in cornea, cancer sunt, & uulnera, [lacuna] pustula, & pustulae albedo.

[43] The translation of the Latin passages is by Francis Newton. The translation of the parallel Arabic passages is by N. Peter Joosse (Universities of Oxford and Warwick), whom we wish to thank for his extensive help with the Arabic original. Emphasis added by the authors.

[44] We owe this explanation to N. Peter Joosse.

[45] From an 1877 Arabic edition of the *Pantegni*, translated here by N. Peter Joosse (Universities of Oxford and Warwick). Al-Maǧūsī, *Kāmil al-ṣina'ah al-ṭibbiyah*, p. 256.

> And those that originate in the cornea are cancer, abscesses, [lacuna], the pustule, and white-surface pustule [glaucoma].

This passage concerns an enumeration of five symptoms or diseases. There is however one such term missing in the Latin: that indicating a growth or tumour. The limited space in the lacuna confirms that we are dealing with one word, and a short one for that matter.[46]

The third example also involves a single word, although here we are not dealing with a technical term but probably with an Arabic word for which the Latin equivalent was unknown to the translator:

> [no. 9, Arabic] And whenever he says 'malicious' or blameworthy, then this points to the fact that it is possible to cure the sick person of his disease, especially when favourable signs are apparent.

> [no. 9, Latin] Cum autem malum [lacuna] dixerit possibile est infirmum sanari si bona signa apparuerint.

> But when he says 'bad' [lacuna] it is possible for the patient to be healed, if good signs are evident.

The lacuna is positioned between the word 'bad' and the remark that it is still possible for a patient to be healed. It is very likely, therefore, that the blank space covered the word that followed 'malicious' in the Arabic text, which acts as an adjective: 'blameworthy'. This is also confirmed by the Latin sentence structure that shows the skipped word was positioned close to 'bad' ('Cum autem malum [lacuna] dixerit'). It seems Geraldus was compensating for the missing second leg of a 'this or that' construction, or perhaps he deemed the chosen word in his exemplar unsuitable.

In the fourth example we see Geraldus working around what appears to be a missing reference. In chapter 26 of book VI (table 2.1, no. 4) we read: 'Defectio vel ex dolore est nimio, cum in interiora corporis calor fugiat naturalis, vel ex defectione virtutis spiritualis, cum arterias dilatare in omnes suas extremitates non possit' (Fainting arises from excessive pain, when the natural heat of the body withdraws into the inner parts, or as a result of a failure of the spiritual force, when it cannot extend the arteries into all its extremities).[47] However,

[46] Al-Maǧūsī, *Kāmil al-ṣinaʿah al-ṭibbiyah*, p. 256. For Latin medical terminology, see Roth, *Klinische terminologie*, p. 397.

[47] On the three types of forces and spirits — the animal, spiritual, and natural — and their functions as given in the various translations of Constantine, see Newton, 'Constantine the

after this MS 73 J 6 reads 'sicut [lacuna] videmus' (just as we see [lacuna]). When we turn to the Arabic text, it becomes clear that the added phrase is the remnant of a more pronounced and extensive guide for the reader, present as follows in the Arabic: 'we will discuss *in the future*, in the location where fainting [*el-ghushi*] is spoken of'.[48] It seems that Geraldus skipped the temporal phrase to later replace it with a reference to the precise location in the text where fainting was discussed. He anticipated he needed about half a line, enough space to write down a book number and chapter title.[49]

In the fifth and last example we can reconstruct what Geraldus likely skipped by comparing the sequence in which information is presented in both Arabic and Latin:

> [no. 8, Arabic] And when the diet *of the sick is one, then the repetition of the loosening is inherent to the system*. It has occurred in this way that a tertian fever, every time nature expels/rejects the bad excess on the day on which it strikes and the surplus is expelled.[50]

> [no. 8, Latin] Si aut dieta [lacuna] aliquando hoc in tertiana est febri cum colericos humores natura expellit in die accessionis.

> If the diet [lacuna] at times this occurs in the case of a tertian fever, when nature expels the choleric humours on the day of its [the fever's] appearance.

In Arabic, the discussed notions cover, in order of appearance: 1) Diet; 2) Repetition of the 'loosening'; 3) Tertian fever. While Constantine's Latin translation is phrased very differently from the Arabic text, it does suggest that the second element (emphasized in the above translation) is the section skipped in MS 73 J 6, given the sequence of the information. Moreover, this space left blank in the Hague manuscript is one of the larger gaps, which shows that Geraldus skipped a substantial passage. Geraldus may have initially skipped this passage because of its opaque nature. Gerrit Bos shows that Constantine

African', especially the chart at pp. 41–42, and Burnett, 'The Chapter on the Spirits'.

[48] Al-Maǧūsī, *Kāmil al-ṣina'ah al-ṭibbiyah*, p. 242. Emphasis added by the authors.

[49] Note that a similar practice is witnessed in the autograph of the mathematical tract *De arte mensurandi*, where the author, Johannes de Muris, left gaps where precise references to chapter and proposition numbers should be placed. The author did not know the chapter numbers offhand and aimed to look them up later; see Victor, 'A Study of Johannes de Muris' Autograph of the *De arte mensurandi*', p. 394.

[50] Al-Maǧūsī, *Kāmil al-ṣinā'ah al-ṭibbiyya*, ed. by Sezgin, p. 434, and the 1877 edition of the same, *Kāmil al-ṣina'ah al-ṭibbiyah*, p. 364, respectively. Emphasis added by the authors.

tended to translate quite literally, producing translations that other scholars deemed 'poor', 'corrupt', and 'incomprehensible'.[51] One can imagine just how incomprehensible the literal translation of this passage into Latin would be.

Comparison with the Arabic original provides a less satisfactory outcome for the remaining three lacunae.[52] Two of these (nos 1 and 3) are not found at all in the Arabic editions, while for the third (no. 7) it is difficult to identify the Arabic passage which corresponds with the lacuna in the Latin passage:

> [no. 7, Arabic] If a person eats food that is fatty and 'imprisoned' in the body, then he follows it with food that is refined or with food that fills the belly. And then the second rots away before that the first one is brought down to the stomach. Concerning the fact that if a person eats food that does not settle, then he follows this with other foods and he does not digest.

> [no. 7, Latin] Aut in substantia cibi crossi sicut caro est uaccina, & panis azymus, quae [lacuna, with strike-out line] aut in ordinatione cibi, sicut cum quis crossum aut stipticum manducaverit cibum, postea subtilem apponat, qui antea corrumpitur quam crossus, a stomacho egrediatur, aut cum cibum accipiat quem antequam digerat alium rursum suscipiat

> Either in the substance of fatty food, such as cows' flesh, and unleavened bread, which [the substance] [lacuna] or in the order of [consuming] the food, as when one eats food that is fatty or styptic [i.e. constipating], let him after that take a fine-grained kind, one that is broken down before the fatty one departs from the stomach, or when he takes food, before he digests it in turn should take another.

In conclusion, while a reconstruction of Geraldus's rationale behind deploying this relatively rare correction technique suffers from the fact that the blanks were never filled in, they do provide sufficient detail to draw some conclusions. First, the majority of the blanks suggest that an intervention was planned in the text Geraldus copied from his exemplar. Considering what we know about problems encountered by medieval translators, Geraldus may have deemed a Latin word or phrase improperly translated, he may have compensated for a Latin transliteration of an Arabic word (such 'code switching' is especially com-

[51] Literal translation is given as one of the features of Constantine's technique in Bos, 'Ibn al-Ǧazzār's *Risāla fi al-nisyān*', p. 216. Other examples of Constantine's tendency to translate literally are discussed in Strohmaier, 'Constantine's Pseudo-Classical Terminology and its Survival', p. 95. This case shows that Constantine was unaware of existing terminology already circulating.

[52] Table 2.1, no. 2 has not been included in this section, because it was found after the research in collaboration with Arabic scholar N. Peter Joosse was concluded.

mon in scientific manuscripts), or perhaps even encountered an original Arabic word or phrase.[53] The alternative seems less likely: that Geraldus meticulously copied blank spaces encountered in his exemplar.

A second important conclusion is that this lacuna technique was a two-step method to achieve the best text possible: first the potential flaw was identified by an educated eye, and then the correction postponed so that it could be verified by an expert eye. In this scenario someone besides the scribe must have also participated in upgrading this *Theorica* copy, and this someone was consulted because he was better suited to correct potential flaws. After all, if Geraldus could correct these himself, he would likely have done so at the very moment he copied down a sentence and noticed issues; there would be no need for the lacuna technique. It is probable that the aim was to consult with Constantine himself, given that the production of MS 73 J 6 happened in Constantine's vicinity and during his lifetime. It is, in other words, probable that Geraldus's interventions reflect, by proxy, how Constantine sometimes struggled to render al-Maǧūsī's Arabic original into Latin.

The third conclusion is related to the observation that there are no lacunae in the 1539 printed edition of the *Pantegni*, not because they were filled with text, but because they have been contracted.[54] This omission of the lacunae reflects the manuscript or manuscripts on which that edition was based.[55] At

[53] Constantine must have encountered substantial difficulties providing Latin equivalents for Arabic terms; see Strohmaier, 'Constantine's Pseudo-Classical Terminology and its Survival', especially p. 91. An example of transliteration (Greek literary terminology into Latin) is discussed in McKitterick, 'Glossaries and Other Innovations in Carolingian Book Production', pp. 46, fig. 17; 47–48. See also Metcalfe, *Muslims and Christians in Norman Sicily*, pp. 127–40. An example of a manuscript in which a term in the original language is found embedded in an otherwise translated text is the translator's autograph of the German vernacular version of *Somniale Danielis*, where 'tempesta[tis]' is scribbled down in a thin pen. Palmer and Speckenback, *Träume und Kräuter*, pp. 53, 132, and illustration 11 inserted between pp. 52–53. For code switching, see Glick, 'Communication', p. 137. See also Lorch, 'The Science of Weights' on how Arabic translators transliterated the names of weights from Greek for lack of proper terminology.

[54] All lacunae are contracted in the Basel edition of the *Pantegni* from 1539; see pp. 40, 47, 131, 164, 225, 256, 278, 279, and 329. The edition is slightly different in no. 9: MS 73 J 6 reads 'Cum autem malum [lacunae] dixerit possibile est infirmum', whereas the edition on p. 329 reads 'Cum autem dixerit possibile est infirmum' with 'malum' lacking. It is also absent in Helsinki, Yliopiston kirjasto, MS EÖ II 14.

[55] For example, BnF, Latin 6887 (*c.* 1100), and Helsinki, Yliopiston kirjasto, MS EÖ II 14, show the same pattern as the Basel edition: most of the gaps were contracted rather than filled in. Yet in two cases in BnF, Latin 6887, lacunae nos 4 and 6, the lacunae fall at the end of

some point in the tradition, probably very early on, a manuscript was produced in which the blanks were simply skipped, so to speak, after which the lacunae-free text (that was missing small pieces) emerged that is now encountered in some manuscripts and the 1539 printed edition. Evidently, the flaws highlighted by the blanks remained unresolved.

Final Assessment

The most important observation resulting from analysis of the lacunae, that MS 73 J 6 presents an incomplete and imperfect text, has implications for our understanding of the manuscript at the heart of this study. As shown, Geraldus actively intervened in the text. However, given that the manuscript was made in Constantine's translation kitchen, one wonders why there was so much to correct at all. Nowhere is the discrepancy between the *Pantegni* in MS 73 J 6, and what one would expect from a book made in the shadow of the translator, clearer than at the end: this *Theorica* copy is incomplete — after all, the text on the five last pages were filled by a later, *c.* 1150 scribe. So much work was still left undone in perfecting this copy, which raises an intriguing scenario worth consideration: could the translation as it survives in this early copy have been taken from Constantine's desk before he had the chance to finish and polish it?

As remote as this suggestion may sound, MS 73 J 6 would not be alone in such a situation. Premature copying of a freshly translated text is encountered, for example, in a fourteenth-century Middle Dutch translation of Jacobus de Voragine's *Legenda aurea*, which was whisked from the translator's desk before he finished editing the final text.[56] More pertinent to the present discussion, a similar scenario lies at the root of two early copies of Constantine's *Isagoge*, both made at Monte Cassino during the translator's lifetime: Monte Cassino, MS 225 (*c.* 1075–*c.* 1090) and Paris, BnF, NAL 1628 (fig. 1.4), a booklet covering fols 19–26 (*c.* 1075–*c.* 1095).[57] Both texts are incomplete, breaking off before the end, although at different points; namely in chapters 86 (Monte

a line, and there a blank space is left. We are grateful to Iolanda Ventura for checking this manuscript and pointing out the possibility of two residual lacunae.

[56] Kwakkel, 'Lost but Not Forgotten', p. 271.

[57] The early version of the *Isagoge* present in these two manuscripts is studied in Newton, 'Constantine the African', pp. 26–40. Note that while Monte Cassino, MS 225 was already established as a product of the abbey, the Cassinese origin of BnF, NAL 1628 is new and is presented in Chapter 1 of the present volume. It is also entirely clear now that the *Isagoge* was one of Constantine's translations.

Cassino, MS 225) and 79 (BnF, NAL 1628). Eventually, the Latin translation consists of one hundred chapters. These premature stops were not dictated by space. Rather, it has been proposed that in both cases 'the scribe copied all the text that was available to him at the time'.[58] One may explain the incompleteness of the exemplar: these two copies have a common ancestor, an 'informal copy' or 'rough *brouillon*' (draft) that came 'from the translator's own atelier'.[59] This draft was either written by the translator's own hand, or, more likely, dictated to someone very close to him.[60] A reconstruction shows how this common source, potentially Constantine's original, presented the text in such an unorganized fashion that it led the scribes of both manuscripts to make the same mistakes; it likely had some of the text to be copied written in the margins or between lines.[61]

From this analysis it follows that copies may have been made of Constantine's draft of the *Isagoge* before the translator had finished his work; not just once, it seems, but twice, and at different moments (considering that Monte Cassino, MS 225 and BnF, NAL 1628 break off at different points). That the process allows copying work to stop prematurely forms an intriguing parallel to what we might reasonably reconstruct happened with MS 73 J 6. However, the similarities between the *Isagoge* and *Pantegni* go even further. It has been shown that a corrector is found on several pages of the Paris booklet. These corrections are substantial in that complete sentences are added in the margins and between lines, as seen in MS 73 J 6. These emendations form the early stages of a 'revision', and it is this revised version, to which the remainder of the completed text was added later, that becomes the 'Vulgate' text of the *Isagoge*, which circulated in the twelfth and thirteenth centuries.[62] In other words, the second striking parallel between BnF, NAL 1628 and MS 73 J 6 is that both contain revisions that have been considered the 'set text' in the later manuscript tradition. They show, above all, a text still in the process of being formed.[63]

[58] Newton, 'Constantine the African', p. 31. Note that the scribe of Monte Cassino, MS 225 writes at the end of his incomplete copy 'Explicit deo gratias', expressing that his copying task was done.

[59] Newton, 'Constantine the African', pp. 37–38.

[60] Newton, 'Constantine the African', p. 31.

[61] Newton, 'Constantine the African', p. 35. For the role of dictation in the creation of a new text, see the discussion of Peter Damian's practice on pp. 150–51.

[62] Newton, 'Constantine the African', pp. 37–38.

[63] It is not clear whether Geraldus's exemplar, Constantine's own copy, did contain the

Close inspection of the marginal revisions in the Paris booklet prompts a stunning observation: as discussed in Chapter 1, the revisions were written down by the very hand that copied the majority of MS 73 J 6: Geraldus. It appears, then, that he had access to Constantine's translations before they were finished. The manuscripts show that he was not only authorized to copy drafts, but was also revising the Latin text under Constantine's direction: note the marginal revisions in the Paris booklet and the attempted revisions in MS 73 J 6. Indeed, all the signs point to Geraldus having collaborated closely with Constantine. We already know from historical sources that Constantine had assistants who helped him: Atto (Hatto, Adto, Azo) and Johannes Afflacius.[64] Atto even changed the wording of Constantine's Latin text. Peter the Deacon tells us that Atto 'took the texts that the aforementioned Constantine had translated out of different languages and put them into Latin in elegant style'.[65] Thus the observations presented in this chapter add significantly to what we already know about Constantine's collaboration with other individuals at Monte Cassino: 1) His circle of assistants is larger than we might have thought, and 2) Constantine had different individuals working on his drafts with different goals, such as polishing it with an elegant style (Atto), and working to improve the accuracy of the translation, perhaps at Constantine's own dictation (Geraldus). It is now time to take a closer look at this inner circle at Monte Cassino that supported the translation endeavours.

words and phrases missing (the lacunae) in MS 73 J 6. But certainly, the Hague manuscript is considerably cleaner than the Paris *Isagoge*, and is largely free of extensive corrections and revisions. It may well represent a version of the text penultimate to the final, approved and completed copy, which would then have been appropriate as a grand dedication copy to be given to Desiderius.

[64] Newton, 'Constantine the African', pp. 23–26; and Green, 'Constantine the African', p. 146.

[65] Newton, 'Constantine the African', p. 24.

Chapter 3

Team Constantine

The coming of so exotic a figure as Constantine to Monte Cassino must have made a vivid impression on contemporaries. Constantine himself emphasized his foreignness by calling himself regularly 'Africanus' or 'the man of Ifrīqya' in his works.[1] His foreignness is yet more emphatically underscored in the Cassinese accounts of Constantine's career. These last are preserved in two forms, or biographies. In addition to the 'biographies', there are other passing allusions to monks associated in some way with Constantine. It is the purpose of the present chapter to examine these several references to Constantine in Monte Cassino sources, so as to shed light on the observations made in the previous chapters. This exploration at times does, necessarily, delve into the nature of these texts themselves. We propose a new assessment of the reliability of the Cassinese sources. The final goal is to relate them to the evidence of the surviving manuscripts of Constantine's works.

The opening page of the Hague manuscript (MS 73 J 6) makes a strangely complex initial impression, already briefly noted, upon the reader. The first column and the upper three-quarters of the second are written in a uniform late Caroline minuscule (by Scribe A, Geraldus) which is tiny but carefully formed

[1] This is discussed by Glaze in the introduction to this monograph. We remind the reader, as Jacquart and Micheau point out, that the name refers to the classical Roman province of 'Africa', that is, modern Tunisia, with the addition of the region of Constantine; its extent is seen in Overview Map I (p. 3) of Talbert, ed., *Barrington Atlas of the Greek and Roman World*; Jacquart and Micheau, *La médecine arabe et l'occident medieval*, p. 107. At Monte Cassino the epithet would have distinguished our Constantine from Constantinus Sardus, who hailed from Cagliari; see Hoffmann, 'Die Kalender des Leo Marsicanus', p. 113 (under 4 July), and p. 133 (with bibliography). But it is probable that Constantine had this full name already in Salerno.

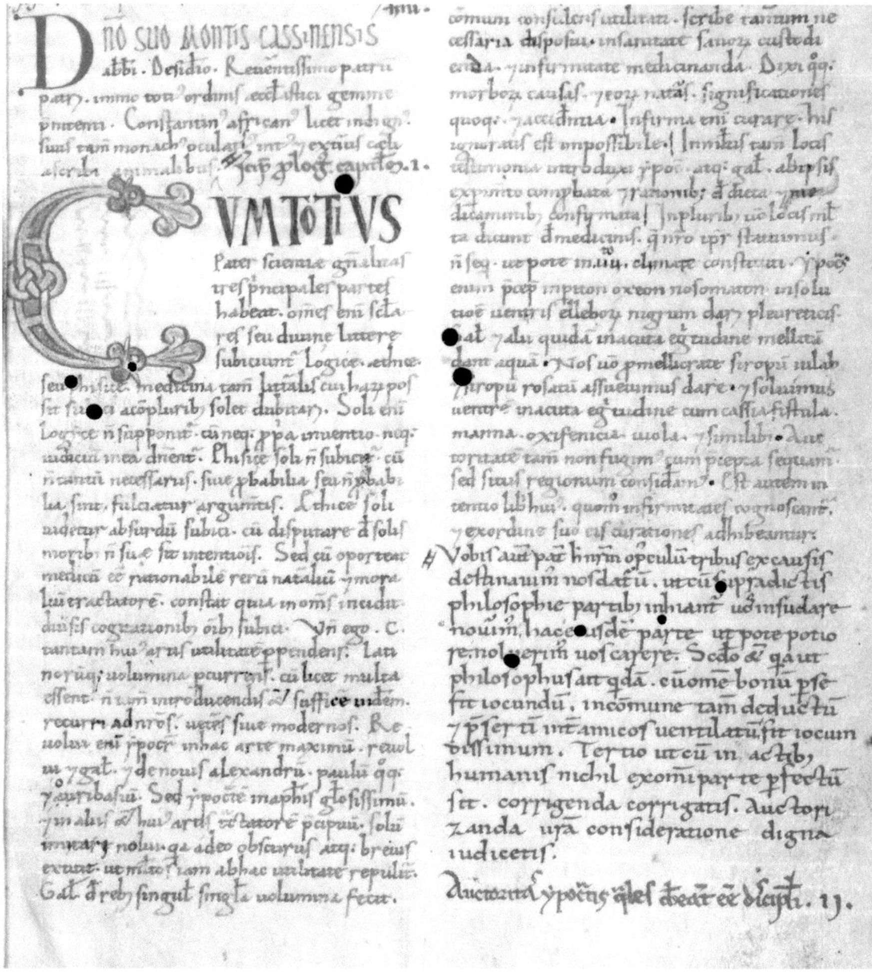

Figure 3.1. Unusual positioning of the 'Vobis autem, pater' part of the Prologue (in red in the original), here called Part C. The Hague, Koninklijke Bibliotheek, MS 73 J 6, fol. 1r (detail). Late 1070s–early 1080s (before 1086).

and clear. On the other hand, the final thirteen lines of the text in the second column are in a completely different, but contemporary, hand with a bolder script-type and larger module. Most remarkably, in contrast to the faded but clear brown ink of the preceding lines, these last lines are written in brilliant red ink (pl. XI).

To add to the page's perplexing mixture, there are small symbols in brown, a 'II' before this last paragraph, and a corresponding 'II' before the main body of the Prologue (beginning 'Cum totius');[2] these are subsequent additions to indicate to the reader that the last paragraph on the page, beginning 'Vobis autem, pater', should in fact stand after the opening address and before the 'Cum totius' text of the first column (fig. 3.1).

The change in hand and in ink corresponds to a definite and demonstrable change in the nature of the text. The long central part of this Prologue to the entire work (see the Latin text and translation in this volume's Appendix C) recounts Constantine's failure to find any Latin medical books suitable for teaching *introducendi*, and his turning back to 'our own people, whether ancient or modern ones'. There follows, from al-Mağūsī, the survey of great Greek medical writers, Hippocrates, Galen, Alexander, Paul, and Oribasius, with critique of their strengths and their failings. This part ends with discussion and examples of medicines prescribed contrary to the practice of those earlier authorities, and the reasons for diverging from them; again Constantine is following al-Mağūsī.

By contrast, the paragraph in red at the end which begins 'Vobis autem, pater' is not based on al-Mağūsī, and its subject is an elaborate, three-fold explanation for the translation's dedication to Abbot Desiderius; his name 'pater' marks the return to him, as the same word had been placed near the opening of the central part of the Prologue. The last part, therefore, corresponds to the formal address to Desiderius with which the text started; the two passages frame the body of the Prologue. The third hand's note, intended to shift this final paragraph, is the result of a misunderstanding of the structure of the Prologue, and it has caused chaos in the manuscript tradition.[3] But why this patchwork effect on the initial page in the Hague manuscript, the earliest extant manuscript of this famous encyclopaedia of medical theory?

Peter the Deacon: Reliability as a Source

The very mention of Peter the Deacon of Monte Cassino's name will raise immediate scepticism in the minds of many scholars. Historians are conditioned by the brilliant exposé of Caspar to expect forgery and fantasy from the brilliant but deeply flawed twelfth-century Monte Cassino scholar. Peter does

[2] The symbol stands before the added title in the latter place.

[3] This was perceived by Malato and de Martini. Constantine the African, *L'arte universale della Medicina*, ed. and trans. by Malato and de Martini, p. 79 n. 2. These scholars understood that the larger Prologue has the frame structure that we are examining in the oldest surviving manuscript, the Hague volume that is the focus of the present study.

however preserve facts about, especially, the eleventh-century monks of the abbey and their writings which would be otherwise lost to us; this has enabled modern scholars to identify a number of these writers' works.[4]

Atto, 'Constantini Africani Auditor'

It was Herbert Bloch who, in his fresh and ground-breaking survey of Constantine's activities, first examined the important figure of Atto. (If our understanding is correct, his name has come down in the transmission spelled variously as 'Atto', 'Adto', 'Hatto', and 'Azo'.)[5] In the treatise *De viris illustribus*, the entry for this personage reads:

> Adto, Constantini Africani auditor et Agnetis imperatricis capellaneus, ea que supradictus Constantinus de diversis linguis transtulerat, coturnato sermone in Romanam linguam descripsit.[6]

> (Adto, *auditor* of Constantine the African and chaplain to the Empress Agnes, took the writings that the aforementioned Constantine had translated out of different languages and turned them into the Roman language in high-buskined style.)

The term 'coturnato sermone', which has puzzled commentators, refers to the exalted style derived from the grand style of tragedy, from *cothurnus*, which is the high boot, or buskin, worn by tragic actors.[7]

[4] An example of such an identification is Alberic of Monte Cassino's treatise on the Eucharist against Berengar of Tours; see Radding and Newton, *Theology, Rhetoric, and Politics in the Eucharistic Controversy*. For other works of Alberic's identified by scholars in the second half of the twentieth century, see the list in Radding and Newton, pp. 55–56 and n. 5. A mathematical treatise on the abacus by Pandulf of Capua has also been identified; see Gibson and Newton, 'Pandulf of Capua's *De calculatione*'.

[5] Bloch, *Monte Cassino in the Middle Ages*, pp. 104, 135–36.

[6] Peter the Deacon, *De viris illustribus Casinensibus*, 24, col. 1035. This text is from Peter's autograph, Monte Cassino, MS 361. The possible implications of the term *auditor* are discussed further in this chapter.

[7] The literal meaning of *cothurnus* would have been known to twelfth-century Monte Cassino writers, including Peter the Deacon, from many classical authors, and the literal meaning of *cothurnatus* from a smaller group, including Seneca, the *Dialogi* II.18.4. The *Dialogi* is one of the rare and notable classical works copied in the Desiderian scriptorium, preserved today as Milan, Biblioteca Ambrosiana, MS C 105 inf. See Newton, *Scriptorium and Library*, pl. 59 and pp. 259–62, 348. The adjective is applied by classical and post-classical writers (in the sense 'concerned with tragic or elevated themes', Glare, ed., *Oxford Latin Dictionary*, *s. v.*); see Martial V.5.8 (Martial, *Epigrams*, ed. and trans. by Shackleton Bailey, I, 356–37), and VII.63.5

It was after the dedication of Abbot Desiderius's new basilica on 1 October 1071 that the German Empress Agnes, widow of Emperor Henry III and mother of his successor the reigning Henry IV, came to visit Monte Cassino, where she remained almost half a year.[8] On the basis of the surviving documentation, Bloch has suggested that she arrived at the abbey 'late in 1072 or early in 1073'; she left before the end of June 1073. In the splendid prose of the *Chronicle of Monte Cassino*, Agnes's visit recapitulates the paradigmatic visit of the Queen of Sheba to King Solomon and his temple. Like Sheba on her visit to Jerusalem, Agnes presented rich gifts to Monte Cassino. The gospel book that she offered has been identified; it remains at the abbey today, as Monte Cassino, MS 437.[9] This is a beautiful volume with script and decoration that testify it was created in England for Judith of Flanders, wife of Earl Tostig. There is evidence in the manuscript that it later belonged to the Empress Agnes, and the chronology fits: it can be conjectured that on her arrival in Germany (1070/71) to marry Duke Welf of Bavaria, Judith presented the beautiful book to Agnes, and this is how it came to Monte Cassino as a gift from the empress in 1072/73.

From contemporary accounts we know something about the empress's entourage at the time of her visit. A letter dated 23 April 1073 from the newly-elected Pope Gregory VII (Hildebrand) announcing his election to Desiderius, asks the abbot to greet the empress on Gregory's behalf and also 'Rainaldus, the venerable bishop of Como' who was Agnes's trusted advisor. It was recently proposed that Rainaldus, or one of his company, gave to, or left at, the monastery an unpretentious volume of the *Vita S. Remigii Episcopi Remensis* (now Monte Cassino, MS 494); the book contains neumes of the Como region and so could well have been brought to the abbey at the time of the visit of the empress and Rainaldus.[10]

Another member of the empress's train is listed beside these in the Subiaco Sacramentary of 1075 (today Rome, Biblioteca Vallicelliana, MS B 24), compiled by the scribe Guitto for Abbot John V. The *Liber vitae* in MS B 24 con-

(Martial, *Epigrams*, ed. and trans. by Shackleton Bailey, II, 128–19); Phocas, *Carmen de vita Vergilii* 123 ('cothurnato [...] versu'), ed. by Riese, p. 132.

[8] *Chronica monasterii Casinensis*, III.29, III.32, ed. by Hoffmann; on the dedication, see III.29, p. 398, on Agnes's visit, III.32, pp. 402–03. For more on Agnes's time in Italy, see Bulst-Thiele, *Kaiserin Agnes*, pp. 83–112.

[9] Newton, *Scriptorium and Library*, pp. 233–40.

[10] Newton, *Scriptorium and Library*, pp. 251–52.

tains a remembrance of Agnes, who had visited that monastery in 1073/74. The community at Subiaco prayed for:

HENRICUS IMPERATOR.
AGNES MATER EIUS.
Rainaldus aepiscopus. Hatto clericus[11]

(EMPEROR HENRY.
HIS MOTHER AGNES.
Bishop Rainaldus. Cleric Atto)

As Bloch was first to observe, 'Hatto clericus' in this context must refer to the figure known, through Peter the Deacon's notice, as Agnes's chaplain. The entry in the sacramentary demonstrates that at the time of Agnes's visit to Subiaco, Atto was still in her service and had not yet taken monastic vows at Monte Cassino. It is probable that, as Bloch suggests, he carried that out only after the empress's death in January 1077.[12]

Atto and the High-Buskined Style

This then is the figure who was an 'auditor' of Constantine's.[13] More importantly, and primarily, he in some way worked on the translations of the North African medical man by contributing his own stylistic polish. After all, this churchman was cosmopolitan in his experience and career, and for some years formed part of the retinue of the book-receiving and book-giving empress. As has been noted within a South Italian context, 'books were the outward appurtenances of learned clerics [of this age]'.[14]

[11] The first three names and titles are in red. The entry 'Hatto clericus' is a contemporary addition in black. See the fundamental study by Schwarzmaier, 'Der *Liber vitae* von Subiaco', pp. 80–147, especially p. 146 and Abb. 2.

[12] It has previously been suggested that Constantine must have arrived in South Italy no earlier than 1077, but new analysis of the Salernitan biography, as well as the textual analyses of the present volume, suggests that the early view of Vera von Falkenhausen may be correct: Constantine may well have arrived prior to Guiscard's conquest of the city. It is clear, however, that he secured the patronage of Guiscard and Prince Richard of Capua almost immediately following the city's conquest, perhaps through the influence of Sikelgaita, Gaitelgrima, Alfanus, and Johannes de Curte. See Newton, 'Constantine the African', pp. 19–26, especially 26; Newton, 'Arabic Medicine and Other Arabic Cultural Influences in Southern Italy in the Time of Constantinus Africanus', pp. 25–55; and this volume's Introduction.

[13] The Latin word 'auditor' is discussed further in the present chapter.

[14] Newton, *Scriptorium and Library*, p. 13.

Peter the Deacon's words on the collaborative assistance that Atto contributed to Constantine's great task of translation leads us to take a closer look at the complex of hands, inks, and styles that make up the Prologue of the *Pantegni* on fol. 1^r of its earliest surviving manuscript, MS 73 J 6. In particular, the alien passage at the end of the Prologue (written in a new hand and a different-coloured ink) draws attention to itself. It reads:

> Vobis autem, Pater, hoc nostrum opusculum tribus ex causis destinavimus nos daturum, ut cum supradictis philosophiae partibus inhianter vos insudare noverimus, hac eiusdem parte utpote potiore noluerimus vos carere; secundo etiam, quia ut philosophus ait quidam, cum omne bonum per se sit iocundum,[15] in commune tamen deductum et praesertim inter amicos ventilatum fit iocumdissimum; tertio, ut cum in actibus humanis nichil ex omni parte perfectum sit, corrigenda corrigatis, auctorizanda vestra consideratione digna iudicetis.
>
> (And I determined to present this my little work to you, O father, for three purposes: [1] so that since I know that you with panting zeal sweat over the three aforementioned parts of philosophy, I did not wish you to be deprived of this part of the same, the very best part. [2] In the second place, besides, as a certain philosopher says, 'While every good thing in and of itself is pleasing, still that which is shared and especially that aired among friends becomes supremely pleasing'. [3] In the third place, since in the doings of human creatures nothing is in every way perfect, so that you might correct what is in need of correction, and might judge deserving of publication what is worthy of your consideration.)

The address to 'father [Desiderius]' marks a change of section. Indeed, the structure of the whole Prologue is now clear:

> Part A. Col. 1, lines 27–32 (in brown-black ink), beginning: 'DOMINO SUO MONTIS'. This is the opening address to Desiderius, who is called, *inter alia*, 'most revered' and 'patrum patri' (father of fathers).
>
> Part B. Col. 1, lines 33–col. 2, line 47 (in the same brown-black ink and hand), beginning: 'CUM TOTIUS, Pater'. This is the long central portion, with its beginning marked by the renewed invocation of the 'Pater' (father, i.e. Desiderius).
>
> Part C. Col. 2, lines 48–60 (in red, in a new hand), beginning: 'Vobis autem, pater'. This is the Prologue's conclusion, with its beginning marked by another appeal to the same 'pater'.

[15] The reading of this first 'fit' in the Hague manuscript is surely an error; we have emended it to 'sit'.

The Prologue's tailpiece, like the opening address, is highly personal and dominated by the figure of the abbot of Monte Cassino. In contrast, the central block, drawn principally from al-Maǧūsī's original Prologue, focuses on the nuts and bolts, the bibliography, as it were, of the field.[16] Brief as it is, the Prologue's final part is rhetorically structured; there are three purposes outlined in this dedication to Abbot Desiderius: (1) the subject of the *Pantegni* is so congenial to his interests, indeed his passionate interests (and the language of panting and sweating brings the grand, and, by suggestion, bejewelled, abbot of the initial address down to the level of the hard-working clerk/scribe or even field-labourer, but also one who is hard-working on behalf of others and of learning); (2) the value of sharing all good and noble things among friends; and (3) the humble plea for the abbot's aid in the editing and publication of this work. The piece is characterized by its formal, three-part structure, corresponding to the Isidorian technical tripartite division of philosophy at the opening of the second part, but, within the conventions, it possesses warmth and a personal tone that is an advance upon the insistence on Desiderius's splendour of the initial address. It is, in short, the work of an artist in rhetoric. Is this not the role that the *De viris illustribus* described Atto as filling?

The fact that the concluding part that so neatly wraps up the Prologue on this page is entered *secundis curis* (as editors used to say), as a separate operation and indeed by a different hand (it is probably an Italian hand, but definitely not Geraldus's), and even in a different colour ink, corresponds to Peter the Deacon's description of Atto's work.

The reasonable conclusion is that the tailpiece was not left out by accident: it is probable that this last part of the page was left blank in order to receive a part of the text later. In fact, it is probable that it had not even been composed when the scribe Geraldus sat down to copy out the first column and the top three-quarters of the second. The part *was* ready, however, when the Hague Rubricator (Scribe B) left his mark on the book: he copied it, after all, when he added the rubrics to the text. The Hague manuscript represents a stage in the initial creation of Constantine's *Pantegni*, a volume, as it were, from his own workshop. As with the lacunae discussed in the previous chapter, we witness how the final text of the *Pantegni* is put together. After all, the part in question was probably only composed after Geraldus had started copying the manuscript. Astonishingly, and before the modern reader's eyes, the part played by

[16] For a comparison of Constantine's Prologue to al-Maǧūsī's, see Jacquart, 'Le sens donné par Constantin l'Africain'.

Atto is explicitly and even (in a literal sense) graphically visible. It is also noteworthy that the new tailpiece, Prologue Part C, directly characterizes the text of the *Theorica* that follows as incomplete and imperfect; this section appeals directly to Abbot Desiderius for his own critical attention and for further support in the completion of the project.[17]

In considering the construction of this tripartite Prologue, one who peruses the Monte Cassino account(s) with care can see a supplement and its function:

***Chronicle* passage on Constantine (*Chronica monasterii Casinensis*, III.35):**	***De viris illustribus* passage on Atto (*De viris illustribus*, chap. 24):**
Constantinus Africanus [...] e Cartagine, de qua oriundus erat, egrediens, Babiloniam petiit, in qua grammatica, dialectica, geometria, arithmetica, mathematica, astronomia, nec non et phisica Chaldeorum, Arabum, Persarum, Saracenorum, Egiptiorum, ac Indorum plenissime eruditus est.[18]	Atto, Constantini Africani auditor et Agnetis imperatricis capellaneus, ea quae supradictus Constantinus de diversis linguis transtulerat, coturnato sermone in Romanam linguam descripsit.[19]
(Constantine the African [...] departing from Carthage, where he was born, made his way to Old Cairo, where he was most completely educated in grammar, dialectic, geometry, arithmetic, mathematics, astronomy, and also in the medicine of the Chaldeans, Arabs, Persians, Saracens, Egyptians, and Indians.)	(Atto, *auditor* of Constantine the African, and chaplain to the Empress Agnes, took the writings that the aforementioned Constantine had translated out of different languages and turned them into the Roman tongue in high-buskined style.)

For the reader who has even a modest awareness of the system of the medieval *artes*, the *Chronicle*'s account of Constantine's education has a glaring gap: in the expected list of the Trivium (grammar, rhetoric, and dialectic) the essential art of rhetoric is here missing! The author of this account (whether Peter's teacher and predecessor Guido, or even Guido's predecessor, Leo Marsicanus)

[17] The incomplete nature of the text is discussed in Chapter 2. Whether Desiderius was also asked to help support the reconstruction of the *Practica* is unclear.

[18] Peter the Deacon, *De viris illustribus Casinensibus*, col. 1035b.

[19] *Chronica monasterii Casinensis*, III.35, ed. by Hoffmann, pp. 411.22–412.4.

understood Constantine's weakness and, by inference, knew that the weakness was made good by Atto's work. Or, put another way, the gap in the *Chronicle* narrative of Constantine was waiting to be filled by the *De viris illustribus* narrative of the work of Constantine's assistant Atto, with his 'coturnato sermone'. The second account supplements the first and answers the question ('What about rhetoric?') that at once arose in the mind of the reader of the first account. We can only conclude that these two accounts form an old, genuine, and mutually dependent Cassinese tradition.

That this tradition is not only genuine but older than Peter the Deacon's works is proved by what Peter did to it. In expanding and rewriting the *Chronicle* account of Constantine for his *De viris illustribus* chapter on him, Peter not only embellished that sober predecessor's work with phrases like 'teacher of East and West, and new, brilliant Hippocrates',[20] and imagined fantastic journeys of Constantine to India and Ethiopia, he also blithely made sure that Constantine had studied all the Trivium ('grammatica, dialectica, rhetorica', he says), as well as a pair of other *artes* inserted near the end ('necromantia, musica phisicaque'). But the addition of 'rhetorica' shows that Peter did not grasp the subtle fit of the two old traditions that he had before him; in the case of the Atto chapter, he preserved that part of the tradition without understanding how it related to the *Chronicle* account.

In summary: the two pieces of evidence fit together like the pieces of a jigsaw puzzle. For the student of the story of Constantine the African, knowing this is useful: (1) Peter the Deacon was not the author of either of these two elements; (2) Peter was not even aware of the delicate pattern of complementarity. In fact, in tinkering with the *Chronicle* passage for his *De viris illustribus* version, he destroyed the complementarity; (3) Therefore, this jigsaw, interlocking complex of narrative comes from an earlier generation; (4) The account must derive from Guido, Peter's predecessor and teacher, or possibly from Guido's predecessor, Leo Marsicanus; (5) In either case, the narrative comes from the period shortly after Constantine's death, and from a writer, or writers, in part contemporary with Constantine or his students; (6) These circumstances lend considerable credibility to the entire narrative of Constantine's coming to Monte Cassino, and his work there. In this respect one may echo the words of Bloch: 'The value of Peter's list is all the greater as it was drawn up only fifty years after Constantine's death'. It can now be said that the original list, in the *Chronicle*,

[20] 'Orientis et Occidentis magister, novusque effulgens Hypocrates'. Peter the Deacon, *De viris illustribus Casinensibus*, col. 1034a.

was drawn up much earlier than that, and Bloch's statement of credibility can be applied to the entire older tradition.[21]

The old bipartite tradition is a single tradition, a genuine tradition, and its story of collaboration between the scientist-scholar and the rhetorical stylist is now borne out by the physical evidence of the opening page of the *Pantegni* in the Hague manuscript; a manuscript miraculously preserved from Constantine's own collaborative workshop. The manuscript in The Hague, with its many lacunae, shows how Constantine's translation was being produced and perfected. That is, the manuscript shows perhaps the final stages of production, where the final touches were executed. Considering what we now know about Atto, he was no doubt involved in helping Constantine render medical texts into Latin. The Hague manuscript is very likely visual evidence of this collaboration. Indeed, historical accounts and manuscript evidence go hand in hand.

Another Early Witness: Paris, BnF, Latin 6887

The Hague volume is not the only early manuscript of the *Pantegni* that presents anomalies in its opening chapter. Paris, BnF, Latin 6887 is an Italian manuscript of the early twelfth century; among surviving manuscripts, it may be second in age to the Hague book that is the principal subject of the present study.[22]

In this manuscript, again, a part of the Prologue is written in red ink, and, just as remarkable, in a module different from that of its main body (fig. 3.2 and pl. X). In the case of the Paris manuscript, however, there are two parts set apart. They are the beginning of the Prologue, or perhaps one should say the address (Part A), and (as in the Hague manuscript) the tailpiece (Part C). In this manuscript as a whole, the text is laid out in a single column throughout. But, at the beginning of each book, the *capitula*, written in brown ink, but with *paragraphoi* for each in green shaded with red, are crowded in a number of informal columns. On this first page there are four columns to accommodate the twenty-five *capitula*. On the right, and under the third column partially, and all the fourth, stands the address. As in the final part of the Prologue in the Hague manuscript, the script of both address and tailpiece in Paris, BnF, Latin 6887 is written on ruled lines, but in larger script, and in red. The parts, therefore, that are so privileged can thus be shown as Parts A and C:

[21] Bloch, *Monte Cassino in the Middle Ages*, p. 129.

[22] On the lacunae in Paris, BnF, Latin 6887, see p. 91 n. 55 in this volume.

Part A: 'To his lord, the abbot of Monte Cassino', etc.

Part B: [Technical Prologue]

Part C: 'And it is to you, O father, that I determined', etc.

In the case of the Hague manuscript, the address has before it the heading, 'Epistola Constantini ad Desiderium abbatem Montis Cassini', and after it the heading, 'Incipit prologus.capitulum .i.'. It is written in the hand of the Hague Rubricator (Scribe B). There is no explicit for the technical Prologue (Part B), and no incipit nor explicit for the tailpiece (Part C). In Paris, BnF, Latin 6887, the technical Prologue has before it the rubricator's 'INCIPIT PROLOGUS', and after it his 'EXPLICIT PROLOGUS'.

In fact, these Parts A and C at beginning and end resemble each other in being composed in the high-rhetorical style ('sermo coturnatus').[23] As regards the writer, the *topos* of humility appears in each; in Part A, 'licet indignus [...] oculatis intus et exterius caeli ascribi animalibus', and in Part C, 'ut [...] corrigenda corrigatis'. As for the addressee, moreover, both speak eloquently in praise of the abbot. His titles are grand: Desiderius's name 'father of fathers' not only echoes the title of al-Maǧūsī's original Persian dedicatee 'Aḍud al-Dawla, called 'Šāhanšāh' (king of kings). The term 'father of fathers' also corresponds to the major theme of Desiderius's praise, which has been explicated in a close reading of the opening poem and opening miniature in the grandest of Desiderius's manuscripts, the lectionary for Sts Benedict, Maur, and Scholastica (BAV, Vat. lat. 1202), called in its facsimile the 'Codex Benedictus'.[24] The epithet 'bright shining jewel of the entire ecclesiastical order' points directly to Desiderius's splendid dress on ceremonial occasions, represented in the same Vatican lectionary and in the fresco that depicts him as donor in the church of Sant'Angelo in Formis. Another study has attempted a reading of the rhetoric of Desiderius's vestments in these paintings and in the verse panegyric of Desiderian poets.[25] Both the address (Part A) and the tailpiece (Part C) breathe the 'high-buskined style' of Atto.[26]

[23] See p. 98 on the meaning of 'sermo coturnatus'.

[24] Newton, *Scriptorium and Library*, pp. 291–307.

[25] Newton, '"Expolitio" per l'Umanesimo', pp. 169–235. See, for summary of this rhetorical study, this volume's Appendix D.

[26] In fact, years before the discovery of this treatment of the tailpiece in the Hague manuscript and of the same treatment of both the opening address and tailpiece in the Paris manuscript, Newton suggested, *apropos* Atto: 'Constantine, who may have come to Italy rather late

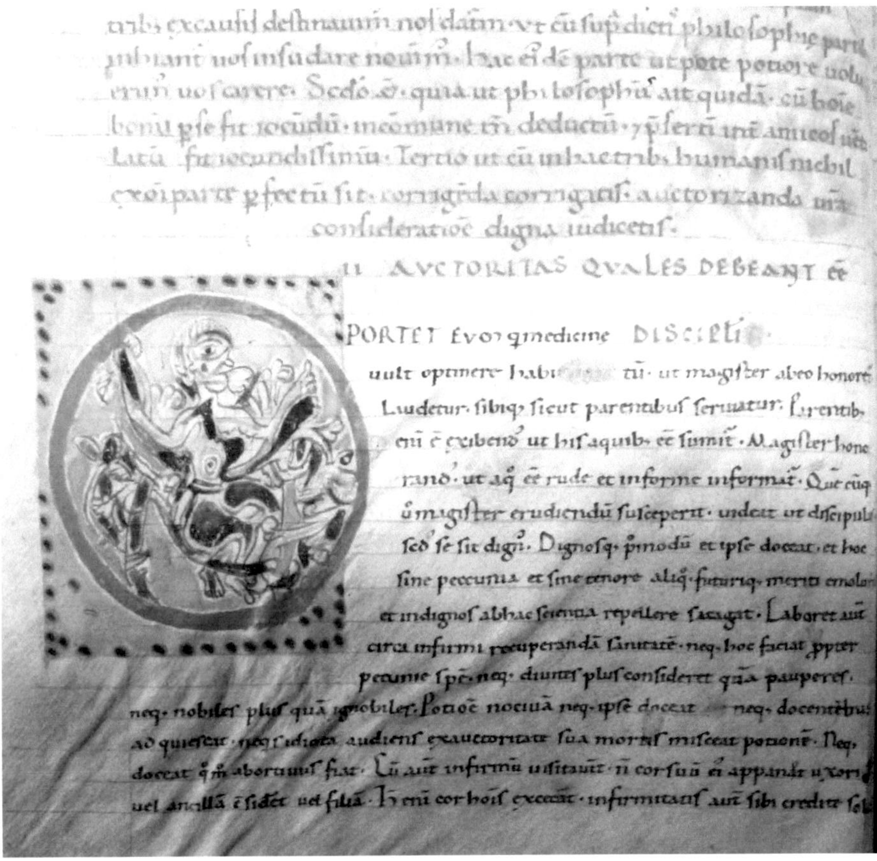

Figure 3.2. Prologue of the Paris *Pantegni*, Paris, Bibliothèque nationale de France, Latin 6887, fol. 1v. *c.* 1100–*c.* 1125.

Paris, BnF, Latin 6887 shows us, even more vividly than the Hague manuscript, the collaboration between Constantine and Atto; the latter's rhetorical handiwork frames the translator's Prologue proper. It must reflect a model also present in manuscripts or a manuscript found in Constantine's workshop at Monte Cassino. It is remarkable that two surviving manuscripts preserve this; such fine points in treatment (distinctions in ink colour and module) would not, in the nature of things, be likely to have survived many generations of copy-

in his life, would have been glad to have someone help him polish the Latin of his translations, and possibly to supply him with quotations from Cicero, as at the opening of the *Viaticum*, or with elegant turns of phrase ("coturnato sermone") about "jewels of the entire ecclesiastical order", and the like'. Newton, 'Constantine the African', p. 24.

ing. For editors of Constantine's work, these manuscripts, quite apart from the grounds of their age, must be studied most seriously for the text that they present.

But there was a downside to this visible evidence of collaboration in the early manuscripts. We have seen that, within a century of its production, a reader added signs (two tilted II marks) to the Hague manuscript to indicate that the tailpiece (Part C) should be read, not at the end of the Prologue, but after the address (Part A); presumably this shift was intended to bring these stylistically congruent and personally similar passages together. But, as Marco T. Malato and Umberto de Martini acutely observed, since Part C, citing the discussion of 'the aforementioned three parts of philosophy', refers to Part B, it cannot have preceded it.[27] The lazy reader who added the marks to rearrange the text had not read it with any care.

The confusion was not confined to this single reader. Many manuscripts have the same misplacement. Only two of Malato and de Martini's manuscripts have the tailpiece in the correct place.[28] The correct order is seen in the Lyon edition of 1515.[29] We shall return in Chapter 5 to the meaning of the situation in the manuscript Erfurt, Universitätsbibliothek, Bibliotheca Amploniana, Cod. Amplon. 4° 184 of the year 1147, which omits both Prologue A and Prologue C.[30]

Theodemar of Hildesheim and Monte Cassino

In the first chapter of this monograph it was demonstrated that The Hague, MS 73 J 6 was produced by a scribe active at the monastery of Monte Cassino in the second half of the eleventh century. A Cassinese document still preserved at the abbey gives us the scribe's name: Geraldus, presbyter and monk (fig. 1.8). This present chapter has shown that, alongside Constantine, the translator/adapter of al-Maǧūsī's work, a second writer provided the rhetorical parts; the introduction and conclusion that frame Constantine/al-Maǧūsī's Prologue to

[27] Constantine the African, *L'arte universale della Medicina*, ed. by Malato and de Martini, p. 79 n. 2.

[28] These two are BAV, Vat. lat. 2455 and Vat. lat. 2456. See Malato and de Martini's comment (p. 79 n. 17); in spite of their observation, they print the Prologue in the order A, C, B.

[29] Isaak ben Salomon Israeli, translated by Constantine the African. *Omnia opera Ysaac*. Although Mark Jordan argues that the Basel printing of the *Pantegni* by Henricus Petrus is more representative of the older and larger manuscript traditions of the text, he does note that Constantine's Prologue was rewritten in a humanistic style, either by Petrus or his deputy; see Jordan, 'The Fortune of Constantine's *Pantegni*', pp. 286–90.

[30] See Chapter 5 of the present volume.

the *Theorica*. Furthermore, this skilled rhetorical writer must be Atto of the high-buskined style that he is credited with in the *De viris illustribus* ascribed to Peter the Deacon. These early manuscripts and Cassinese tradition tell the same story.

That same Cassinese tradition provides further evidence regarding the history of Constantine's collaborator which has never been exploited before. Alongside his *De viris illustribus*, the short biographies of the figures in the history of Monte Cassino famous for outward historical or literary achievements and works, Peter the Deacon left in the same manuscript (Monte Cassino, MS 361), a parallel set of biographies of Cassinese monks noted for spiritual eminence, entitled *Ortus et vita iustorum cenobii Casinensis*. This interesting and important work has been made available to scholars in a meticulous edition and full commentary by R. H. Rodgers.[31]

One aspect, previously understudied, of these two important and parallel works that have come down to us in Peter's hand, is the possibility of duplication. The author himself acknowledges at least once in the *De viris illustribus* that one of the monks at Monte Cassino had two names; chapter 29 of that work begins, 'Benedictus qui et Guaiferius, Salernitanus'[32] (Benedict, also called Guaiferius, from Salerno), and proceeds to list this writer's works. The immediately interesting aspect here is that the same figure is the subject, under the name 'Guaiferius', of *Ortus et vita*, chapter 48.[33] Aided by Peter's explicit statement, scholars have had no difficulty in understanding the Benedict of the *De viris illustribus* and the Guaiferius of the *Ortus et vita* as a single historical figure. Scholars have also been aided by the fact that Benedict/Guaiferius was an eminent writer of the Desiderian age with his writings still preserved together in a manuscript retained at the abbey (Monte Cassino, MS 280), a friend of the literary giant Albericus,[34] and the subject of a notice in the *Chronicle of Monte Cassino*.[35]

Another doublet is more obscure and has not been recognized by historians. It is Lawrence, monk of Monte Cassino and afterwards archbishop of Amalfi.

[31] Peter the Deacon, *Ortus et vita*, ed. by Rodgers.

[32] Peter the Deacon, *De viris illustribus Casinensibus*, col. 1037a.

[33] Peter the Deacon, *Ortus et vita*, ed. by Rodgers, pp. 70–71, and notes on pp. 156–57.

[34] See the discussion of Albericus's *Lexicon prosodiacum* in Chapter 1 of the present monograph. The same manuscript, Monte Cassino, MS 280, also preserves the texts of Alfanus, archbishop of Salerno.

[35] *Chronica monasterii Casinensis*, III.65, ed. by Hoffmann, p. 443.20–25.

De viris illustribus, chapter 6, contains a short biography of this scholar and poet who, as we now know, was at the abbey by the time of Abbot Theobald, probably even by 1021; he was made archbishop of his native city in 1029. After 1039, by reason of the hostility of Duke Waimar, ruler of Amalfi, he went into exile, first in Florence and, in his last years, in Rome. Iotsald tells of the close friends he had there, including the saintly Odilo of Cluny. So close were they that, after Odilo's return to Gaul and death, a miraculous event attended Lawrence's own death, in March, 1049. Iotsald recalls:

> Succedente vero Quadragesima, domnus Laurentius archiepiscopus, de quo supra diximus, Romae moritur. Aderat devotus in exequiis ejus quidam clericus, Albero nomine, natione Teutonicus, genere nobilissimus, patri Odiloni dum viveret familiarissmus, qui cum domno papa Leone, sibi proximo parente, Romam advenerat ea tempestate. Is itaque, memorato archiepiscopo defuncto et ad ecclesiam deportato, lassitudine cogente, se sopori dedit in quodam ejusdem ecclesiae angulo, cum subito adhuc pene vigilanti, Odilo vir beatus apparuit. Cui ille tremens et pavidus amicabili voce diceret: Domine, quando huc et cur advenisti? Ad exequias, inquit, fratris nostri domni Laurentii archiepiscopi veni: quibus expletis, hinc recedens quin viderem te praeterire nolui. His dictis, visio disparuit. Ipse vero postmodum haec nobis et pluribus aliis in veritate narravit.[36]

> (Now in the Lenten season that followed, the lord Lawrence Archbishop of Amalfi, whom I have mentioned earlier, died in Rome. In devout attendance at his funeral was a certain cleric, Albero by name, of German origin, of the noblest descent, a close friend of father Odilo while he lived, who had come to Rome with the lord Pope Leo, his close kinsman, at that time. So, when the aforesaid archbishop died and was brought to the church, [Albero] overwhelmed by weariness, was preparing to sleep in a certain corner of that same church, when suddenly there appeared to him (still, though barely, awake) the blessed Odilo. Trembling and afraid, he said to him in a loving tone, 'Lord, when did you come here, and why?' 'I have come', he replied, 'for the funeral of my brother lord Lawrence the archbishop. And when that was over, as I was leaving, I could not pass by without seeing you'. With that, the vision disappeared. Albero himself afterwards told this story to me and to many others in all truth.)

A striking parallel to this last tale is found in the *Ortus et vita*, chapter 63:

> Leo quidam Amalphitanus in Casino monachus fuit, qui ad finem uite non leuiter egrotans, se custodientibus fratribus aquam petiit, quoram unus cum aliquantulum in hauriendo moratus bibendam aquam ei obtulisset, ille renuit dicens, 'Nolo hanc

[36] Iotsaldus, *Vita S. Odilonis*, cols 913c–14a.

> aquam, quoniam Odilo Cluniacensis abbas statim huc ueniens aquam michi detulit, meque sitientem refecit;'quod audientes illi mirati sunt, statimque predictus frater e mundo recessit.[37]

> (A certain Leo of Amalfi was a monk at Monte Cassino. And at the end of his life, being very ill, he asked the brothers who were caring for him for water. One of them, after some short delay in drawing the water, brought it and offered it to him to drink, but he refused it, saying, 'I don't want this water; Abbot Odilo of Cluny came at once and brought me water and relieved my thirst'. They were amazed to hear that, and at once the aforesaid brother departed from this world.)

In this case, it is recorded in non-Cassinese sources that the Archbishop Lawrence was born with the name Leo.[38] The two accounts refer to only a single figure, and the deathbed stories are but a single story, with the dead saintly Abbot Odilo of Cluny the consoling visitor, once as the Amalfitan lay dying, and again at the service after the Amalfitan's death. In both cases, that of Benedict/Guaiferius of Salerno and that of Leo/Lawrence of Amalfi, it is, naturally, the *Ortus et vita* that preserves the miraculous story.

It may be proposed that there is yet another new doublet discoverable in Peter's autograph texts, and this one involves the figure Atto. We have already examined the brief notice of Atto in the *De viris illustribus*. One of the longer biographies in the *Ortus et vita* is that of Theodemar (chapter 49, following that of Guaiferius). The account begins:

> Theodemar was born in the Alemannic province and was chaplain to the Empress Agnes. So then, when, forsaking and despising the pomp of the world, he was making his way to Monte Cassino, he came to the River Liri outside Ceprano; when he had crossed it, a wave seized his servant and began to drag him under. When he observed this, he at once fell to praying on the spot, and, as soon as he rose from prayer, a wave cast the servant out upon the bank. And when he had reached Monte Cassino, he put on the habit of a holy life. And what a perfect religious life his was, and how pleasing to God, will be made clear in what follows.[39]

At this point, the sceptical, positivist historian may say, 'But wait! Never mind the silly miracle. What's important is that Atto was the empress's chaplain, who

[37] Peter the Deacon, *Ortus et vita*, ed. by Rodgers, p. 94.30–38.

[38] For a thorough discussion of Leo/Lawrence, see Braga, 'Lorenzo d'Amalfi', especially p. 92.

[39] The complete transcription of chapter 49 on Theodemar by Rodgers (Peter the Deacon, *Ortus et vita iustorum cenobii Casinensis*, chap. 49, pp. 71.8–73.23) is given along with a translation in this volume's Appendix D.

travelled with her, and it was Atto who afterwards settled down at Monte Cassino and became a monk'. But once again, the Cassinese tradition offers biographies of two monks, with quite different names, whose narratives are doublets.

In this case, there is an even more remarkable fit later in the series of miraculous events surrounding Theodemar. The author continues:

> In the city of Salerno a certain countryman had a son who was lame, and he took him to the Abbas de Curte [the abbot of the court] and asked him to confer some remedy upon him who was lame. But the abbot saw the man of God, Theodemar, approaching and thrust the boy down in front of him and began to beg him to raise him up from the ground. Then the man of God, who had no idea what was going on, stretched out his hand and grasped the boy, saying, 'Rise up'; and the boy at once stood up.[40]

At first glance, this story seems to present nothing remarkable. It is certainly not the inexplicable healing that is striking in the series of miracles associated with Theodemar. The holy man was surrounded, as it were, by such supernatural happenings. The arresting element is the presence of the Salernitan personage known as the 'abbot of the court'. This is the constant epithet of Johannes, the brother of Prince Gisulf II, the last Lombard ruler of the city of Salerno. According to a Salernitan source, he played a key role in the reception of Constantine the African at Salerno.

This source is the account of Magister Mattheus F[errarius] of Salerno preserved in an early-fourteenth manuscript in Erfurt, Universitätsbibliothek, Bibliotheca Amploniana, Cod. Amplon. 8° 62. Mattheus tells of the arrival of Constantine in Salerno and how at 'the court of St Peter' (today the church of San Pietro a Corte, near the harbour) Constantine was first recognized for his excellence in urine analysis by 'peroptimus medicus, frater principis, qui "Abbas de Curia" nuncupabatur' (the preeminent physician, brother of the prince, who was called 'abbot of the court'). This interesting personage forms a key figure in the fundamentally important assessment of Constantine the African's career by Bloch, and our knowledge of him has been greatly expanded by the research of Eliza Glaze.[41] It is now clear that the 'abbot of the court' played a critical part in the reception of Constantine in South Italy. Yet, until the addition of this piece

[40] See Appendix D.

[41] Glaze, 'Salerno's Lombard Prince', where the evidence for Johannes de Curte's activities are assembled from the Salernitan biography of Constantine, archival and epigraphic documentation at Monte Cassino, and the early twelfth-century Salernitan pharmaceutical treatise, the *Antidotarium Nicolai*.

of evidence, there seemed to be no mention of him in the Monte Cassino narrative about Constantine.

The career of Theodemar recapitulates the career of Atto in three fundamental aspects:

(1) Atto was chaplain to the Empress Agnes	(1) Theodemar was chaplain to the Empress Agnes
(2) Atto retired to Monte Cassino, became a monk there	(2) Theodemar retired from the world, became a monk at Monte Cassino
(3) In South Italy Atto was linked to a leading medical personage: he helped Constantine the African in translating medical works.	(3) In South Italy Theodemar was linked to a leading medical personage: he was known to the 'abbot of the court', foremost helper of Constantine the African in establishing himself in Italy.

The presence of the third element in the two stories is astounding; it ties both figures closely to Constantine, all the more so as, in the case of Theodemar, the name of the preeminent physician, the 'abbot of the court' is quite gratuitous and unnecessary to the account. As in the case of Leo/Lawrence, where folk-memory recalled and preserved a link with Odilo of Cluny, so in the case of Atto and Theodemar, that same type of traditional memory recalled a link with the leading medical innovators Constantine and his close friend, the 'abbot of the court'. Atto and Theodemar are a doublet; they are one and the same figure.

There are at least two ways in which the identification presented here assists the historian in drawing a picture of the arrival, reception, and work of Constantine. If this reconstruction is accurate, our independent pieces of evidence confirm one another. The new evidence drawn from the *Ortus et vita* corroborates the tale told by Mattheus F[errarius] in the Erfurt manuscript and the evidence amassed by Bloch and Glaze of the importance of the 'abbot of the court'. Besides, the link of Theodemar as Atto allows us to confirm details in the career of this figure. It was in 1072/73 that the empress and her entourage paid the almost six-month visit to Monte Cassino. The Subiaco Sacramentary confirms that Atto/Hatto (a.k.a. Theodemar) was still in the service of the empress in 1074, at the time of their visit to that abbey. Bloch conjectured that it was after the empress's death in 1077 that Atto came to Monte Cassino. And the discovery of the doublet helps: according to the account in the *Ortus et vita*, Theodemar (Atto) performed his only miracle that is dated to the time of the Eucharistic Controversy, that is, in late 1078 or early 1079; the affair was settled in the Lenten synod of February 1079.

And, finally, it appears that, thanks to recognition of the doublet, we know where Theodemar (Atto) came from in Germany. Forty years ago, a suggestion of major importance was made by Rodgers, who first identified the Theodemar, chaplain to the empress, 'from the province of Germany' with the Thietmarus of Hildesheim named in the *Chronicle* of that cathedral centre: 'Tiethmarus presbyter Hildeneshemensis canonicus postea monachus in Monte Cassino'[42] (Thietmar priest and canon of Hildesheim, afterwards a monk at Monte Cassino). Atto/Tiethmarus/Theodemar would have had an education in a great German archiepiscopal centre and left a strong impression there; this entry in the Hildesheim record is longer than any other in the list of 'presbyteri' in which it stands (and only one other comes close to it in length). Similarly, as we have noted, the entry for Theodemar in the *Ortus et vita* is among the longest of the brief biographies in that work. This figure made an impression upon his contemporaries, both in his chapter of canons in Germany and in his cloister in South Italy.

To this one may add that Atto/Theodemar's origin at, and probable continued connection with, Hildesheim could help explain why by the 1140s Hildesheim is documented as possessing an astoundingly rich collection of Constantine's translations and other Salernitan medical works.[43]

Joannes Medicus

In fact, the *De viris illustribus* knows a further monk connected, and closely, with Constantine. It is 'Joannes Medicus', in chapter 35 of that work:

> Joannes Medicus, supradicti Constantini Africani discipulus et Casinensis monachus, vir in physica arte disertissimus ac eruditissimus; post Constantini sui magistri transitum aphorismum edidit physicis satis necessarium. Fuit autem supradictis imperatoribus. Obiit autem apud Neopolim, ubi omnes libros Constantini sui magistri reliquit.[44]

[42] *Chronicon Hildesheimense*, ed. by Pertz, p. 849.11.

[43] A rich array of medical texts known by the monk Northungus at St Michael's, Hildesheim by 1140 is revealed in Wack, ''al-ʿAbbas al-Maǧūsī and Constantine on Love'. A bit later, Bishop Bruno of Hildesheim deposited a remarkable cache of medical texts at Hildesheim Cathedral before departing for the Holy Land. For the list of texts and the diffusion of Constantine's works into Northern Europe, see Glaze, 'The Perforated Wall', chap. 5 and table 1, pp. 280 and 285.

[44] Peter the Deacon, *De viris illustribus Casinensibus*, col. 1042c.

> (Johannes the Physician, a student of the aforementioned Constantinus Africanus, and monk at Monte Cassino, a man most skilled and most learned in the art of medicine, after the death of his teacher Constantine, published the *Aphorisms*, a work that is really necessary for physicians. And he lived under the aforementioned emperors. He died in Naples, and he, also there, left behind all the books of Constantine, his teacher.)

There is an important contrast between Atto and Johannes.[45] Both are addressed in Constantine's prefaces as 'my son', but, whereas in Peter's biography Johannes is described only as a student of Constantine's, Atto was an *auditor*, meaning, seemingly, that he took dictation from the master and thus assisted directly in producing manuscripts. Then too, Johannes is a medical man, while in Atto's case, the attribute that is specifically mentioned is his rhetorical skill or his 'high-buskined style'. Both ask Constantine for a translation, but the generalist Atto asks for 'something of Galen's', while the specialist Johannes asks precisely for a work on the different varieties of fever. And it is more difficult to be specific about the date of Johannes's arrival at Monte Cassino; was he perhaps the great translator's student even before the master came to the abbey? One thing, at the very least, seems clear: thanks to a most valuable observation of Hartmut Hoffmann's, it is clear that before the death of Abbot Desiderius in 1087, Johannes had presented a valuable chasuble ('Planeta Ioannis medici') to Monte Cassino;[46] in a passage in its *Chronicle*, which we may call the Treasure List of 1087, the objects of great value that Pope Victor III (Desiderius) left in the abbey are listed.[47] It is a reflection of the house's language habits that the same verb is used of Victor's *Nachlass* of precious items in the Cassinese sacristy ('dereliquit') and of Johannes's *Nachlass* of all the books of his master Constantine that he left at Naples ('reliquit'). (One would dearly love to know to whom or in what *fondo* the latter were left.)

[45] It seems prudent to restrict the discussion of Johannes to the two Monte Cassino documents referring to him, and for purposes of this present study to ignore the 'Ioannes Afflacius' evidence and that for the Johannes of the siege of Majorca. Bloch, *Monte Cassino in the Middle Ages*, p. 102 and n. 3. See also the Introduction of the present volume.

[46] *Chronica monasterii Casinensis*, III.74, ed. by Hoffmann, p. 456.21–22, and Hoffmann's note on p. 611.

[47] Newton, *Scriptorium and Library*, p. 260.

Two Teams at Monte Cassino: Desiderian and Oderisian Eras (1058–1105)

It is time to sum up in one place what can be discovered about the various figures who collaborated in the task that Constantine set himself, of translating and adapting a vast body of Arabic works, and other medical texts in Latin. The following discussion highlights important products of Monte Cassino's scriptorium in the Desiderian and Oderisian eras, and places the work of Team Constantine within the wider context of the impressive output of the great abbey. The broader team of scribes at Monte Cassino, and the elite group of Team Constantine are part of the same, yet nuanced, narrative. A discussion of Team Constantine (indented and in bold, below) differentiates these exclusive scribes and their work, while at the same time it weaves their achievements into the broader tapestry of book production (within normal margins, below) at Monte Cassino.

> **Geraldus was present at Monte Cassino as early as 1061 when he wrote, in Beneventan, the text of the document for Traetto, and signed it as witness in Caroline minuscule.**[48]

As the sequence has been reconstructed, this occurred in the early Desiderian years when the master scribe Grimoald was writing his magnificent homiliaries preserved as Monte Cassino, MSS 104 and 109 (the latter containing Grimoald's portrait).[49] Those volumes, formerly dated to the Theobaldan era (1022–*c.* 1030), are, in the present authors' opinion, certainly later than that, and the beautiful Exultet Roll (BAV, Vat. lat. 3784), also in his hand, is dated to the Desiderian era by all scholars.

> **Subsequently, in part-Beneventan, part-Caroline minuscule, Geraldus made a rough copy of the *Lexicon prosodiacum* (Monte Cassino, MS 580), Alberic's book for students of verse composition.**[50] **From this early date (perhaps even in the 1060s) Geraldus was then assisting in the production of house texts; in this case he was working closely with Albericus, the celebrated master of rhetoric at Monte Cassino.**

[48] See pp. 42–43.

[49] Newton, *Scriptorium and Library*, pp. 34–51. Grimoald's work has recently, on the basis of the decoration, been reassigned the traditional date, 'sec. XI in.'; see Orofino, *I codici decorati dell'Archivio di Montecassino*, II.2, 179–233, and Tavv. CIX–CXLIX.

[50] See pp. 38–40.

A lectionary (Monte Cassino, MS 453), to be dated in the *quinquennium* of the building of Desiderius's new basilica (1066–71), shows the most exquisite care in its production,[51] and in a brief passage shows an early specimen of the superb but non-Cassinese Beneventan of the *Dialectica* Scribe. The decorative style of this master, as well as his penmanship, is seen in two Exultet Rolls (Pisa, Museo Nazionale di San Matteo, Exultet Roll 2, and the fragmentary Monte Cassino, Exultet Roll 1).[52] The fully developed new Beneventan script of the Desiderian period (the classic Cassinese style) appears in the era of the basilica's dedication (1 October 1071) in such manuscripts as the *Homiliarium* in Monte Cassino, MS 98 and the slightly later *Homiliarium* in Monte Cassino, MS 99, dated to 1072.[53] Both contain finely drawn pen-and-ink miniatures celebrating the great feasts marked in the readings. A lectionary rich with miniatures in full, vivid colours is BAV, Vat. lat. 1202, which was almost certainly produced for the additional chapel and atrium dedications of 1075. Albericus's most prestigious assignment was his collaboration with Desiderius in the writing of the Abbot's *Dialogi de miraculis sancti Benedicti*, completed in about 1076. The handsome copy of that text in stately Beneventan is preserved as BAV, Vat. lat. 1203.

It is conceivable that Geraldus also worked on drafts or early stages of that text. As for another workhorse scribe, called here the Bodleian Juvenal Scribe, he was a collaborator in the production of an important medical text, the Copenhagen Pseudo-Soranus, probably before 1070.[54]

It was almost certainly upon the death of the Empress Agnes in 1077, or just after, that Atto/Theodemar arrived at the abbey. In the winter of 1078/79 he is attested as supporting Desiderius and Alberic's stand, with Pope Gregory, against Berengar of Tours.

The victory over Berengar (February 1079) was celebrated at the abbey by the production of a superb volume (now BAV, Ottob. lat. 1406) of logical texts penned and decorated by (this is his name-volume) the *Dialectica* Scribe.[55]

51 Newton, *Scriptorium and Library*, pp. 56–57, 114–18.

52 Newton, 'Un *codex Casinensis nobilissumus* di testi classici'.

53 On these masterpieces, Newton, *Scriptorium and Library*, pp. 62–70; and Orofino, 'Miniatura a Montecassino'.

54 See pp. 40–41.

55 See Newton, 'Un *codex Casinensis nobilissumus* di testi classici'.

As far as can be determined, the late 1070s saw the beginning of the scriptorium's intense production of medical texts.[56] Certainly the Hague *Pantegni* dates from before May 1086, when Desiderius, accepting the election, assumed the papal name of Victor III. The scribe is Geraldus, and Atto/Theodemar composed the rhetorical passages that frame, fore and aft, Constantine's Prologue (Part B), which is translated almost wholly from al-Maǧūsī's Arabic Prologue. The end-piece (Part C) is written by a contemporary Italian scribe. This seems to be the period (late 1070s or first half of the 1080s) when Paris, BnF, NAL 1628, an early Latin adaption of the *Isagoge* (Ḥunayn's Arabic text) was produced by the scribe of the Bodleian Juvenal.[57] The Paris text was perhaps transcribed from wax tablets, and it was Geraldus who then, possibly at Constantine's dictation, added textual suppletions in the margins.[58] The presence in NAL 1628 of these two scribes, documented as having worked at Monte Cassino, proves that the *Isagoge* was produced there; it also strongly implies that Constantine was the author of the translation/adaptation. Both manuscripts vividly demonstrate a stage of Constantine's effort as work-in-progress, and perhaps more importantly, as work-in-collaboration: the creation of an entire team. Perhaps one might even call it a dedicated team; it is not too fanciful to imagine Desiderius commissioning an experienced member of the scriptorium, such as Alberic, to assemble and oversee the *équipe* that set about this grand undertaking.

It was indeed a grand undertaking in part because it was not restricted to Constantine's new texts. The Scribe of the Bodleian Juvenal also copied, in this same era, the important text of Paul of Aegina, book III; the copy survives at the abbey as Monte Cassino, MS 351.[59] He also had a hand in the production of an extraordinarily valuable collection of gynaecological, pharmaceutical, and other medical treatises, today Copenhagen, KB, GKS 1653 4°.[60] Geraldus also contributed to the crafting of this book; again, a vivid demonstration of the team at work. The manuscript is certainly a product of Monte Cassino in this period. In terms of the 'team' concept, two 'workhorses' were involved.

Another member of the team, Johannes Medicus, presented a handsome vestment to the abbey before the death of Desiderius in 1087; perhaps Johannes

[56] See p. 47, Table 1.1.

[57] See pp. 35–37.

[58] The production stages of Constantine's translations are discussed in greater detail in Chapter 5.

[59] See pp. 155–56.

[60] See pp. 40–41.

was already a monk by then. He was Constantine's 'discipulus', and to him the distinguished translator/adaptor dedicated three of his treatises.

The opening of the period of Abbot Oderisius (1087–1105) saw a continued emphasis on recovery of ancient texts. There are fewer large liturgical manuscripts produced, but the workmanship of such small breviaries as Paris, Bibliothèque Mazarine, MS 364 is exquisite.[61]

Alongside the fine liturgical books, our Team Constantine continues. This is probably the era in which the Scribe of the Bodleian Juvenal produced his namesake manuscript (Oxford, Bodleian, Canon. Class. Lat. 41, with the thirty-four 'Winstedt lines'.[62] It is also the period when Monte Cassino, MS 333, the textually superior of only two surviving manuscripts of the Maximus Confessor text translated by John Scotus Eriugena, was produced in a Beneventan hand with marginal *scholia* in the clearly distinguishable Caroline minuscule of Geraldus, the scribe of The Hague, KB, MS 73 J 6.[63]

[61] See Newton, *Scriptorium and Library*, pp. 341–42, pl. 42.

[62] On the 'Winstedt lines', see Chapter 1, p. 55–56.

[63] See pp. 37–38.

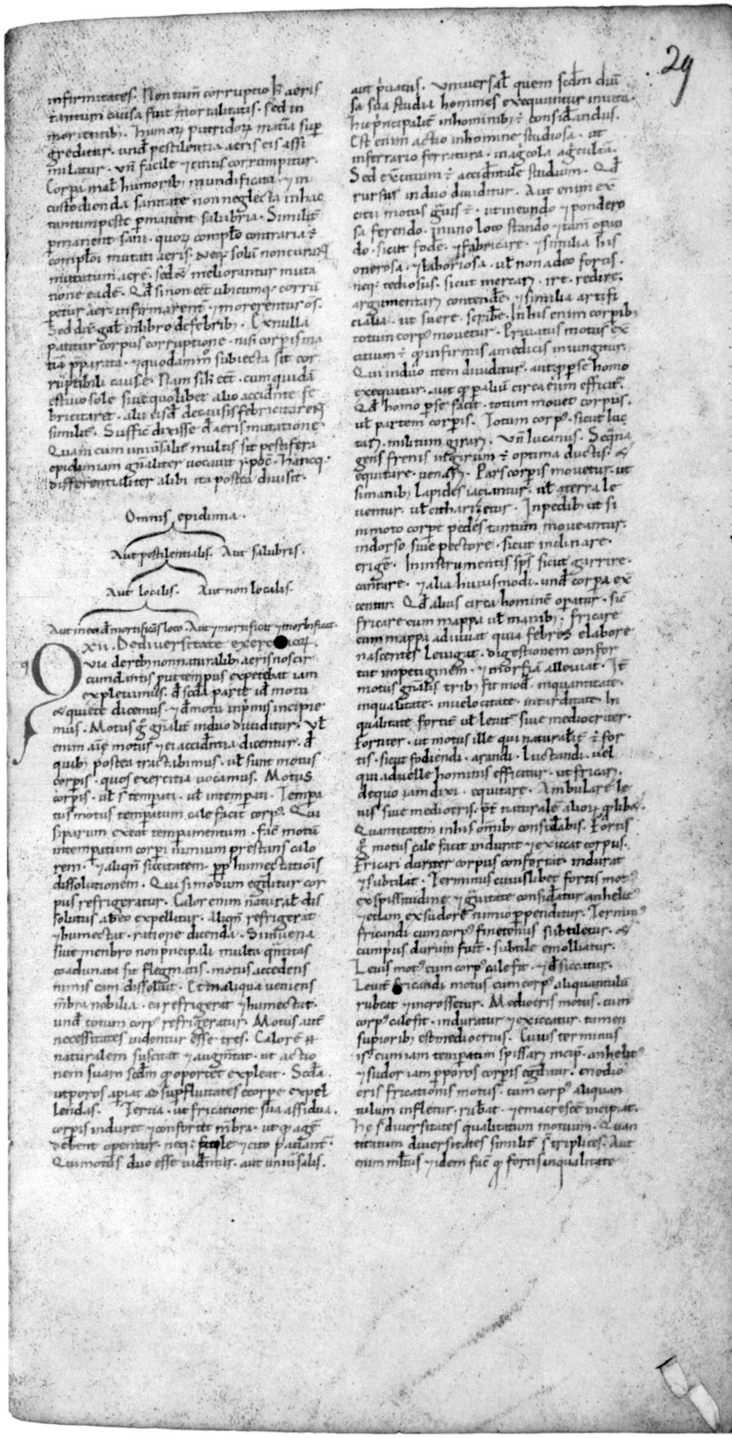

Figure 4.1. Narrow page, showing diagram and bookmark (lower corner), The Hague, Koninklijke Bibliotheek, MS 73 J 6, fol. 29[r]. Late 1070s–1080s (before 1086).

Chapter 4

Using the Manuscript

A reader of the *Pantegni* could learn from its pages how physical marks on the outside of the body indicated illnesses hidden inside; likewise the codicologist may use those same pages as material attributes of that same book's inner workings. Scribes did not choose randomly for a particular set of codicological and palaeographical traits. Rather, the cultural background of the reader influenced the manuscript's design (monastic readers sometimes had different preferences from lay readers or students) as well as the setting in which the book was produced (monastic book production operated under a different set of rules from production in a commercial environment).[1] Because of such forces at play in the choice of codicological and palaeographical features, the ultimate physical appearance of a manuscript can become key in answering what is arguably one of the most important questions the codicologist can ask of a book: how was it used? The physical evidence hidden in the book itself, from layout and quire construction to dimensions of the page and the type of binding, is particularly important; even if a scribe tells something about himself and his manuscript in the rare instance that he added a colophon to his work, he does not usually indicate how he anticipated the manuscript would be used.[2] This chapter therefore aims to 'diagnose' The Hague, MS 73 J 6 and reconstruct from the manuscript's physical features (as described in Appendix A) how the scribe anticipated it would be used by the reader. One of the most important aspects of this reconstruction is the unusual dimensions of the page: it is remarkably narrow (fig. 4.1). This is another of the enigmas with which this study began.

[1] Kwakkel, 'Decoding the Material Book'.

[2] Less than 20 per cent of surviving manuscripts hold such a colophon. See Overgaauw, 'Where Are the Colophons?', especially pp. 85–89. The study is based on 4127 manuscripts.

Book Design

An important stage in the Hague manuscript's production, and one of the first choices Geraldus made at the outset of this project, was to determine what dimensions MS 73 J 6 would have. The dimensions that were ultimately chosen for a book are telling, of course, about the environment and circumstances of its use. A manuscript with small dimensions may be made that way, for example, because it was meant to be a portable object, as in the case of some thirteenth-century Paris Bibles of smaller format used by ambulant Dominican friars.[3] Very large manuscripts, by contrast, were sometimes shaped that way for display purposes or because they were intended to be used, at some distance, by multiple individuals at the same time, such as a choir. Giant Bibles, made to impress while displayed, frequently exceed a height of 500 mm, as do Antiphonals from which monks sang the Office.[4] The dimensions are particularly telling when this information is paired with another aspect of a manuscript's design, namely the manner in which the text was laid out on the page (*mise en page*). Margins that were made wider than usual may indicate that the user wished to add additional information to the book, such as notes or glosses. In other cases, large margins point to an atmosphere of prestige and plenty that a patron wished to communicate through the spaciousness of the page; not strapped for resources, he or she could afford to waste space. If a page was prepared to receive reading aids, for example, with an extra ruled line added in the top margin to hold a running title, this may indicate that the manuscript was designed for optimal searching of its contents. The most striking observation related to the design of MS 73 J 6 is the unusual page dimensions chosen by the scribe.

Even before one opens the red box in which the codex is currently kept, it is apparent that this is a remarkably narrow object. The manuscript measures 235 mm high and 128 mm wide. In relative terms, the proportions of the page add up to 1 (height) to 0.54 (width), which is to say that the width is little over half of the manuscript's height. A relative width as narrow as 0.54 is quite unusual. A quantitative study of 390 medieval manuscripts by J. P. Gumbert suggests that the majority have a relative width between 0.67 and

[3] For more on portable Paris Bibles, see Chapter 5, 'Portable Bibles of the Thirteenth Century', in de Hamel, *The Book*, pp. 114–39; and Light, 'The Bible and the Individual'.

[4] Examples are found in Chapter 3, 'Giant Bibles of the Early Middle Ages', in de Hamel, *The Book*, pp. 64–91; Yawn, 'The Italian Giant Bibles'; and Boeren, Korteweg, and Piket, *Catalogus van de liturgische handschriften van de Koninklijke Bibliotheek*, pp. 131–32 (Antiphonals).

0.72 of the height, roughly the proportions of our modern book.[5] A much larger quantitative study by Carla Bozzolo and Ezio Ornato, which specifies results by century, shows that the broadest medieval books were made in the ninth and tenth centuries, when the average width ratio was 0.74.[6] Indeed, it is not difficult to find books from this period that exceed the medieval average. The Stiftsbibliothek in St Gall has a number of volumes with a relative width of around 0.85, while the Stiftsbibliothek in Einsiedeln contains a square manuscript with a relative width of 1.0.[7] Bozzolo and Ornato's study shows that after the tenth century the average relative width of manuscripts hovered around 0.7, confirming Gumbert's estimates. In the eleventh century, when MS 73 J 6 was produced, the average width of the page was 0.69,[8] substantially wider than the *Pantegni* copy in The Hague: according to contemporary norms this manuscript is almost 40 mm (or 17 per cent) too narrow.

Although medieval scribes likely proportioned their manuscripts intuitively (experience and muscle memory driving the hand that cut the sheets), the fact that medieval books are commonly similarly proportioned, and that these proportions follow a temporal pattern, suggests that scribes obeyed certain rules. A ninth-century manuscript from Tours that outlines in detail how the page ought to be proportioned shows that these rules were sometimes written down. The tract states, for example, that the page is to be five parts high and four wide (thus 0.8), that the lower and outer margins should be one part, and the top margin two-thirds of a part.[9] The eleventh-century rules were apparently slightly different, because a width of 0.69 (the average for that period) results in a height of five parts and a width of three and a half, not four. That the scribe

[5] Gumbert, 'The Sizes of Manuscripts', table 1 at p. 278 and p. 279. This study is based on dated parchment manuscripts from the eighth through thirteenth centuries. In the present chapter, the relative proportions of books will be expressed by stating the width as a ratio to height (set as 1).

[6] Bozzolo and Ornato, *Pour une histoire du livre manuscript au moyen âge*, pp. 296–98. Their analysis is based on 6200 manuscripts.

[7] Examples from the Stiftsbibliothek of St Gall include: Cod. Sang. 10 (tenth century) at 182 × 149 mm (0.82); Cod. Sang. 48 (*c.* 850) at 225 × 185 mm (0.82); Cod. Sang. 18 (*c.* 1000) at 240 × 200 mm (0.83); Cod. Sang. 106 (ninth century) at 255 × 215 mm (0.84); and Cod. Sang. 63 (*c.* 900) at 223 × 192 mm (0.86). The square manuscript is Einsiedeln, SB, Cod. 324 (1154), which measures 160 × 160 mm (tenth century). Digital facsimiles of these manuscripts can be found online at e-codices.

[8] Bozzolo and Ornato, *Pour une histoire du livre manuscript au moyen âge*, pp. 287–310.

[9] Lemaire, *Introduction à la codicologie*, p. 127; Rand, *The Earliest Book of Tours*, p. 88.

of MS 73 J 6 breaks with the guidelines of his time is significant to the present study, firstly, because there are relatively few books that narrow made before 1300. Among the 390 manuscripts ranging from the eighth to the thirteenth centuries assessed by Gumbert, only five (or 1.3 per cent) have a relative width of 0.57 or less. While this type of manuscript, sometimes called a 'holster book',[10] gained popularity after paper was introduced to book production, particularly among humanists, it seems that only in exceptional cases did medieval scribes before 1300 opt for books with dimensions like those of MS 73 J 6.[11] Second, the dimensions of MS 73 J 6 are significant because there is evidence that such narrow manuscripts were indeed conspicuous to the eyes of medieval readers as well. This is demonstrated, for example, by inscriptions found in two manuscripts from Nieuwlicht Charterhouse in Utrecht, now Utrecht, UB, MSS 102 and 159. In MS 102, Hector van Moerdrecht (d. 1465), a local Carthusian, remarked about the dimensions of the book:

> Item epistule pauli cum glosa interlineari [...] non ex toto quas antea habuimus, secundum quas libri ceteri formati sunt ut fieret unum volumen. et commodius ligarentur. licet non sit bona formacio cum sit longa et non secundum exigenciam eius lata.[12]

> (The Epistles of Paul with interlinear gloss [...], which we previously did not have in their entirety, in conformity with which the rest of the books were formed, so that it might be made into one volume and bound more conveniently, although it is not a good format since it is tall and not as broad as it should have been.)

Hector felt that the book's format ('formacio') was not quite right because it was 'tall and too narrow'. The manuscripts that contain these notes are a thirteenth-century copy of the Pauline Epistles measuring 250 × 160 mm (0.64),

[10] Pamela Robinson defines the 'holster book' as an unusually long, narrow book designed to be held easily in one hand or slotted into a holster or book-satchel on a saddlebag; see 'The Format of Books', p. 54. Robinson also applies the term to manuscripts that are only slightly narrower than the norm, as her example of BL, MS Egerton 2951 shows (175 × 118 mm, 0.67).

[11] There is a case of an English scribe, called Rate, who owned an entire collection of paper holster books described in Boffey and Thompson, 'Anthologies and Miscellanies', pp. 298–99. Examples of parchment humanist manuscripts in holster format include, from the British Library, MSS Egerton 1148 (155 × 85 mm, 0.55), Harley 3722 (225 × 135 mm, 0.6) and Harley 5761 (140 × 75 mm, 0.53), all with works by Petrarch. A curious case is presented by a book of hours, MS Harley 2924, from *c.* 1510–*c.* 1520, which measures 170 × 80 mm (0.47).

[12] Cited from Gumbert, *Die Utrechter Kartäuser*, p. 139 (Utrecht, UB, MS 159 contains a slightly variant note, see p. 141); for MS 102, see pp. 138–39, for MS 159, see pp. 140–41.

and a fourteenth-century manuscript of works by Bernard of Clairvaux measuring 260 × 165 mm (0.63).[13] Curiously, both manuscripts are only slightly narrower than the norm, namely by 15 mm (6 per cent) and 17 mm (7 per cent), respectively. Hector's remarks suggest, then, that books that deviated even marginally from the norm stood out. Evidently, a manuscript as narrow as MS 73 J 6 (which deviated much more from the norm) must have been quite conspicuous to medieval eyes.

Given these considerations, the question of why Scribe A (Geraldus) opted for such a narrow format becomes pressing. This query can best be addressed by broadening our view to include other manuscripts that break as dramatically with the rules of medieval book production. Appendix E presents eighty such holster books selected from a variety of inventories and manuscript catalogues. The corpus is limited to books written before *c.* 1200 that have a relative width of 0.60 or less. This proportional limit is imposed to stay deliberately clear of the lower end of the spectrum of regular widths, defined by Gumbert as 0.67; this allows us to focus on books that were intentionally made differently, and exclude those that may have been accidentally made slightly narrower than usual, or trimmed considerably during binding. Three groups of manuscripts among the eighty offer insight into why texts were sometimes presented in holster format.

The first of these three groups consists of books with bindings which are decorated with ivory carvings. Appendix E contains a small but significant number of manuscripts that are fitted with ivory plaques (nos 1, 3, 7, 15, and 61). The first among them is the narrowest manuscript in the corpus, St Gall, SB, Cod. Sang. 360, the *Hymni (XXVII) Sangallenses in processionibus*.[14] This spectacularly narrow book measures 255 × 80 mm, which results in a relative width of 0.31. When the codex was made around 1150, it was fitted with a wooden box which protected it from the elements as it was carried around in processions. When the book was needed, it was simply taken from its wooden container. On both covers of the box an ivory plaque was affixed, as well as gold and gems, now gone.

Another manuscript at the lower end of the table in Appendix E is Berlin, SBPK, MS theol. lat. fol. 323 (no. 7). This codex contains the *Vita secunda*

[13] Utrecht, UB, MSS 102 and 159. For the former, see Gumbert, *Utrechter Kartäuser*, pp. 138–39, 322–23; for the latter, pp. 141, 326; and for more on Hector van Moerdrecht, p. 90.

[14] Duft and Schnyder, *Die Elfenbein-Einbände der Stiftbibliothek St. Gall*, pp. 129–46; and the facsimile and description online in e-codices.

of St Liudger and measures 300 × 125 mm (0.42). When the book was made around 1100, it was also fitted in a book box with two ivory plaques. However, with their late antique origins these carvings are much older than the ones from the *Hymni Sangallenses*.[15] London, BL, MS Harley 5431 (no. 3), measuring 230 × 85 mm (0.37) and containing the Rule of Benedict, may have also had ivory plaques embedded in its binding.[16] These examples show how manuscripts were sometimes made narrow so as to match the size of the ivory plaque or plaques that would be fitted onto its binding or storage case. In other words, the width of the book followed the width of the ivory carving (which in turn was limited by the diameter of the tusk). Scholars have already explained the narrow dimensions of the Berlin *Vita secunda*, the London Rule of St Benedict, and other ivory-covered manuscripts, in this way.[17]

A similar example from the more proportionate end of the spectrum is St Gall, SB, Cod. Sang. 53, a gospel book prepared for liturgical use made around 895 (no. 61). The ivory diptychs used on this codex, which measures 395 × 230 mm (0.58), are not part of a wooden storage case but were attached to the actual binding of the manuscript. A revealing piece of evidence is provided by Ekkehart, monk and historian of the Abbey of St Gall (d. 1022). In his *Casus Sancti Galli*, Ekkehart describes how Salomon, bishop of Constance and abbot of St Gall (d. 919) relieved Hatto, archbishop of Mainz, of treasure chests kept at the abbey for safe-keeping in retaliation for Hatto's theft of the abbot's jewelled cup. Among these treasures were two ivory plaques, one carved and one plain, which had once been waxed and used as writing tablets. Ekkehart claims that they had belonged to Charlemagne, and were indeed the very ones mentioned by the emperor's biographer Einhard.[18] Salomon decided

[15] For the box and its decoration, see Kinney, 'A Late Antique Ivory Plaque'.

[16] For St Gall, SB, Cod. Sang. 53, see Duft and Schnyder, *Die Elfenbein-Einbände der Stiftsbibliothek St. Gall*, pp. 55–94. For London, BL, MS Harley 5431, see 'Treasures Known and Unknown in the British Library: Tall Narrow Books' in the British Library's online Catalogue of Illuminated Manuscripts.

[17] Kinney, 'A Late Antique Ivory Plaque and Modern Response', p. 464: 'it seems likely that the manuscript was proportioned to the diptych'. For the Rule, see the previous footnote. On the relationship between manuscript dimensions and their ivory plaques from the Carolingian period, see Nees, 'Early Carolingian Manuscripts and Ivories'.

[18] Einhard, writing during the reign of Charlemagne's son Louis the Pious, recounts how Charlemagne kept tablets and blank sheets under the pillows of his bed so that he might practice his writing in spare moments, although he never succeeded in learning to write. See chapter 25 of Einhard, *The Life of Charlemagne*, trans. by Turner.

that the shells of these tablets, which together formed a diptych, would be used to decorate a book, and had the abbey's monk-artist Tuotilo carve one plaque with a scene from the miracles of the abbey's namesake.[19] The scribe Sintram was assigned to produce this book, and doing so, Ekkehart tells us, he made sure that the height and width of the pages would match that of Charlemagne's diptych ('Quibus longioris et latioris moduli Sintrammum nostrum scribere iussit evangelium'). Ekkehart calls the gospel book that is the result of Sintram and Tuotilo's labour the 'Evangelium longum', which is how Cod. Sang. 53 is still known today.[20]

Ekkehart's designation is important because it shows how the physical format of MS 73 J 6 will have been perceived in the century in which the object was produced, namely as tall or long. It is unlikely, however, that the *Pantegni* was produced as a holster book because it was to be fitted with ivory plaques. After all, as the five examples in Appendix E show, books with such furnishings were made 'prominent' in other respects as well, for example in the quality of their parchment, decoration, and script. By contrast, MS 73 J 6, which has a mediocre writing support, is written in a medium-quality script and contains only one decorated initial (a rather unimpressive one, at that), is hardly the high-end book fit to bear precious ivories.

A second group of manuscripts provides insight into the rationale behind the production of holster books: codices used by solo singers during Mass. Particularly illuminating is St Gall, SB, Cod. Sang. 359 (no. 15), a tenth-century cantatorium that measures 280 × 125 mm (0.42). Cantatoria contain the chants executed by a solo singer at the ambo between the lections at the beginning of Mass.[21] Ease of handling was a crucial consideration in the design of this type of liturgical manuscript. Reflecting on how a cantatorium is used, Amalarius of Metz (d. 780) states: 'Cantor, sine aliqua necessitate legendi, tenet tabulas in manibus' (the cantor, without any necessity of reading, holds the tablets [that is, the cantatorium in ivory plaques] in his hands).[22] Although they were customarily ivory-bound like the first group,[23] there was another cru-

[19] For this story, and on Tuotilo's carving, see De Wald, 'Notes on the Tuotilo Ivories in St. Gall'.

[20] Duft and Schnyder, *Die Elfenbein-Einbände der Stiftsbibliothek St. Gallen*, pp. 18–22 (quotation at p. 20).

[21] Palazzo, *A History of Liturgical Books*, pp. 74–75.

[22] Huglo, 'The Cantatorium', pp. 95–96.

[23] Huglo, 'The Cantatorium', pp. 100–01.

cial motivation for their dimensions besides the width of the ivory plaques: unlike the musical manuscripts used by a choir, a cantatorium was not placed on a lectern but was held up by the cantor, so that the luxurious binding, and the symbolic performance of singing the sacred text it held (although the words were surely memorized by the cantor) could be displayed.[24] Practically speaking, because of the weight of these bindings, it was likely that the dimensions were limited (in effect narrow), allowing the cantor to hold it steady, open, and upright, possibly even in one hand.

Moreover, in her brief assessment of holster books, Robinson emphasizes that such a narrow format was convenient because 'the reader can support the back of the book with one hand while turning the page over with the other'.[25] In other words, if held at the outer edges as is customary, the weight of the book is borne by the fingers and thumb, whereas the holster format shifts it to the palm of the hand. This balance enabled by the narrow format is echoed in the practical use of cantatoria, the majority of which are, in fact, holster books.[26] Likewise another musical manuscript that was held by soloists: the troper. Surviving tropers from before 1200 are all holster books, including the three in Appendix E (nos 19, 21, and 28).[27] Thus the cantatorium and the troper highlight the correlation between a book's slender dimensions and the ability to use it, without the support of a lectern, in one's hands. A similar claim has been made with respect to chant manuscripts from the High Middle Ages, many of which are also narrow books made in such a way as to enable soloists to hold them upright in their hands.[28]

The largest group of holster books in Appendix E, thirty-four in total, are those containing classical texts from Ancient Rome and Greece. The majority

[24] In monasteries, the cantor would perform this role from the choir with the Gradual. In Frankish imperial chapels and cathedrals, however, this role took on a performative element, and was carried out at the ambo where it could be seen. See Huglo, 'The Cantatorium', pp. 97–98.

[25] Robinson, 'The Format of Books', p. 24.

[26] See the cantatoria, and their dimensions, listed in Huglo, 'The Cantatorium', Tables 3.1a and 3.2 at pp. 96 and 99; and Gamber, *Codices liturgici latini antiquiores*, II, 500–03 (explicit verdict about their narrow dimensions at p. 500).

[27] For the dimensions of tropers, see Huglo, 'The Cantatorium', table 3.1b at p. 97 (all ten tropers listed are holster books). For tropers as soloists' manuscripts, see Cyrus, *The Scribes for Women's Convents*, pp. 100–01. A detailed example is discussed in Grier, *The Musical World of a Medieval Monk*, pp. 20–21.

[28] Palazzo, *A History of Liturgical Books*, p. 69. See also Escudier, 'Les manuscrits musicaux'.

of these manuscripts contain texts by classical authors from the golden age to Late Antiquity: Statius (five manuscripts), Horace (four), Ovid (four), Virgil (three), Cicero (two), Lucan (two), Priscian (two), Prudentius (two), and Terence (two), followed by single manuscripts for Asterius, Flaccus, Justinus, Sedulius, and Vegetius.[29] Three further manuscripts contain ancient philosophy, namely Porphyry's *Isagoge* (no. 30), Plato's *Timaeus* (no. 33), and Boethius's *Consolatio philosophiae* (no. 11).[30] At first sight one might be inclined to reduce the correlation between the holster format and the dominance of their classical contents to the literary form of classical verse texts. Many are written in hexameters, after all, and such narrow text columns would produce either a page with much 'white' if presented in a single-column layout, or with a textblock that was slightly too wide if copied in two columns (unless the overall size of the manuscript was substantial, or the script particularly minute). It would make sense, the sceptical reader might say, if scribes chose the single-column layout using narrower than usual pages so as to economize on parchment. It is unlikely, however, that this is the true motivation. Firstly, as discussed above, holster books stood out as unusual to contemporary readers, which makes it improbable that scribes chose this format unless called for by a specific use. Secondly, thirteen of the thirty-four classical manuscripts in Appendix E are prose texts, and three others are partially prose, suggesting that the text format had likely little to do with the scribe's choosing to make a narrow book.[31]

Holster Books and Education

In fact, the explanation for the correlation between form and content is found in the manner in which classical texts were used. What binds these thirty-four texts is their common context of use: education. It is widely known that classical texts were popular teaching instruments in the medieval classroom, both in monastic and cathedral schools, as well as in the later universities.[32] This rela-

[29] Appendix E, nos 8, 12–14, 16, 17, 23–27, 32, 34–36, 43, 46, 47, 50, 57–60, 62, 66, 67, 70, 74, 77, 78, 80, 41, 68, 45, and 48.

[30] The Boethius codex (no. 11) also holds non-classical texts (sermons; Ephraim the Syrian) and the manuscript with Plato also holds Cicero's *Somnium Scipionis* (which means Appendix E contains thirty-five texts, bound in thirty-four manuscripts).

[31] In prose are nos 11, 30, 33, 35–37, 42, 45, 47, 48, 57, 66, 68, 77, and 78; in prose and verse, nos 55, 59, and 60, in prose and with musical notation, 63.

[32] Kwakkel, 'Manuscripts of the Latin Classics', pp. 14–16.

tionship between genre and use shows just how closely the largest group of holster books in Appendix E is affiliated with education. There are, moreover, primary texts in which masters explain what literature they use in the classroom; the classics are prominently present. Alexander Neckham (1157–1217), who taught in Paris and Oxford, emphasizes that the young student should read Horace, Virgil, Ovid, and Statius as an essential part of his training in grammar. These four are notably the most popular authors among the thirty-five classical texts listed here as holster books.[33]

Conrad of Hirsau (1070–*c.* 1150), in his dialogue between master and pupil, discusses the importance of certain classical texts and authors in the classroom. The pupil encourages him to 'explain briefly and in summary form what we must look for in each of the school authors who are used in training the blossoming minds of beginners'.[34] Conrad starts with the 'lesser authors' and then moves on to 'the major ones', so as to 'give milk to little babies and solid food to those who have been weaned'.[35] Thus he first discusses Aesop, Avianus, Sedulius, and Juvencus, whom he designates as 'for the young', 'to educate young beginners', and for the 'young in the Church'. He then moves on to Horace, Juvenal, Homer (probably the *Ilias Latina*), Persius, Statius, and Virgil.[36] A century earlier, Gerbert of Aurillac (d. 1003), head of the cathedral school of Mainz, had read and taught ('legit itaque ac docuit') rhetoric with the help of Virgil, Terence, Juvenal, and Persius.[37]

The importance of classical texts for medieval education is also apparent from library catalogues. In monasteries, these texts are generally listed in the catalogue of the cloister school rather than that of the main library, where they are presented under the heading 'libri liberales', 'libri saeculares', or, most commonly, 'libri scholastici'.[38] A catalogue from Tegernsee Abbey made around 1150 shows that their schoolbooks included such classical authors as Virgil, Horace, Lucan, Ovid, and Martianus.[39] In the monastic schools, texts by ancient authors

[33] For Neckham, see Reynolds, '"Let Him Read the Satires of Horace"', p. 22. Neckham listed books used in Paris classrooms: see Haskins, 'A List of Text-Books from the Close of the Twelfth Century'.

[34] Minnis and Scott, *Medieval Literary Theory and Criticism*, pp. 39–64 (quotation at p. 40).

[35] Minnis and Scott, *Medieval Literary Theory and Criticism*, p. 40.

[36] Minnis and Scott, *Medieval Literary Theory and Criticism*, pp. 49, 51, and 54, respectively.

[37] Bowen, *A History of Western Education*, p. 45.

[38] Leclercq, *The Love of Learning and the Desire for God*, p. 114.

[39] Glauche, *Schullektüre im Mittelalter*, p. 93. Glauche discusses numerous examples of

were commonly used in the teaching of the Trivium. Some were suitable for the study of grammar (Horace and Priscian), while others were a good fit for rhetoric lessons (Cicero's *De inventione* and the *Rhetorica ad Herennium*, both originally designed as school manuals), or dialectic (Cicero's *Topica*).[40] For the latter topic a number of philosophical texts were also used, such as Porphyry's *Isagoge*, Aristotle's *Categoriae* and *De interpretatione*, and Boethius's *De differentiis topicis*.[41] A similar trend is seen in cathedral schools, where from the eleventh century the Trivium was likewise actively taught. The manuscripts in Notre Dame Cathedral, for example, are divided up into 'divini libri' and 'libri gramatice artis', and the latter category, listing schoolbooks, included classical authors as well as books on arithmetic and the *computus*.[42] The latter were used in the Quadrivium, as was some ancient philosophy, including Plato's *Timaeus* and its commentary by Calcidius, and Cicero's *Somnium Scipionis* (both on astronomy and probably for this reason united in one volume, Appendix E, no. 33).[43] It was not unusual in this period for books of medicine inherited from antiquity to be listed in monastic and cathedral inventories among the works of classical authors; for example, the medical poem of Quintus Serenus might be followed by other medical texts.[44]

While not all classical manuscripts in Appendix E were certainly made or used for education, it is reasonable to assume that a substantial number were produced with this purpose in mind.[45] Indeed, five of these manuscripts were most certainly produced for in-class use by the magister. Suzanne Reynolds's study of glossed Horace manuscripts focuses on three manuscripts that were,

classical texts used in an educational setting, pp. 62–100.

[40] Evans, *Old Arts and New Theology*, pp. 21–24. See also Reynolds, '"Let Him Read the Satires of Horace"', p. 24.

[41] Evans, *Old Arts and New Theology*, pp. 22–23.

[42] De Bruyne, 'Le plus ancien catalogue des manuscrits de Notre-Dame de Paris', p. 485. For the assumption that the 'libri gramatice artis' are instructional books, see Lendinara, 'Instructional Manuscripts in England', p. 80.

[43] Evans, *Old Arts and New Theology*, p. 24; see also Glauche, *Schullektüre im Mittelalter*, pp. 62–100.

[44] Glaze, 'The Perforated Wall', table 1.

[45] About the difficulties of determining whether a manuscript is a schoolbook, see Lendinara, 'Instructional Manuscripts in England', p. 71; and Reynolds, 'Glossing Horace', pp. 103–05. Munk Olsen implies that most manuscripts of the twenty-nine most popular classical texts in the eleventh and twelfth centuries were made for teaching purposes. Munk Olsen, 'The Production of Classics in the Eleventh and Twelfth Centuries', p. 2.

as evidenced by the type of glosses they contain, used by schoolmasters.[46] Curiously, all three are holster books: Paris, BnF, Latin 8216 (no. 29), Cambridge, Peterhouse College, MS 229 (no. 35), and London, BL, MS Harley 3534 (no. 46). The Harley manuscript was in part copied by a master, while a second scribe, perhaps a pupil, copied the remainder of the book under his supervision. Masters in monastic schools doubled as the head of the scriptorium, which made such a collaboration a relatively easy undertaking.[47] The Peterhouse manuscript contains two layers of glossing, which were added by two different individuals: one in the second half of the twelfth century (who may have been a schoolmaster) and one in the first half of the thirteenth century (who was probably a schoolmaster).[48] The Paris manuscript, finally, combines both Horace and, presented as gloss, the *Verba preceptiva*, a grammatical text associated with the school of Ralph of Beauvais. The blend makes this book ideal for teaching and is perhaps 'the best example of a Latin classic as a classbook'.[49] Past research has tied two other manuscripts to schoolmasters: St Gall, SB, Cod. Sang. 833, a copy of Porphyry's *Isagoge* made *c.* 1100, which lists the names of four teachers who used the book in the early twelfth century (no. 30); and Leiden, UB, BUR Q 1, a copy of Lucan's *Pharsalia*, which was donated to Egmont Abbey around 1100 by the schoolmaster Baldewinus (no. 67).[50]

These five examples are particularly revealing. Firstly, they emphasize the correlation between holster books and education as such, but also suggest that the holster format was desirable for books specifically handled by magistri while teaching. Second, the three manuscripts studied by Reynolds are heavily glossed by magistri, who relied on these 'teaching notes' while using the book. Furthermore, the teachers likely copied the books themselves, which means that these glosses may be regarded as an argument in favour of the inference presented above: the holster format was chosen for a purpose beyond the verse nature of the text. That is to say, the individuals who produced these books for in-class use could have extended the available blank space by making the page wider, thus producing a standard-size book (with relative dimensions of 0.7),

[46] Reynolds, 'Glossing Horace'.

[47] Reynolds, 'Glossing Horace', pp. 108–09 (for BL, MS Harley 3534); Eder, *Die Schule des Klosters Tergernsee*, pp. 69–71 (for the role of a master in the scriptorium).

[48] Reynolds, 'Glossing Horace', pp. 110–13.

[49] Reynolds, 'Glossing Horace', pp. 113–16 (quotation at p. 116).

[50] See the description of St Gall, SB, Cod. Sang. 833 in e-codices; and for Leiden, UB, BUR Q 1, Gumbert, 'The Irish Priscian in Leiden', especially p. 295.

but chose not to. This strongly suggests that the immediate reason for keeping the book so narrow, to easily use it for teaching, was demonstrably more important than the text's literary format.

We do not have to look far to explain why this narrow format was chosen for teaching texts, because the reason for the use of holster books during Mass likewise applies here. Schoolmasters benefitted from the holster format just as much as soloists did, in that it 'freed' the book from the lectern and allowed the teacher to hold the object for a considerable time, supporting the spine with one hand and turning the page with the other, while walking around the classroom. This format also left one hand free for relaying non-verbal information to students by means of gestures with the right hand, which was a very common practice in the medieval classroom.[51] A book placed on a lectern also left one hand free for gesturing, or even both hands if the object was large enough that the pages remained open alone, but the holster book enabled the reader to move around with the book at the same time.[52] Manuscripts designed to be placed on a lectern were too large and heavy to be comfortably mobile frequently or for long. In short, the real benefit of the holster format was combined in two features: it provided ease of handling to the reader and portability to the book.

Iconographical evidence supports the image of masters holding their textbooks in one hand while teaching, although in illustrations they are still more commonly placed on lecterns.[53] In a French manuscript from the early fourteenth century, for example, Aristotle is depicted as a teacher, holding a manuscript in one hand while pointing at a book held by the student sitting in front of him with his other hand.[54] Hand-held books also feature in some twelfth-century images in which Grammar is personified as a teacher. On fol. 15^{v} of Florence, Laurenziana, MS San Marco 190, Grammar instructs the students before her. While they hold wax tables (for notetaking), Grammar holds an open book in her right hand.[55] Bethesda, US National Library of Medicine, MS 78, a medical manuscript with the *Articella* made in Paris *c.* 1210–*c.* 1230,

[51] O'Boyle, 'Gesturing in the Early Universities', p. 264.

[52] For the use of lecterns, see Dillon, *Medieval Music-Making*, pp. 99–107.

[53] The image of a book on a lectern was commonly used by late medieval illustrators to connote learning and teaching. Examples are found in Dillon, *Medieval Music-Making*, pp. 99–100.

[54] Oxford, Bodleian, MS Canon. Class. Lat. 288, fol. 1^{r}.

[55] Cleaver, 'Grammar and her Children', fig. 5. Cambridge, UL, MS Gg.2.32, fol. 1^{r} also shows Grammar holding an open book, this time in her left hand (Cleaver, 'Grammar and her Children', fig. 8).

shows on its first page a teacher holding up an open book with his left hand. He points out a passage to a student, who also holds wax tablets, poised to take notes.[56] Perhaps the most illustrative example is the famous depiction of Hugh of St Victor on fol. 3^{v} of Oxford, Bodleian, MS Laud Misc. 409. In this French manuscript from the 1190s, we see Hugh teaching in the school at St Victor. In his left hand he holds a book, which rests on his palm. His right thumb rests on the edge of the right-hand page of the open book, ready to turn it. The student in front of him similarly holds a book. An apparently early example of such an image, dated to 1156/57, is found in a historiated initial on fol. 174^{v} of Avranches, BM, MS 159. It contains two scenes featuring books. In one, two scholars seemingly debate before an audience, a book placed on a lectern between them. Sitting below them on the lip of the initial, a tonsured monk and a smaller, untonsured man, perhaps a young novice or student, interact over a narrow book. The monk, balancing it on his left palm, holds it out towards the student and gestures to it with his right hand, while the student reaches towards it, perhaps gesturing in discussion.[57]

As for soloists in the Mass, the holster book was a good fit for teachers as it guided the pressure of the book's weight away from fingers and thumb and into the palm, making it easier to hold for an extended period, such as the duration of a lecture. This may well explain another notable feature of the thirty-four classical holster books in Appendix E: they consist of considerably fewer folia than average medieval manuscripts. Roughly two-thirds (twenty-three books) contain one hundred folia or less, while one-third (twelve books) have fifty folia or less. Moreover, some of the bulkier ones are composite and consist of several parts that were bound together after their initial period of use. The manuscript with the most folia, London, BL, MS Harley 3859 (no. 47), contains eight contemporary booklets with the same origin, some of which are very thin. As is shown by the individual foliation sequences in the codex, its eight parts were used in smaller segments of forty-one, one hundred and sixty-two, forty-seven, and thirty-two leaves.[58] Another hefty volume of 216 folia, the Priscian

[56] Bethesda, US National Library of Medicine, MS 78, fol. 19^{v} shows a master with a closed book under his left arm interacting with two students. Judging from their hand gestures, the two are in discussion with their teacher.

[57] Other examples of masters holding a book while teaching are found in New Haven, Harvey Cushing/John Hay Whitney Medical Library, MS 28, perhaps made in Bologna around 1300, at fols 320^{r}, 343^{r}, and 407^{r}. The illustrations show Rāzī, Ibn Buṭlān, and others lecturing to students.

[58] See Munk Olsen, *L'Étude des auteurs classiques latins*, I, 215. Individual foliation

commentaries in Durham, Cathedral Chapter Library, MS C.IV.29 (no. 45), were likely divided into four different booklets consisting of fifty-four, eighty-two, fifty-eight, and twenty folia.[59] The limited number of folia made holster books even lighter than did their restrained width, which further increased the ease of using them.

The Vossius collection in Leiden University Library contains several holster books with classical contents, including some that are quite narrow, such as VLQ 42 (255 × 125 mm, 0.49, Virgil), VLQ 81 (230 × 115 mm, 0.50, Lucan), VLO 51 (205 × 105 mm, 0.51, Ovid), and VLO 77 (173 × 90 mm, 0.52, Lucius Florus). Some of these were probably designed for teaching. Clearly a teacher's copy, VLQ 73 contains Ovid's *Fasti* (fig. 4.2). With measurements of 240 × 120 mm, it has a relative width of just 0.5. It contains only forty-eight leaves, which made it light enough to hold in one's hand for a long time. Moreover, it is unlikely that a book this thin was bound with wooden boards, which would have also limited its weight. Ovid was particularly popular in teaching the Trivium, and the manuscript holds an *accessus*: an academic prologue that highlights to the student such things as the intention of the writer, the life of the poet, the title of the work, the quality of the poem, and the style of writing.[60]

Before returning to MS 73 J 6, the absolute dimensions of holster books must be briefly addressed. It appears that the holster format is less common in manuscripts of somewhat smaller proportions. For example, there are only four manuscripts listed in Appendix E that are less than 190 mm high: nos 28 (179 × 90 mm, a troper), 14 (184 × 82 mm, Horace), 63 (180 × 105 mm, astronomy), and 68 (170 × 100 mm, a gloss on Priscian). Furthermore, among the 182 surviving manuscripts produced at Monte Cassino under Desiderius and his successor Oderisius (between 1058 and 1105) there are fourteen hol-

sequences are found in fols 42–204 (parts II–V); fols 205–51 (part VI); fols 253–85 (parts VII–VIII). Three parts are described in Munk Olsen: part III, fols 169–73 (I, 215); part VI, fols 205–52 (II, 500); and part VIII, fols 286–365 (II, 832).

[59] Although the booklets are in the same hand, blank leaves suggest the following division: fols 1–54 (fol. 54^{r-v} blank), fols 55–136 (fol. 136^{v} blank), fols 137–95 (fols 194^{r-v} and 195^{r-v} blank), fols 196–215. Other manuscripts with substantially more than one hundred leaves are similarly divided. For example, St Gall, SB, Cod. Sang. 380, containing a calendar, *computus*, troper, and sequentiary, has 195 folia, and can be divided thus: pp. 3–17 (7 fols), pp. 18–27 (5 fols), pp. 28–117 (45 fols), and pp. 118–387 (136 fols).

[60] For the manuscript, see De Meyïer, *Codices Vossiani latini*, II, 173–74, and for the *accessus*, Minnis, *Medieval Theory*, pp. 15–72.

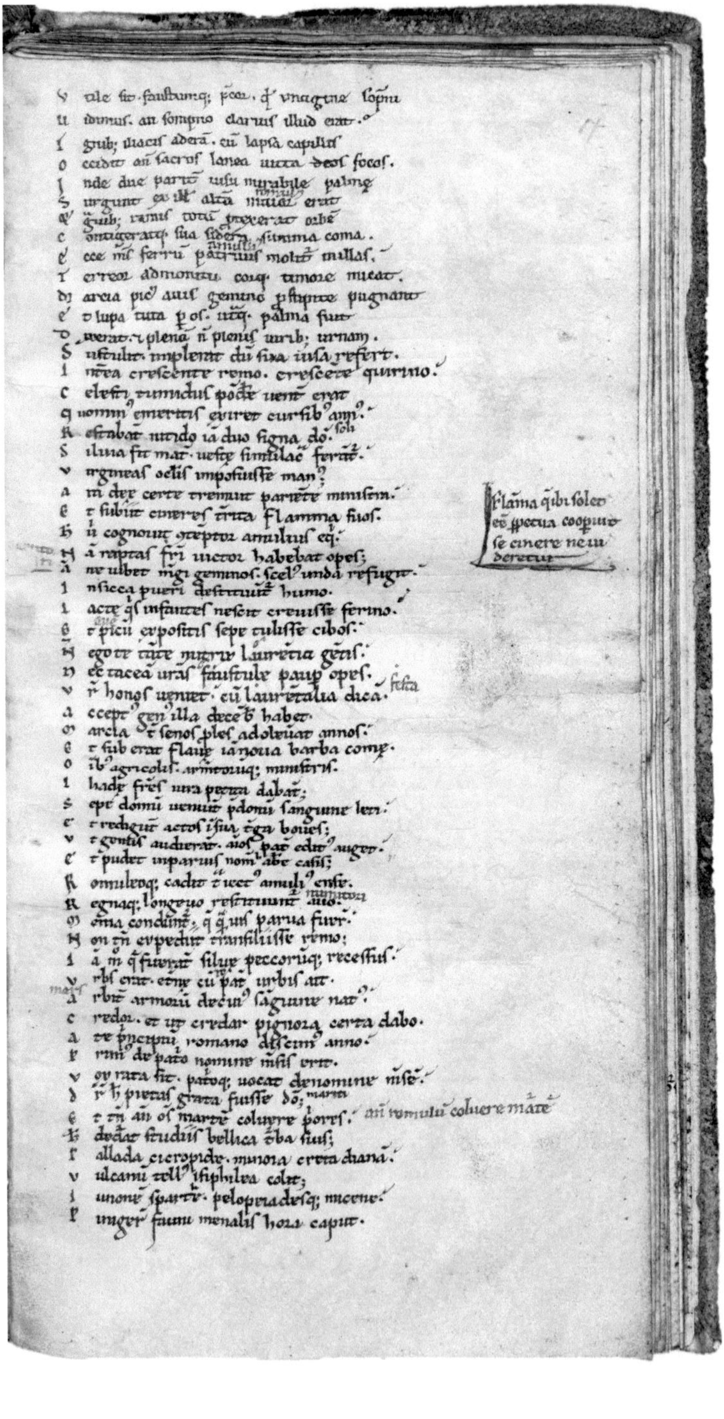

Figure 4.2.
Holster book with Ovid's *Fasti*. Leiden, Universiteitsbibliotheek, MS VLQ 73, fol. 17r. *c.* 1100–*c.* 1150.

ster books.[61] Only one of these, to use the same limits as before, is less than 190 mm high.[62] Scribes apparently saw no need to adopt a holster format for books smaller than 170 mm, which is the height of the smallest manuscript encountered here in holster format (no. 68). The explanation is straightforward: the drive behind the holster format was anticipated hand-held use. Books less than 170 mm high did not need to be presented in a holster format, because at normal proportions they were already easy to handle. If formatted according to the eleventh-century norm, that is, with a relative width of 0.69, the page would measure 117 mm wide. Books this narrow offered the same effect as holster books of taller dimensions, namely a balance and weight that could be held open in one's hand with ease. The advantage of using a holster book over smaller books of regular proportions is that the former holds more text per page (they have, after all, substantially more space on the north–south axis). This ultimately helped reduce the total number of leaves and thus the book's overall weight.

Handling the Manuscript

Returning to MS 73 J 6, in all likelihood Geraldus designed the book the way he did so it could be held in one hand as it was read, instead of being placed on a lectern or desk. Particularly striking, in this respect, are the parallels provided by cantatoria and tropers. Indeed, the physical features of MS 73 J 6 are well suited for hand-held use. Because of the small script and layout in two columns, the entire *Theorica* fits on only eighty-nine folia, making it both thin and light:

[61] These fourteen are: BAV, Vat. lat. 3262 (Ovid, *Fasti*, relative width 0.46; Newton, *Scriptorium and Library*, fig. 204); Milan, Biblioteca Ambrosiana, MS C 90 inf. (Seneca, *Dialogues*, 0.53; Newton pl. 59); Monte Cassino, MS 293, part II (Jerome, *Adversus Iovinianum*, 0.53; Newton pl. 149); BAV, Vat. lat. 3253 (Virgil, *Georgica*, 0.57; Newton pl. 203); Monte Cassino, MS 105 (Homiliary, 0.57; Newton pl. 95); Naples, Biblioteca Nazionale, MS IV F 3 (Ovid, *Metamorphoses*, 0.57; Newton pl. 197); Monte Cassino, MS 451 (*Ordo Romanus*, 0.57; Newton pl. 179); Florence, Laurenziana, MS Plut. 66.21 (Justinus, *Epitome*, 0.57; Newton pl. 52); Monte Cassino, MS 520 (*Octateuchus*, 0.58; Newton pl. 19); Monte Cassino, MS 571 (Bible, Prophets, 0.58; Newton pl. 18); Monte Cassino, MS 108 (Homiliary, 0.59; Newton pl. 98); Wolfenbüttel, Herzog-August Bibliothek, Cod. Guelf. 52.5 Aug. 4° (Lucan, *Bellum civile*, 0.59; Newton pl. 212); Monte Cassino, MS 351 (Paulus Aegineta, *De curatione totius corporis*, 0.60; Newton pl. 165); and Monte Cassino, MS 170 (Augustine, *De disciplina Christiana*, 0.60; Newton pl. 124).

[62] Wolfenbüttel, Herzog-August Bibliothek, Cod. Guelf. 52.5 Aug 4° (Lucan, 185 × 110 mm). See Newton's *Scriptorium and Library*. Thanks are owed to Julie Anne Somers for collating the dimensions of Monte Cassino manuscripts as an intern in Leiden (2012).

it weighs only 463 grams.[63] Because of its dimensions, thickness, and weight, the codex is excellently balanced and can be held up with little effort. However, a pressing question remains: does this imply that the manuscript was made for educational purposes? This medical text would become popular in education, as discussed in the Introduction, but was this function intended from the very outset of its transmission at the Abbey of Monte Cassino? This might initially seem implausible, given that no evidence has been brought forward that medical teaching occurred in the abbey, despite its fame for providing medical texts that would ultimately prove popular in classrooms.

It is appealing to imagine a magister teaching students from MS 73 J 6, but the medical nature of its contents requires us to consider another scenario as well: that it was handled by a physician as he practised his profession. The well-known illustration cycle in the abovementioned Bethesda, US National Library of Medicine, MS 78 demonstrates that medical books were indeed used in this way. Of the twelve decorated initials pertaining to medicine, five have scenes in which a physician interacts with a book. For example, fol. 32^{r} shows a physician standing next to the patient's bedside with a book in his left hand. He looks at the pages while his right hand points (or perhaps moves) towards the patient's exposed chest.[64] This scene elaborates another situation for which a medical book might be designed for hand-held use: attending at a patient's bedside. A similar depiction is found in the well-known Paneth Codex (New Haven, Harvey Cushing/John Hay Whitney Medical Library, MS 28). In a historiated initial on fol. 560^{v} we see a master physician gesturing to a patient, who is drinking from a goblet, with his right hand, while holding a book in his left hand. An illustration in a copy of Gariopontus's *Passionarius* made *c.* 1100 (Milan, Biblioteca Ambrosiana, MS D 2 inf., fol. 2^{r}) shows an older bearded man and a younger man, presumably master and student, sitting before a patient. The young man looks toward the older man, from whom he is likely receiving instructions. In this scene, the physician holds up the open book in one hand and points at the pages with his other. The overall message of these depictions is that therapeutics should be based upon literary texts, grounded in theory, and not upon purely empirical traditions.

[63] The book is presently bound in an eighteenth-century binding without wooden boards, which may well reflect the medieval situation. Books this thin were not commonly bound with wooden boards. It is probable that MS 73 J 6 was fitted with a limp cover. For limp bindings from this period, see Thomson and others, 'Technology', pp. 107–08.

[64] Digital images and a description of Bethesda, US National Library of Medicine, MS 78 can be found on the Library's website in a dedicated section entitled 'The Articella'.

Moreover, the common denominator in these scenes depicting physicians with hand-held books is that they are situated not in the classroom but in the patient's home. While they may depict idealized situations, their iconography reflects a practical truth of medicine in any era: the physician, through the very nature of his work (including treating patients too sick to move) had to bring himself, and any books he wished to consult, to the patient. Naturally, smaller manuscripts were more convenient for this purpose than larger ones. It is striking, in this respect, that during the later Middle Ages physicians used particularly small manuals for such *in situ* consultation, which came in the form of a girdle book (so small they could be hung from one's belt) or a *vade mecum*, an almanac with folding leaves. For example, a fifteenth-century scientific girdle book in the Bodleian Library measures just 100 × 65 mm (Oxford, Bodleian, MS Ashmole 6). A slightly larger (but still small) *vade mecum* can be found in London, BL, MS Harley 5311, which measures 180 × 80 mm when folded, but 340 × 230 mm unfolded.[65]

However, despite the fact that medical books were sometimes on the move, it is unlikely that MS 73 J 6 was designed for use at the patient's bedside. This is apparent from two traits of the manuscript. First, with its dimensions of 235 × 128 mm the codex is no match for late medieval girdle books, which were much smaller. MS 73 J 6 is portable, but it is likely that a scribe who knew the book would be predominantly used on location by a physician would have opted to make it much smaller than it is. Another argument against the portable use of MS 73 J 6 relates to its contents. The manuscript's text is the first part of the *Pantegni*, the *Theorica*, which deals with the theoretical dynamic of medicine. The kind of practical knowledge that would be useful when dealing with a sick patient is found only in the *Practica*, no part of which is found in MS 73 J 6.[66] Alternatively, a copy of the *Viaticum*, Constantine's translation of Ibn al-Ǧazzār's *Kitāb Zād al-musāfir* would have been eminently suitable for any bedside practitioner.[67] In sum, there was no need for a practitioner to take

[65] Nine examples are mentioned in Voigts, 'Scientific and Medical Books', pp. 356–57, 392 n. 40.

[66] It appears that Constantine did not translate this part of al-Maǧūsī's text. Rather, the complete *Practica* is a 'pastiche from a variety of different sources'. Green, 'Constantine the African', p. 146. See also Wack, 'ʿal-Maǧūsī and Constantine on Love'.

[67] A fragmentary copy of the *Viaticum* copied in Cassinese Beneventan does, in fact, survive from the final decades of the eleventh century; see Long and Irving, 'An Early Fragment of Constantine the African's *Viaticum* in Beneventan Script'.

the *Theorica* to the patient, and the manuscript's size suggests that it was not intended for that purpose.

It seems most likely, therefore, that the manuscript was designed for an educational setting. More precisely, it was in all likelihood made for use by a master. This is primarily supported by the strong link between the holster format and education, as demonstrated by the five master's manuscripts discussed above, as well as the known educational context in which the *Theorica* functioned. The earliest evidence for such use dates from the first half of the twelfth century, when scholars affiliated with the nearby medical school at Salerno consulted the text, in part to design an *accessus* style for their early commentaries on components of the *Articella*, and more particularly to improve their understanding of the *Isagoge*.[68] Around the same time, the text was available and used by scholars associated with the cathedral school of Chartres, including William of Conches. That magister, grammarian, and 'physicus' frequently refers to the *Pantegni* in his *De philosophia mundi* (*c.* 1125–*c.* 1145) and *Dragmaticon* (*c.* 1144–*c.* 1149), providing explicit references to 'Constantinus' and '*Pantegni*'.[69] A little later, between *c.* 1150 and *c.* 1170, a Salernitan master named Marius used the *Pantegni* 'extensively and beyond question' for his *De elementis*. Marius used Constantine's discussion on the nine complexions and the viridal soul of plants (and perhaps some other passages as well).[70] In all of these cases, the *Theorica Pantegni* was used to conceptualize broader philosophical theories; those seeking therapeutic guides had to look elsewhere.

In addition to placing the manuscript in the hands of a teacher as far as its format and contents are concerned, one piece of evidence not yet discussed shows how well MS 73 J 6 accords with what little we know about magister manuscripts used in the school of Monte Cassino. As Diane Warne Anderson has shown, the collection of texts in BAV, Ottob. lat. 1354, a codex produced in Monte Cassino around 1100, are all affiliated with the famous school of Alberic of Monte Cassino. They include Priscian on Virgil's metrics (fols 1^{v}–16^{r}), an abacus treatise (fols 54^{v}–55^{v}), Bede's *De metrica arte* (fols 57^{v}–65^{v}), the *Lexicon prosodiacum* (fol. 71^{r}-84^{v}), and Alberic's *De longitudine et brevitate principa-*

[68] Kristeller, 'The School at Salerno', pp. 154–55; Jordan, 'Medicine as Science'; Dronke, *A History of Twelfth-Century Philosophy*, p. 413; and Jacquart, 'La medicine entre théorique et pratique'.

[69] Ronca, 'The Influence of the *Pantegni*'; O'Boyle, *The Art of Medicine*, p. 101 n. 64.

[70] Dales, 'Marius "On the Elements"', pp. 211–12; Thomson, '"Liber marii de elementis"'.

lium sillabarum (85r–90r).[71] In their study of the abacus treatise, Craig Gibson and Francis Newton agree with Anderson that the text collection was designed for students (they define the codex as a '*livre d'étude*' and 'schoolbook'). They also take it a step further and demonstrate that this specific copy was a 'personal collection' made and used by 'almost certainly a teacher of grammar' at Monte Cassino. This is apparent, for example, from the cross-references added by the teacher to 'remind himself and his pupils of earlier treatment of the questions in this collection'.[72] Thus BAV, Ottob. lat. 1354 is a valuable asset to this study, because it shows us what a near-contemporary magister book looked like at Monte Cassino.

Striking material parallels with the Hague manuscript are instantly apparent in the Vatican magister book, further tightening the potential ties of MS 73 J 6 to the school at Monte Cassino. First and foremost, the Vatican manuscript is also a holster book. With dimensions of 180 × 100 mm the book is somewhat smaller than MS 73 J 6, which measures 235 × 128 mm, but its relative width is nearly identical (0.56 compared to the 0.54 of the Hague manuscript). Apparently, the unidentified teacher of grammar who used BAV, Ottob. lat. 1354 also favoured teaching with a narrow book in his hand. The second parallel is that the pages of the Vatican manuscript also contain an unusually high number of lines. As discussed in Chapter 2, MS 73 J 6 has sixty-two lines per page, resulting in the very modest average line height of 3 mm. At fifty-two lines per page, the average for BAV, Ottob. lat. 1354 is 2.8 mm, nearly identical. In other words, like Geraldus, the scribe who copied the Vatican manuscript packed an unusual amount of text onto the page, thus reducing the number of folia needed to contain the volume (not only stretching resources, but limiting, as much as possible, the book's weight). Another draw for the teacher may have been that this practice reduced the frequency with which pages had to be turned. Also notable is that the scribe of the Vatican manuscript, like Geraldus, maintained the regular space allotted for writing. That is to say, that despite the attempt to include a high volume of lines within the regular textblock, both scribes left the marginal space intact. It is striking that both books have a similar percentage of upper/lower and side margins: in MS 73 J 6 they are respectively 20 and 23 per cent (which leaves 38 per cent of the page blank), while for BAV,

[71] Anderson, 'Medieval Teaching Texts', p. 195 (including the identification of Alberic as author of the treatise on syllables).

[72] Gibson and Newton, 'Pandulf of Capua's *De calculatione*', pp. 295–301; quotations at 295, 298, and 300. The Monte Cassino connection was first suggested by Gehl, 'Vat. Ottobonianus lat. 1354', p. 297.

Table 4.1. Medical manuscripts in holster format made prior to *c.* 1200.

	MS	Date	Origins
1	Zurich, Zentralbibliothek, MS C 128	1075–1100	Italy, Beneventan zone
2	London, BL, MS Sloane 2426	1150–1200	Southern France
3	London, BL, MS Sloane 1621	1075–1100	England (Bury St Edmunds)?
4	The Hague, KB, MS 73 J 6	1075–85	Italy, Monte Cassino
5	Paris, BnF, Latin 7029	1075–1100	Italy
6	Orléans, Médiathèque, MS 301 pp. 128–248	1075–1100	Italy, Monte Cassino
7	Berlin, SBPK, MS lat. fol. 74	*c.* 1169	France
8	Vienna, Österreichische National-bibliothek, Cod. 253	1175–1200	Southern England?
9	London, BL, MS Harley 5228	1175–1200	England
10	BAV, Pal. lat. 1163	1150–1200	Germany
11	Mantua, Biblioteca Comunale Teresiana, 111 (A.IV.51)	1150–1200	Southern France
12	Paris, BnF, Latin 11223	1150–1200	Unknown
13	London, BL, Harley 4348	1150–1200	Germany
14	Glasgow, UL, Hunter 320	1100–1200	Unknown
15	Utrecht, UB, MS 687	1150–1200	France
16	Arezzo, Biblioteca della Città, MS 246	1050–1100	South Italy
17	Cambridge, St John's College, MS D.4 part II (fols 105–147)	1100–1150	Italy?
18	Cambridge, St John's College, MS D.4 part III (fols 149–181)	1075–1125	Italy
19	Milan, Biblioteca Ambrosiana, MS D 2 inf.	1075–1100	France
20	BAV, Vat. lat. 4418	1075–1100	South Italy
21	Monte Cassino, MS 351	1070–90	Italy, Monte Cassino

Contents	Dimensions (w:h)
Gariopontus, *Passionarius*	205 × 102 mm (0.50)
Medical compendium	225 × 118 mm (0.52)
Acephalous antidotarium; *De urinis mulierum*; and other texts	202 × 110 mm (0.54)
Constantine the African, *Theorica Pantegni*	235 × 128 mm (0.55)
Portions of the early *Articella*; excerpts from Constantine the African, *Viaticum*	204 × 112 mm (0.55)
Constantine the African, *Viaticum*[73]	237 × 131 mm (0.55)
Stephen of Antioch, *De regali dispositione*; Constantine the African, *Practica Pantegni*	200 × 110–20 mm (0.55–0.60)
Hippocrates; miscellaneous	214 × 125 mm (0.58)
Medical miscellany	215 × 125 mm (0.58)
Constantine the African, *Viaticum*	225 × 130 mm (0.58)
Stephen of Antioch, *De regali dispositione*, part I (books I–V)	234 × 137 mm (0.58)
Constantine the African, *Theorica* and *Practica Pantegni*, book I	240 × 140 mm (0.58)
Honorius of Autun?, *Apex physicae*	185 × 110 mm (0.59)
Medical miscellany	195 × 115 mm (0.59)
Gariopontus, *Passionarius*	200 × 120 mm (0.60)
Gariopontus, *Passionarius*	222 × 134 mm (0.60)
Herbarium	240 × 145 mm (0.60)
Muscio, *Gynaecia*; Theodorus Priscianus, *De genecia*; Constantine the African, *De matrice* (chap. 34 of the *Theorica*)	240 × 145 mm (0.60)
Gariopontus, *Passionarius*	255 × 155 mm (0.60)
Gariopontus source texts	270 × 163 mm (0.60)
Paulus Aegineta, *De curatione totius corporis*	285 × 170 mm (0.60)

[73] This manuscript's *Viaticum* segment is said to be from Monte Cassino during Constantine's lifetime by Irving and Long in their recent article, 'An Early Fragment of Constantine the African's *Viaticum* in Beneventan Script'. Orléans, MS 301 is a composite of booklets. Its first half varies in genre, but its last half is decidedly medical; in addition to the *Viaticum*, it also holds medical recipes, an excerpt of the *Antidotarium magnum* (as indicated by its incipit), and Constantine's *Liber graduum*.

Ottob. lat. 1354 the margins take up 19 and 25 per cent (leaving 40 per cent of the page blank).[74] A further similarity between the two books is their script. The scribe of the *Vaticanus* also copied the book in Caroline minuscule and, similarly, did so in a low-quality script with tiny letters to accommodate the high number of lines on the page.[75]

Another manuscript surviving from a Monte Cassino classroom is Monte Cassino, MS 580, Alberic's *Lexicon prosodiacum*, also copied by Geraldus (fig. 1.6).[76] The *Lexicon* combines an alphabetical wordlist excerpted from the works of eleven classical authors (pp. 1–68), with passages in which these words are found (starting at p. 69). Each word in the first part is preceded by a number, which corresponds to the appropriate verse in the second part. The various length of words (their number of syllables) could thus be assessed in their original context. Anderson argues that this treatise was likely produced in the school of Alberic as early as the 1060s or 1070s, probably by the great teacher himself. While Monte Cassino, MS 580 contains a teaching text and was made in close proximity to its author, who was a teacher himself, it is (perhaps surprisingly) not a holster book. Measuring 140 × 95 mm, its relative dimensions are 0.68, which is close to the normal proportions of the eleventh century (0.69). As discussed, however, due to their limited width, such small books shared the same benefits that made holster books so convenient in 'performance' settings like the Mass and classroom: they were light, and the weight of the book rested on the palm of the hand, not on the fingertips and thumb. They, too, were therefore easy to handle. This benefit is employed again in late medieval books of hours and psalters made for private devotion, which were also held in the user's hands.

Other medical holster books survive, showing that MS 73 J 6 is not an isolated case. If we take the relative width of 0.6 as a cut-off point, as before, twenty-one others may be pointed out (table 4.1).[77] The majority originate from the

[74] These are simple but effective calculations based on a comparison of dimensions of the page and writing space. The textblock of BAV, Ottob. lat. 1354 is 145 × 75 mm, and that of MS 73 J 6 is 189 × 28 mm. The two present a notable difference, however, in *mise en page*: the Vatican manuscript is copied in one column and the Hague manuscript in two.

[75] The script of BAV, Ottob. lat. 1354 is distinguished by the scribe's tendency to enlarge Tironian 'et' when presented as the first word of a sentence.

[76] For this manuscript, see Chapter 1, at pp. 38–40.

[77] This list is by no means complete, and my search for medical holster books has not been systematic. Discussions with colleagues helped us create this modest table. Eliza Glaze identified nos 1 and 12 as holster books, and Monica Green helpfully pointed me towards nos 2, 3,

eleventh century, and all of them are of modest size, their height ranging from 200 to 245 mm. Based on the discussion in this chapter it seems probable that many of these medical holster books would have been used for teaching purposes.[78] Curiously, table 4.1 includes two medical holster books from *c.* 1050–*c.* 1100, in addition to MS 73 J 6, that were produced by scribes accustomed to writing in Beneventan (although not at Monte Cassino) who opted instead to copy in Caroline minuscule (of, again, low quality): Zurich, Zentralbibliothek, MS C 128 (no. 1) and Arezzo, Biblioteca della Città, MS 246 (no. 16), both containing Gariopontus's *Passionarius*.[79]

There are three other narrow medical books that are worth consideration, because they only slightly exceed the chosen cut-off point of 0.6 relative width to height. Two of these contain works by Constantine: Durham, Cathedral Chapter Library, MS C.IV.12 (*Viaticum*, England, 1100–50, 255 × 140 mm, or 0.62) and Florence, Laurenziana, MS Antinori 20 (*Theorica*, Italy?, early thirteenth century?, 238 × 165 mm, also 0.62). A third, Glasgow, University Library, Hunter 404, was produced at Naples in the tenth century and concerns a collection of various medical texts, including excerpts attributed to Galen and Hippocrates. It measures 280 × 175 mm (0.63) and contains accents pointing to oral use (likely, given its dimensions and contents, in a classroom setting).[80]

Conclusion

With consideration of evidence from BAV, Ottob. lat. 1354, and several other holster books, including medical volumes, it is reasonable to propose that the most likely use setting for MS 73 J 6 was the school of Monte Cassino. Pope Victor II's claim in 1057 that Monte Cassino was a 'principale gymnasium' (foremost training ground) expresses just how important the abbey was as an educa-

and 5. Others have been located by calculating the height–width ratios of suitably dated manuscripts in Beccaria, *I codici di medicina del periodo presalernitano*, and by searching major online catalogues for medical manuscripts of holster book proportions. The dates of these manuscripts are often our own and may deviate from those existing in secondary sources.

[78] See pp. 132–36.

[79] Glaze, 'Gariopontus and the Salernitans'; see Appendix 1 for the manuscripts, including the script of Zurich, Zentralbibliothek, MS C 128. Images provided by Glaze show that the scribe of Arezzo, Biblioteca della Città, MS 246 uses the Beneventan '**ri**' abbreviation. Monte Cassino, MS 351 was copied in *c.* 1070–*c.* 1090 at Monte Cassino. This is a new discovery and contrasts the statement at Newton, *Scriptorium and Library*, p. 376.

[80] See Beccaria, *I codici di medicina del periodo presalernitano*, pp. 243–46.

tion centre.[81] Teaching at the abbey went far beyond the scope of usual monastic training, as was indeed expressed by Pope Victor II's words. It was particularly well known for its training in the Liberal Arts: when Archbishop Pandulf mentions the education of John of Gaeta (Pope Gelasius II), who was trained in Monte Cassino by Alberic in the 1070s, he emphasizes that the young man was educated in the Liberal Arts by 'men most expert in all fields'.[82] The emphasis on the Arts can also be observed in the interests of the master in charge of the school during the reign of Desiderius: Alberic of Monte Cassino (d. 1105). Celebrated as one of the eminent scholars in the Arts in Central and South Italy, he authored many texts himself, including on grammar and rhetoric.[83]

The Hague *Pantegni* would not be out of place in the classroom of Alberic nor any contemporary teacher within the abbey's walls. Even prior to Desiderius's abbacy, Lawrence of Amalfi, a monk and magister of Monte Cassino, had compiled a magnificent handbook of the Liberal Arts, Venice, Biblioteca Nazionale Marciana, Lat. Z 497. In it, following the Trivium (grammar, rhetoric, dialectic), medicine stands next in line before music, geometry, arithmetic, and astronomy.[84] In the twelfth century, medicine was not only the domain of aspiring physicians, but it was also studied by students and teachers in other disciplines because of its theoretical properties. John of Salisbury, for example, applied information from the *Pantegni* to his political works and pedagogy. For him, it was not the medical facts that mattered, but the metaphors they provided as well as the distinction between theory and practice, which was introduced to the West in Constantine's *Pantegni*.[85] Indeed, much of the early reception of Arabic medicine in the West, some scholars have stressed, was not focused on medical knowledge as such, but on the life-related information that medicine provided. Works like Constantine's *Isagoge* and *Pantegni* were read for the *res naturales* they discussed.[86] In other words, when scholars such

[81] Newton, *Scriptorium and Library*, p. 274.

[82] Newton, *Scriptorium and Library*, pp. 274–75 (quotation at p. 274). In 1088, the future Gelasius had already left for Rome; Schwaiger, 'Gelasius II'.

[83] For Alberic and his school, see Bloch, 'Monte Cassino's Teachers and Library', pp. 585–86; Anderson, 'Medieval Teaching Texts', pp. 192–93; Lanham, 'Alberic of Monte Cassino'; Radding and Newton, *Theology, Rhetoric, and Politics in the Eucharistic Controversy*.

[84] See Newton, 'Tibullus', pp. 275–77. It is this article that first identified Lawrence as the compiler of the book, and the manuscript therefore reflects his teaching.

[85] Shogimen and Nederman, 'The Best Medicine?', pp. 65–66.

[86] Köhler, '*Homo animal nobilissimum*', pp. 142–62, 315. The theoretical properties of the *Pantegni* and *Isagoge* are discussed at p. 151.

as John of Salisbury and William of Conches picked up the *Pantegni*, they did so because the text provided a handle for exploring the nature of things. In his *Speculum doctrinale*, Vincent of Beauvais (d. 1264) deems medicine, which he called 'medicina secunda philosophia', the crown of the Liberal Arts because it unites them.[87] There are, moreover, visual representations of medicine's place in the hierarchy of knowledge. In twelfth-century iconography we see Medicine placed among the Liberal Arts; one such example is found in New York, Morgan Library and Museum, MS 982 (Salzburg, *c.* 1150–*c.* 1160). The recto of this singleton depicts Philosophy nourishing the seven Liberal Arts, while the verso features four scenes portraying the Liberal Arts. Arithmetic, Astronomy, and Music are accompanied by the personification of Medicine. This figure may be Aesculapius, the Greek god of Medicine; he mixes a remedy with mortar and pestle while his teacher, the centaur Chiron, offers him herbs.[88]

Are we to regard MS 73 J 6 as a teaching manual in the *artes* programme at the school of Monte Cassino? It is appealing to imagine the *Theorica*'s use in the manuscript's birthplace in the same way that it was used by John of Salisbury around the middle of the twelfth century. With whatever intention the unidentified master at Monte Cassino held MS 73 J 6 in his hands, whether as an Arts or a medical teaching text, it is striking that there are many other holster books from the abbey that were almost certainly made for teaching purposes, including several classical texts of Ovid, Seneca, Virgil, and Lucan, all of whom were familiar faces in the medieval classroom (see the manuscripts listed in Appendix E). Evidence suggests, in other words, that MS 73 J 6 was designed to be held aloft in the palm of a teacher's hand: education was probably the early and intended role of the Hague *Pantegni*.[89]

[87] Schuler, '*Medicina secunda philosophia*', p. 178. Vincent states: 'Quaeritur autem a quibusdam, quare inter ceteras liberales disciplinas medicinae ars non contineatur. Propter hoc scilicet, quia singulares continent causas ista vero omnium'. For Vincent's use of the *Pantegni*, see pp. 180–82.

[88] These images can be found in the exhibition catalogue, *Pen and Parchment*, ed. by Holcomb, pp. 97–100. The identification of Aesculapius and Chiron has not been previously observed; for a comparable scene in a ninth-century Beneventan manuscript (Florence, Laurenziana, MS Plut. 73.41, fol. 23[r]) harking back to antique models, see Jones, *Medieval Medicine in Illuminated Manuscripts*, p. 63, and discussion in Voigts, 'The Significance of the Name Apuleius in the *Herbarium Apulei*'. The most thorough analysis of the Liberal Arts personified and portrayed in medieval hierarchies of knowledge remains d'Alverny, 'La sagesse et ses sept filles'.

[89] The matter of teaching medical subjects in Monte Cassino is further explored in Chapter 5 (see pp. 161–70).

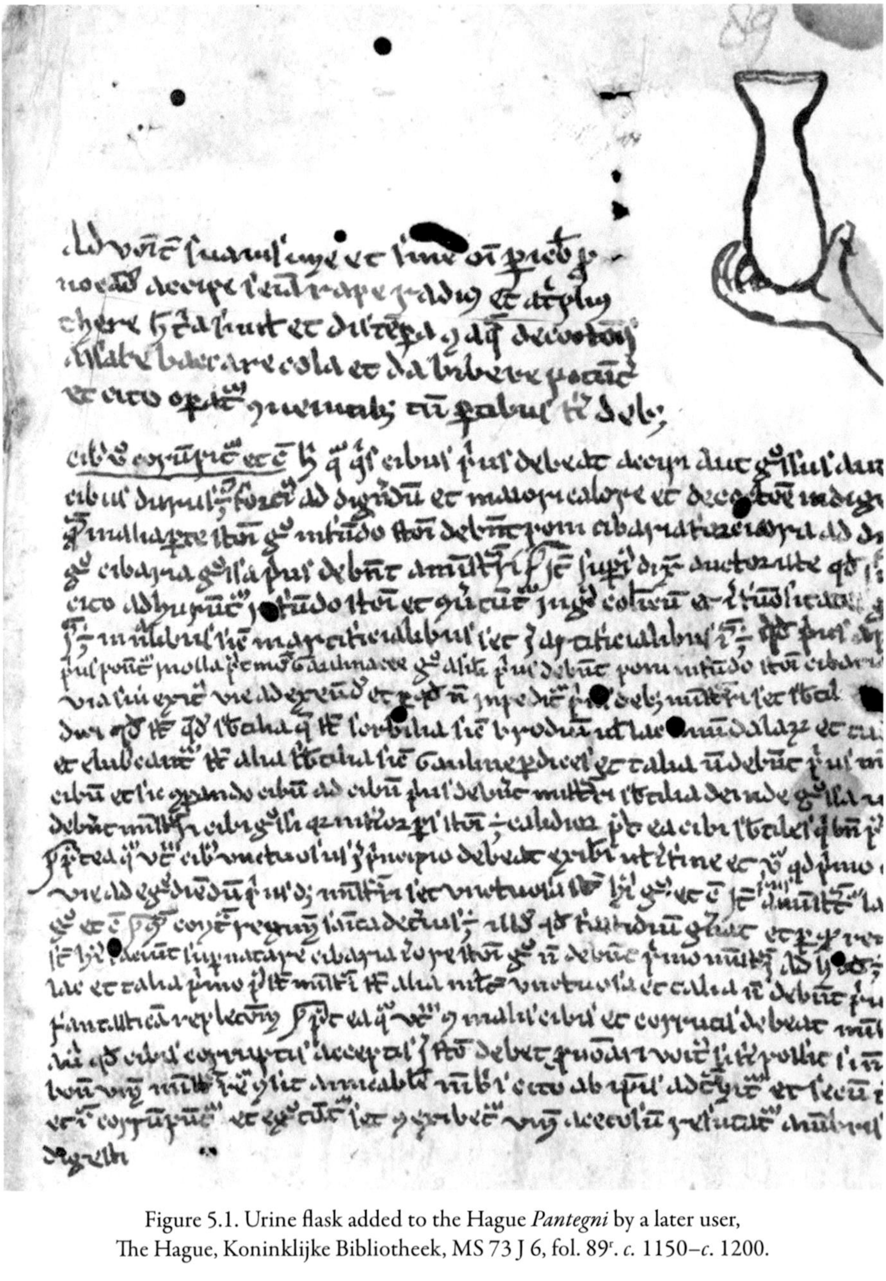

Figure 5.1. Urine flask added to the Hague *Pantegni* by a later user, The Hague, Koninklijke Bibliotheek, MS 73 J 6, fol. 89r. *c.* 1150–*c.* 1200.

Chapter 5

Implications and Complications

The present chapter puts the findings from the previous four chapters in perspective and queries how they add to our understanding of the translation of medical texts in the late eleventh century in South Italy.

Translating Medical Texts in Late Eleventh-Century South Italy

The first question to address appears to be deceptively simple: how did one make a translation from one language into another in the eleventh century? Constantine's task in translating medical texts was complicated by at least three factors. The tradition of translating from Arabic to Latin was very young. Practically, this meant that there may not have been Latin equivalents yet for all Arabic words.[1] A related issue concerns the kind of texts that he translated. As far as scholars have thus far demonstrated, he was altogether engaged in translating highly technical scientific texts from Arabic into Latin.[2] In this domain, of course, the lack of equivalent words in Latin at times may have been particularly apparent. The scope of Constantine's translation enterprise will inevitably have necessitated finding a way to deal with gaps in his Latin knowledge, but also to establish logistics for overcoming this issue.

[1] Strohmaier, 'Constantine's pseudo-Classical Terminology'. Previous scholars have pointed to Constantine's use of terms derived from Arabic, such as *nucha* and *sifac*. But as Strohmeier shows, much of the terminology Constantine used was inspired by classical terminologies, a tradition established early by Ḥunayn ibn Isḥāq. See Glaze, 'Speaking in Tongues' on the ways in which Constantine's chosen terms for diseases, anatomy, physiology, and pharmacy were used already available in older Latin texts, like Gariopontus of Salerno's *Passionarius*.

[2] Francis Newton hopes to discuss translations of medical texts from Greek into Latin in this era in a subsequent study.

Before turning to the manuscript evidence, it makes sense to examine the practice of composing texts in general during this period. In the very first stages of composition, authors are known to have made notes, sometimes on small scraps of parchment. Bernard Itier of Limoges (d. 1225), for example, used parchment off-cuts for composing his extensive historical works.[3] A key element, however, of the ultimate production of a text was its oral delivery to someone who transcribed a draft, often on wax tablets.[4] An insightful account of this process is seen in a letter of Peter Damian. His dictation was taken down on wax tablets by a scribe, and then the draft produced from these tablets was subsequently presented to him for approval on parchment scraps.[5] Peter's tale goes like this:

> Hic autem quid nobis acciderit, silentio praetereundum esse non ducimus. Nam hucusque scribentibus dominica festivitas supervenit, emergentibusque negotiis a scriptione diutius exteriorum nos sollicitudo compescuit. Tunc iuvenculus quidam, Sylvester nomine, qui haec non quidem me dictante scribebat, sed, ut digne me praedicem, tabulis descripta in scedulas transferebat, tanta maligni hostis arte delusus est, ut in lacrimas repente prorumperet, et vix nocte vel die praeter horas soporis et cibi sese a lacrimarum inundantia cohiberet.[6]
>
> (At this point I do not think I should pass over in silence what happened to me. For as I was writing this, down to this point, the Sunday feast intervened and as problems of business came up a concern for outward matters kept me from writing any longer. Then a certain quite young man, Sylvester by name, who was writing out this [letter] not at my dictation, but (to give a proper picture of myself) transferring what was already written down on tablets to parchment scraps [*scedulae*, for *schedulae*], was so deceived by the craft of our wicked enemy [the devil], that he suddenly burst out crying, and could scarcely restrain himself from floods of tears, night or day, aside from the hours given to sleep and food.)

So, first dictation was taken down upon wax tablets, then the text from the initial wax tablets was transferred onto scraps of parchment. At this moment

[3] d'Alverny, 'L'écriture de Bernard Itier'.

[4] For a survey of writing materials, see Bischoff, *Latin Palaeography*, pp. 7–19; on the dictation stage, and the practices of individual authors, see Clanchy, *From Memory to Written Record*, pp. 120–26; also Burnett, 'Give Him the White Cow', pp. 13–15.

[5] See Peter Damian, *Letters: 1–30*, ed. and trans. by Blum, pp. 15–16 (translation modified). For the practice of taking down dictation on wax tablets, see Burnett, 'Give Him the White Cow', pp. 13–15.

[6] Peter Damian, *Die Briefe des Petrus Damiani*, IV.3, ed. by Reindel, *epistula* 153, p. 42, lines 19–26; Reindel, 'Studien zur Überlieferung des werken des Petrus Damiani', p. 52.

the suggestible young scribe Sylvester, copying Peter Damian's lengthy discussion of contrition and penitential tears, fell into uncontrollable weeping. Peter is careful to specify parenthetically that he was not present (the author had no need to take part at this stage in the composition process) and so was not to blame for Sylvester's breakdown; it was the devil who brought it on. Peter's introduction of a pre-emptive self-exculpatory clause suggests that he had perhaps caused such problems with inexperienced youths before; but, whether the responsibility lay with Damian, Sylvester, or the devil, the modern scholar of medieval manuscripts is deeply grateful for this careful technical account of the copying process. After this stage described vividly by Peter, the author corrected the *schedulae*. Then a neat copy of this text, written on good parchment, was subsequently sent out to its destination. Dictation also seems a common scenario with respect to other authors, including Hildegard of Bingen and Thomas Aquinas. As a woman writing books, Hildegard chose to represent herself with wax tablets in hand and a scribe-assistant at her side.[7]

It is useful to remember that Peter Damian, who gives us this account of his own methods of composition and recording of texts at Fonte Avellana, was closely connected with Monte Cassino. He was a friend of the leaders of that house, especially of Abbot Desiderius and its most distinguished scholar in Peter's time, the rhetorician Alberic. Alberic corresponded with Peter before the latter's death in 1072, and a tie between the two monasteries, even a connection between their scribes, remained after that. A team of Monte Cassino brothers travelled to Fonte Avellana in the years immediately following, to copy Peter's works from the exemplars lovingly preserved by the Fonte Avellana monks; the copies they made are today Monte Cassino, MSS 358 and 359.[8]

Another distinguished monk, a Monte Cassino brother of the younger generation, also helps deepen our understanding of how the abbey's authors composed and brought their works to the point of diffusion. It was in the year of Peter Damian's death that we first hear of the activity of Leo Marsicanus, the

[7] Torrell, *Saint Thomas Aquinas*, I, 241–42. Albert Derolez demonstrates that a surviving draft copy of Hildegard's masterpiece, the *Liber divinorum operum*, reveals at its opening various editorial amendments to improve the text. The numbering of the text's chapters, and final chapter table were produced at the very end of the finishing process; see Derolez, 'The Genesis of Hildegard of Bingen's *Liber divinorum operum*'. On Hildegard and her scribes, see Newman, ed., *Voice of the Living Light*.

[8] See Newton, *Scriptorium and Library*, pp. 76–77. On the exemplar from which they were copied, see Peter Damian, *Liber Gomorrhianus*, ed. by D'Angelo, pp. 16–18, 47, 126 n. 94, and 184.

future chronicler of the abbey, in the Monte Cassino scriptorium. In that year, 1072, Leo's uncle, Johannes Marsicanus, formerly archpresbyter of the Marsian church, entered the monastery of Monte Cassino as monk, and, to mark this event, a beautiful lectionary (now Monte Cassino, MS 99) was produced in the Cassinese scriptorium.[9] Young as he was (between the ages of twenty-two and twenty-six), John's nephew Leo was given the responsibility of overseeing its production (it was his *studium* that saw it through to completion), as the verses below the dedication scene on page 3 inform us: the miniature shows Johannes brought before St Benedict by Abbot Desiderius. Johannes holds the jewelled volume in his hands while his nephew, like Sylvester a *iuvenculus*, kneeling at Benedict's feet presents the book's *manutergium* (protective cloth). This same Leo lived to become keeper of the abbey's books (*bibliothecarius*) and was chosen by Abbot Oderisius (Desiderius's successor) to compile the *Chronicle* of the monastery, one of the masterpieces among medieval monastic chronicles.[10]

It is this task which provides us, alongside Peter Damian's account of the earliest stages, an intimate look at the next stage of the authorial/scribal process. The Munich manuscript of Leo's *Chronicle* (Munich, Staatsbibliothek, Clm 4623, fols 85^{r}–189^{v}) shows Leo's autograph marginal and interlinear revisions to his draft text. It was the late Hartmut Hoffmann who made the brilliant identification of Leo's hand in the manuscript.[11] Anna Maria Fagnoni followed in Hoffmann's footsteps with a profound and sensitive analysis of the stages of Leo's revisions and corrections. Fagnoni says:

> From a philological point of view the work possesses most notable interest: not only for the existence of three successive redactions, and not only because it is a matter of an autograph, but above all because the sum total of the interventions permits us, though with difficulty, to see the 'working out' of the *Chronicle* in its continual making and unmaking, in many directions and with many resumptions, so as to enable us to follow Leo in his work, and perhaps to guess at the reasons that motivate it.[12]

[9] On this manuscript and Leo Marsicanus, see Newton, 'Leo Marsicanus and the Dedicatory Text and Drawing in Monte Cassino 99'. It is worth noting that the cost of the manuscript's production was borne by Johannes Marsicanus, as a rich gift to the abbey and to St Benedict. Lohrmann moreover shows Leo as the Scribe in Charge, i.e. director of the scriptorium; Lohrmann, *Das Register Papst Johannes' VIII (872–82)*.

[10] The masterly edition of the *Chronica monasterii Casinensis*, is that edited by Hoffmann.

[11] Hoffmann, 'Studien zur Chronik von Montecassino', pp. 136–38.

[12] 'Dal punto di vista filologico l'opera è di notevolissimo interesse: non solo per l'esistenza di tre successive redazioni, non solo perché si è di fronte a un autografo, ma sopratutto perché

Taken together, Peter Damian's brief description of how he begins to commit a new composition to writing, and Leo Marsicanus's painstaking revisions to his own work in the *Chronicle*, provide unusually clear insight into the practices of authors and scribes in the age of Constantine the African, and in his own region of Central and South Italy.

If we translate these practices to Constantine's situation, a particular theoretical scenario emerges. In terms of the oral delivery, it is important to realize that Constantine's situation is different from that of other medieval Latin authors: he came from a region where Latin was not the dominant language of learning. It is entirely possible, therefore, that the dictation process was not one-sided, but that some sparring occurred with the scribe who received and wrote down the text, probably on wax tablets. Because Constantine's native language was not Latin, and because the *Pantegni* is as much an adaptation as a translation of al-Maǧūsī's original, some polishing may have been required which may not have been necessary in the case of fluent Latin authors such as Thomas Aquinas. Consequently, in this first stage when the dictation was taken on wax, there may have been discussion about the newly translated text. In other words, Constantine may have had help at the level of composition, just as Michael Scot, another prolific Arabic–Latin translator, did over a century later.[13] When the dictation was completed, the text was copied from the wax tablets onto parchment, or perhaps first onto parchment scraps. Peter Damian's case teaches us that the text would now go back to the author for review: Damian, after all, received his original dictation written down on scraps. In Constantine's case, and with such a complicated text, there may have been multiple stages of review at this point. Only after review would the text have been copied onto its more permanent home, that is, quires of parchment. Importantly, at the end of the composition process at least three copies of the text had been made: one

la massa aggrovigliata degli interventi ci consente, pur con difficoltà, di vedere l'elaborazione della cronaca nel suo farsi e disfarsi continuo in più direzioni e a più riprese, così da rendere possibile seguire Leone nel suo lavoro, e forsè di congietturare le ragioni che lo muovono'. Fagnoni, 'Un cronista medievale al lavoro', p. 53. Fagnoni's decoding of that evidence of 'successive redactions' and the continual making and unmaking of a text has profound implications for our understanding of Constantine and his team's many challenges in producing not just the *Pantegni*, but an entire corpus of medical texts in translation.

[13] Kwakkel, 'Behind the Scenes of a Revision'. Another example of the process of medieval composition (although not of a translation) is found in the work of John of Salisbury (Clanchy, *From Memory to Written Record*, p. 127); the *notarius* to whom John dictated a letter that criticized the style of his opening.

in wax (to be copied on scraps), one on parchment scraps (to be reviewed by the author), and one final version on parchment quires. Under normal circumstances, this last copy would be used for producing additional copies of the text, when required.

This overview shows that an author or translator was assisted by at least one other person, who received the oral delivery and transcribed it on wax, then transferred it onto scraps, and ultimately copied it into quires. However, these stages of writing could have also been undertaken by multiple persons, in which case there would be a modest team of assistants. So how did this process work in the practice of Constantine? Fortunately, findings in previous chapters allow us to paint a vivid picture of 'Team Constantine', for a team it was in this case; each member is profiled in Appendix F's Glossary of Scribes. That his translations were a team effort is clear from the magnitude of the undertaking itself.[14] After all, we are talking about at least twenty-four works between *c.* 1077 and (at latest) 1098/99. With more than one text per year, the translation undertaking would have to have been an efficient one, probably with specific tasks appointed to certain individuals; the case of Geraldus in fact suggests this as well. The previous chapters have identified two instances where Geraldus not only copied the Latin text of Constantine's translation, but also assisted in fine-tuning the translation. After all, in the Paris *Isagoge* we see Geraldus entering suppletions in the margins that are editorial in nature, and probably at Constantine's dictation. Similarly, in the Hague *Pantegni* he leaves lacunae in the text where he thinks it needs expanding or completing. Geraldus's tasks show him working very closely with Constantine, and under his direction.

Another member of Team Constantine is the 'Bodleian Juvenal Scribe'. The identifications announced in this book show him as a workhorse of the Cassinese scriptorium, especially in the domain of the *artes*. Even before Constantine's arrival, the Bodleian Juvenal Scribe was involved in copying medical texts. His script suggests that he may have been active as early as the 1060s. He first appears on our horizon in the Copenhagen Pseudo-Soranus (Copenhagen, KB, GKS 1653 4°), which is of this age. This important medical manuscript is the final copy, and shows a number of scribes at work, including a Caroline hand (which among other tasks, enters headings for chapters and headings for the foetal images). Here, too, we see a team working on a medical manuscript, but in the early Desiderian period. Another early *artes* production of the Bodleian Juvenal Scribe is the Eton manuscript (Eton, College Library,

[14] Regarding the economic factors, see pp. 182–89.

MS 150), which contains the earliest surviving copy of the *Ecloga Theoduli*, in a sylloge that includes also the *Bucolics* of Virgil, Maximian, Statius's *Achilleis*, the *Remedia amoris* and *Heroides* of Ovid, and Arator's *Historia apostolorum*: a newly developed anthology of reading texts that served both grammar and rhetoric. It is an early elementary-school text that would spread throughout Europe.

As far as medical texts are concerned, the Bodleian Juvenal Scribe's hand is present in another significant book. He copied the *De curatione corporis* of Paul of Aegina (book III of his *Pragmateia*), at some time in the later Desiderian period (Monte Cassino, MS 351). This is a new identification, like all other scribal identifications in this monograph, which helps build this scribe's profile, and more specifically his involvement with medical texts.[15] In addition to his distinctive Beneventan, this manuscript includes the striking marginal Greek medical terms with yellow wash. Given that it appears that these terms are also written by the Bodleian Juvenal Scribe, it follows that the latter had some understanding of Greek. It suggests that he, like Geraldus, was an educated scribe.

It was the Bodleian Juvenal Scribe who copied the Paris *Isagoge* (Paris, BnF, NAL 1628, fols 19–26). This little gathering, merely a booklet, is hugely instructive. That is because the text is so bad; it remained uncorrected and even incomplete.[16] Basic editorial decisions had not yet been made; on fols 20r–26v there are often sizable spaces left for chapter headings (never supplied), while on the first leaf (fol. 19r–v) no such space appears. Some sentences without initial letters mean that the rubricator never did his work. In other sentences, however, the text scribe did not even save space for the initial; he instead simply continued from the preceding sentence, omitting that first letter.[17] He added unnecessary abbreviation strokes or omitted them altogether, tended to skip a letter or a syllable, and misread the abbreviations in his exemplar. Furthermore, on fol. 20r he wrote the meaningless 'digeria' for 'digerit'; that is, although a Beneventan scribe himself, he confused the letters

[15] One of the authors of the present book, Francis Newton, has undertaken a complete survey of classical texts from eleventh-century Monte Cassino.

[16] Newton, 'Constantine the African', p. 29. The facts remain as stated in that discussion, but as will be seen, the author no longer considers this scribe an 'unintelligent' scribe. His task in the Paris *Isagoge* was simply to transfer the extremely rough text from the wax tablets to parchment, without intervention on his part.

[17] For example, at fol. 19v, line 18, the scribe wrote the nonsensical 'embrorum'; Geraldus inserted the initial 'M' above the word, because there was no free space on the line.

a and **t** (see fig. 1.4, line 9, last word). Now that we know that this is a highly skilled scribe, who wrote a beautiful non-Cassinese version of Beneventan, and who was responsible for learned text and paratext in the Bodleian Juvenal and Monte Cassino, MS 351's *De curatione corporis*, we must acknowledge that there is nothing 'crude' or 'unintelligent' about him; it was, we can now see, the inchoate state of his exemplar that accounts for his mistakes. The exemplar was in a cursive Beneventan (proven by the confusion of **a** and **t** just mentioned) which must have been the initial setting-down of the text, almost certainly on wax tablets, at Constantine's dictation. In Paris we see the first transfer of text, from wax-tablets to parchment, by a craftsman-scribe, but one whose only task was to produce quickly a rough, non-cursive version (the first version on parchment) of the words Constantine had dictated to the wax-tablet writer.[18] The intelligent and learned scribe of the Bodleian Juvenal, if he had paused in this process with the *Isagoge* to give any thought to the mishmash that he was leaving on the parchment, might, like Peter Damian's 'kid named Sylvester', have burst into non-stop crying. The modern scholar, however, rejoices in the survival of this witness to a crucial, early stage in the production of this medical text.

It was someone else who would take the text further and on to the next stage. We see, for one, Geraldus in the margin of the Paris *Isagoge* and between the lines, adding the translator's second thoughts (fig. 1.4). We may assume that the marginal suppletions in the Paris manuscript were produced through a comparison with the Arabic original. Some of these suppletions and changes between the lines or in the margins were necessitated by a later decision to include additional passages from the Arabic original.[19] In other words, these suppletions involved knowledge of Arabic and, more importantly, must have been instigated by Constantine.

Remarkably, we are shown how the team progressed in improving the *Isagoge*, because of a surviving manuscript that shows a further stage just after the first review and correction of Constantine's text. The manuscript in question, Monte Cassino, MS 225, contains a slightly unfinished text; that is, it is

[18] The implication of Peter Damian's passage discussed above may be that Sylvester had taken down the dictation on wax tablets and was now also responsible for transcribing his rough work onto *schedulae*. In the Paris case the wax-tablet scribe and the parchment scribe may have been different persons; the difficulty of transcribing another's rough notes, rather than one's own, into a fair copy would perhaps account for the poor quality of the text (as suggested to us by Jenneka Janzen, Leiden University).

[19] See for further details Newton, 'Constantine the African', pp. 31–33.

not quite the same text that we find later in the *Isagoge* tradition.[20] However, MS 225 does include, as part of the original text, the marginal and interlinear suppletions added to the Paris *Isagoge*. In other words, Geraldus's efforts at improving the translation would become part of the *Isagoge* as it would be disseminated throughout Europe. Team Constantine appears, at least for the most part, to have produced the versions of these texts that would be sent out from Monte Cassino into the world. This was not a theoretical exercise, but one aimed at producing correct translations that could be used by readers beyond their own circle, and in many cases, far beyond the circle.

It is notable that, while a similar attempt to improve the translation can be observed on the pages of the Hague *Pantegni* in the form of the lacunae, this being one of our enigmas, in this case the potential flaws were not corrected. Apparently, then, while the team aimed to receive input from Constantine (who, almost certainly, would be the person to supply the improved readings, as he had done in the case of the *Isagoge*), it was never provided. We have seen that Geraldus and Constantine likely interacted during the production of the latter's translations. Why was the same thing not done for the Hague *Pantegni*? Was the translator unavailable? Was the improvement project abandoned? Did the competition of other texts in the translation pipeline crowd out further work on the *Pantegni*? Or did Geraldus do the best he could but the exemplar was simply incomplete? Geraldus did not copy the complete *Theorica* in this manuscript; he skipped the final five pages of the last book, which were eventually filled in by Scribe C *c.* 1150, in order to provide subsequent users of the Hague manuscript with the full copy of the *Theorica*. However, the observation that the rubrics for the last book were already available in Latin (they are present, after all, in the *capitula* list written by the eleventh-century rubricator on fol. 78^{r}) suggests that this last book had already been translated by Constantine. Furthermore, Geraldus stopped his work at exactly the foot of fol. 85^{r}, at the end of this last line, and in the middle of a sentence.[21] It is clear that a decision regarding the mechanics of production was made to stop the copying process at this point. This shows the rapid, but to our eyes somewhat abrupt, turning from one stage of the copying process to the next.

[20] The text found in the later manuscripts is longer, meaning that more text was likely added at a later stage, presumably by Constantine.

[21] Note that the rubrics are missing in the final pages copied by Geraldus (the last rubric by Scribe B is at fol. 78^{r}). The rubricator's work, which of course followed the text scribe's work at an interval, seems likely to have ceased at the same moment that Geraldus's work stopped.

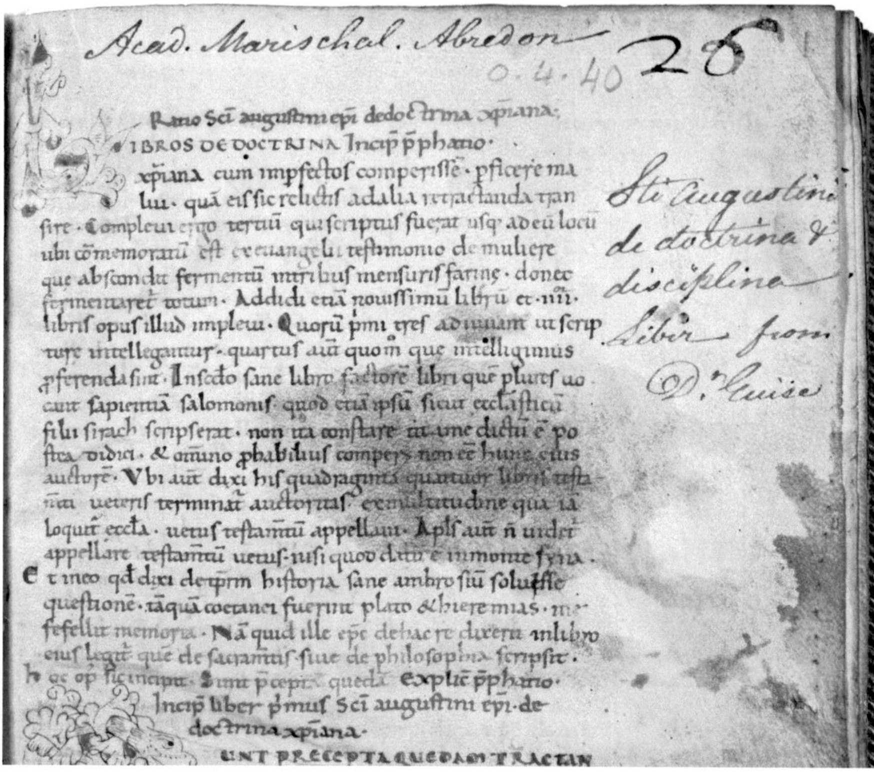

Figure 5.2. Hand of the Hague Rubricator, Aberdeen, University Library, MS 106, fol. 1r. *c.* 1075–*c.* 1100. Augustine, *De doctrina Christiana*.

We will leave this matter for now and turn to another important member of the team: Atto/Theodemar, whose work with Constantine was remembered vividly in the Cassinese tradition. He too had direct access to Constantine. He wrote, or rewrote, the prologues to Constantine's translations, in the 'high-buskined style', according to Peter the Deacon.[22] The Prologue of the *Pantegni* consists of a central section largely translated from the Arabic text of al-Mağūsī (Part B). To the beginning of this, Atto/Theodemar added a laudatory rhetorical address to Desiderius (Part A) and a tailpiece rounding out the whole with complimentary praise also addressed to the abbot (Part C). With this, the Prologue comes full circle, compositionally. The Hague manuscript shows us that Part C ('Vobis autem') was composed later, namely after the other two parts had already been copied on the first page of the book. Atto and Constantine

[22] Peter the Deacon, *De viris illustribus Casinensibus*, col. 1035b.

were, presumably, still working on that last part of the Prologue together, as Geraldus was copying the *Pantegni*. This shows not only that Atto/Theodemar, too, had direct access to Constantine, as indeed one would already assume based on the task assigned to him according to Peter the Deacon, but it also reveals the assembly line production of Team Constantine: various stages of processing a translation were undertaken at the same time.

In a sense, Part C of the Prologue is the only lacuna in the manuscript that was filled in post-production. The scribe who did so is the one who executed the rubrication in most of the manuscript (named Scribe B, or the Hague Rubricator, in Chapter 2). It is clear that his task of adding short rubrics was supplemented with copying a substantial amount of text (when compared to the length of rubrics), namely the 'Vobis autem' Prologue Part C at the end of fol. 1^{r}. There is an instance where we see the Hague Rubricator at work copying even more text in a medical book. The Padua manuscript (Biblioteca Universitaria, lat. 892; fig. 5.5 and pl. XV) of Constantine's *De febribus* is probably also entirely his handiwork.[23] The Hague Rubricator was, moreover, responsible for an important part of a non-medical book. The manuscript in question is Aberdeen, UL, MS 106, containing Augustine's *De doctrina Christiana* (fols 1^{r}–55^{r}), Alberic's treatise on the Eucharist (fols 55^{v}–64^{v}) and the accompanying dossier of edited passages, and Haimo of Auxerre's *Commentarius in cantica canticorum* (fols 65^{r}–89^{v}). The Hague Rubricator is found at the opening of the Augustine text (fig. 5.2 and pl. XII), of which he copied fols 1^{r}–20^{v}, line 19 (last word *narrata*), and in the Alberic treatise, of which he copied fols 55^{v}–62^{v}, line 10 (last word *meum*).

This new identification adds to our understanding of this member of Team Constantine. In the first place, it adds further evidence that the Hague Rubricator can be tied, as expected, to Monte Cassino; the treatise of Alberic was produced at the abbey, and the incipit of his treatise is written in the Cassinese style of Beneventan.[24] Moreover, the identification of the scribe of Aberdeen, UL, MS 106 with the Hague Rubricator shows that he was regarded as part of the team that focused on copying the work of house authors, in one case that of Constantine the African, and in the other that of Alberic. The implications and complications of the enigmas of the Hague manuscript set forth in the preface to the present book, and the solutions proposed for them in

23 We are grateful to Raphaela Veit for bringing this manuscript to our attention during her presentation at the 2016 International Medieval Congress in Kalamazoo. On this manuscript, see also pp. 180–81.

24 Radding and Newton, *Theology, Rhetoric, and Politics in the Eucharistic Controversy*, especially pp. 32–34.

this work, lead to a longer perspective and enable us to broaden the story of this text to its inception in the harbour city where Constantine first found refuge on European shores.[25] But we must first address the basics.

Remarkably, in completing the final part of the Prologue, the Hague Rubricator executes a task that one would expect Geraldus to have carried out. Why add the text in conspicuous red, if the scribe was present, ready to copy it in the same hand and colour as the rest of the manuscript? Was Part C done in red deliberately, so as to make it stand out? To complicate matters, in Paris, BnF, Latin 6887, not only Part C of the Prologue but also Part A is in red ink. In fact, as Jacquart observes, this separates the central text by al-Mağūsī from the framework that the new Parts A and C create for it.[26] For whatever reason the red was used, deliberately or not, the fact that the task was assigned to the rubricator shows that Geraldus's role in the production of this book was fulfilled after he had copied the main text: the rubrication, after all, was usually done after completion of the main text. He did not return to the lacunae, nor did he copy the last part of the Prologue. He probably moved straight on to another task within the overarching medical project. The fact that the main text, copied by Geraldus, and the rubrication of that text both break off and remained unfinished, but that the Hague Rubricator came back and added in his red ink this final flourish that is Prologue Part C, indicates that this production stage of the *Theorica* was complete enough, and it was time to move on to a final or dedication copy. It is likely that both Prologue Parts A and C of this dedication copy, which is unfortunately lost but which stands between the Hague manuscript and Paris 6887, would have been copied in red.

Crucially, the Paris *Pantegni* manuscript shows, in a sense, how the process could produce a book that was incomplete. Not only were there some nine problems that remained unsolved in the Hague manuscript (lacunae that were left blank), but there were also five pages at the very end of the text that remained to be copied. In the Paris *Isagoge* we see a similar phenomenon. Here there were no lacunae in the text. However, additions were to be made, and these suppletions are found in the margins (in Geraldus's Caroline minuscule). There are, however, blank spaces left for the large initial letters at the beginning of some chapters, and quite sizable spaces left for chapter headings. In fact, there is no rubrication whatsoever. In that sense the process was stopped before

[25] See pp. 7–8.

[26] 'Par ces rubriques, se trouvent ainsi distingués ce qui suit (même de loin) le texte d'al-Mağūsī et ce qui est propre à Constantin'. Jacquart, 'Le sens donné par Constantin l'Africain', p. 73 n. 5.

the stage entrusted to the rubricator. The *Isagoge* text itself was not yet complete, and thus not ready for rubrication. Here the assembly line skipped a different step, and more than one; these skipped steps were earlier in the process of text production and revision than what we find in the virtually completed Hague manuscript, but here, too, they represent a case of abandonment, in a sense. These are rare examples of surviving manuscripts where the texts themselves stood at different stages of completion.

As we have noted, both the Aberdeen and the Hague manuscripts show the Hague Rubricator as a scribe involved in the production of books that contained new works from house authors. Both Constantine and Alberic were Monte Cassino's intellectual leaders in medicine and theological debate. The medical texts produced by Constantine are evidently part of a broader range of intellectual interests pursued at Monte Cassino at that very moment. The medical landscape was cultivated by a group of experienced men, who were working closely together, and who were assigned very specific tasks within each stage of production. While the actual tasks varied among their products, it appears that Geraldus, one of the main figures of this study, undertook several of those products: at one point he left blank spaces while the translator worked out the problematic readings (in the Hague *Pantegni*), and at another point he added suppletions provided by Constantine to a text copied by another scribe (in the Paris *Isagoge*). At the same time, however, Geraldus is involved in other writing tasks in the scriptorium: he is not exclusively assigned to Team Constantine, but it is demonstrable that he was called upon when something needed to be done in the context of Constantine's medical productions.

Teaching Medicine at Monte Cassino

An important observation to address here is the key conclusion of Chapter 4, that MS 73 J 6 was likely produced for educational purposes. It is, to be sure, understood that the most intellectually vibrant of the great eleventh-century monastic houses were engaged in teaching the *artes*, and that this instruction included medicine. There is, however, a paucity of specific evidence available to the modern student. This is where the Hague manuscript proves to be particularly significant, as a tool for teaching at Monte Cassino. This argument is best supported by the narrow format of the manuscript. From this assessment the question arises of whether the book was likely used for teaching within the walls of Monte Cassino. In other words, is this specific manuscript evidence of medical teaching in the abbey? To date, Monte Cassino has been credited with the production of medical texts, but not with actually using them in education, even though Constantine's works were clearly used for this purpose elsewhere, including in the nearby school at Salerno from the second quarter of the twelfth century (if not earlier). While medical education is not usually discussed in relationship with Monte Cassino, there is a case to be made to assert just that.

First, there can be little doubt that teaching was an ongoing function of the monks at Monte Cassino.[27] Evidence shows that the educational programme consisted, in large, of the Liberal Arts, as would be expected. In the first golden age of Monte Cassino culture, the Carolingian era, Paul the Deacon is the outstanding figure, who is known to have been resident at Monte Cassino in 775–95 (except for four years spent at Charlemagne's court). His learning and teaching are undoubtedly reflected in the magnificent Paris, BnF, Latin 7530, with its riches in the fields of grammar and rhetoric.[28] Other Monte Cassino manuscripts survive from the ninth century; in fact, it has not been observed, but it can be argued that the books that survive from the later Carolingian period from the abbey are principally books of the *artes*, both from the Trivium and Quadrivium (e.g. Monte Cassino, MS 332, Martianus Capella), such as astronomy (MS 3), grammar (MSS 218, 299, 401, 402), and medicine (MS 69 and, slightly later, MS 97).[29] It is clear that the tenth century continues the tradition in the period of the monks' exile in Capua and after the restoration of the mother house in 950.

The eleventh century sees the second golden age of Monte Cassino, evidenced in the quantity and contents of the books produced. The greatest Cassinese scholar of the beginning of this period is Lawrence of Amalfi, monk of Monte Cassino from 1022 to 1029 under Abbot Theobald, later archbishop of his native city of Amalfi, who, exiled to Florence and Rome in the 1040s, is said by tradition to have taught Hildebrand (the later Pope Gregory VII).[30] He was a learned man, admired by contemporaries for his command of Greek as well as Latin.[31] The surviving monument of his teaching is Venice, Biblioteca Nazionale Marciana, Lat. Z. 497 (1811), a magnificent codex containing Lawrence's hand-

[27] The classic discussion is that of Bloch, 'Monte Cassino's Teachers and Library'.

[28] Holtz, 'Le Parisinus Latinus 7530'. The manuscript is dated 779–97.

[29] For Monte Cassino, MS 69, see Beccaria, *Codici di medicina*, pp. 293–97; Jeffrey Doolittle of Fordham University is engaged in an extensive study of this manuscript. For MSS 69 and 97, see Beccaria, pp. 297–303, and the Introduction to the present volume.

[30] The modern scholarship on Lawrence begins with Holtzmann, 'Laurentius von Amalfi'. For his works, see *Laurentius, monachus Casinensis Archiepiscopus Amalfitanus*, ed. by Newton.

[31] His annotated Greek psalter survives and deserves further study; it is BAV, Vat. gr. 619. See Newton, '"Expolitio" per l'Umanesimo', p. 171 and Tab. 2.

book of the Liberal Arts, which has the further interest of having been part of the Lateran Library of the popes.[32] This volume is organized around the *Artes liberales* in the following order: grammar, rhetoric, dialectic, medicine, music, geometry, arithmetic, and astronomy. It is medicine that concerns us here; in the Venice manuscript, the topic of medicine consists of the treatise *Sapientia artis medicinae* and selections from Isidore's *Etymologies*, book IV.

Furthermore, the four letters of Lawrence contained in the Venice manuscript include one addressed to the famous medical writer and teacher Gariopontus of Salerno. The fact that he wrote to Gariopontus, and the inclusion of a reference to diet, shows that Lawrence had an interest, as a teacher, in medicine.[33] It is relevant that John O. Ward has shown that the Venice manuscript contains a commentary on Cicero's *De inventione* that reflects Lawrence's classroom teaching at Monte Cassino in the 1020s.[34] Lawrence's activities prove that medicine was included in the programme of teaching the *artes* at Monte Cassino in the first half of the eleventh century, although in truth, medicine is represented by only two texts in Lawrence's anthology. The tradition says that Lawrence continued teaching in Rome in the second half of the 1040s, in the closing years of his life. The Venice manuscript, however, was not one that a teacher could hold in one hand as he lectured before his students. It consists of 202 folia measuring 390 × 250 mm. Its magnificent proportions make it a most fitting memorial to a scholarly archbishop, and a stately possession to adorn the library of a pope.

This brings us to the middle of the eleventh century. It has been noted in the Introduction that the youthful Desiderius and his close friend Alfanus, when they first appeared on the larger stage of history, visited Pope Victor II in Tuscany in 1055, accompanied by medicines and medical books.[35] One of these books may have been Alfanus's translation of the *Peri physeos anthropou* of Nemesius of Emesa. This can be said to have set the theme of the golden age of Abbot Desiderius (1058–87), the 'bibliophile abbot'. This is precisely how he is portrayed in the famous miniature in BAV, Vat. lat. 1202, of the year 1075.

[32] The manuscript was first identified as Lawrence's handbook of the Liberal Arts by Newton; see his 'Tibullus in Two Grammatical *Florilegia*'. It contains an *ex libris* of the Lateran library.

[33] On Gariopontus, see the Introduction to this volume, and the published studies of Eliza Glaze.

[34] Ward, 'Lawrence of Amalfi', with edition of the text on pp. 323–40.

[35] Newton, *Scriptorium and Library*, pp. 12–13.

Learning and books are a running theme in the poetry of Alfanus (d. 1086), Desiderius's 'eulogist' in a series of poems, including the one in the Vatican manuscript. In 1057 the same Pope Victor II spoke of Monte Cassino as 'principale gymnasium' (the foremost training ground), showing just how important the abbey was considered to be as a centre of education.[36]

It is against this backdrop that we should view Constantine's coming to Monte Cassino and his installation as instigator and executor of the great translation project which introduces twenty-four, and no doubt more, Arabic medical works to the West. In fact, it is Desiderius's close friend Alfanus who summed up the abbot's programme of teaching in two stanzas from his Poem 39. His description of a vision of paradise culminates in the appearance of a group of saints who shine like jewels (carbuncle, sapphire, jasper, sard, and others). Then follow the two stanzas:

> Cernit insignes legis suae dogmate | inter ignitos et condensos lapides | nitore miro coruscare pariter; | miratur opus et laudat artificem. | Inde scholarem rimatur originem. || Accedit Maurus, Honoratus, Placidus | et Constantinus, Faustus et Simplicius. | Beato Patri omnes ita referunt: | 'Quos sic miraris ex Casino prodeunt: | hos expolivit noster Desiderius'.[37]
>
> ([St Benedict] sees, among the glowing and thickly gathered gems, figures outstanding in the study of his Law [the Rule of St Benedict] shining with a marvellous light; he wonders at their workmanship and praises the workmen. Then he asks what school has shaped them. || Maurus, Honoratus, Placidus, and Constantinus, Faustus and Simplicius, all answer the blessed father in this fashion: 'These, whom you so much admire, come from Cassino: These are those jewels whom our Desiderius polished'.)

The books produced under Desiderius bear witness to an intense interest in the *artes*, both the Trivium and Quadrivium. The revival of learning broadly involved the copying and reading of classical texts, some of which had not been copied or read for centuries. These would inevitably form part of the teaching at the school of Monte Cassino. Witnesses of this movement are the textually unique copies of Tacitus and Apuleius (bound together in Florence, Laurenziana, MS Plut. 68.2), Seneca's *Dialogi* (Milan, Biblioteca Ambrosiana, MS C 90 inf.), and Cicero's *De natura deorum* (Leiden, UB, BPL 118). Charles

[36] Newton, *Scriptorium and Library*, p. 274. The expression, 'the bibliophile abbot' is from Newton's discussion.

[37] Lentini and Avagliano, *I Carmi di AlfanoI Arcivescovo di Salerno*, p. 191, lines 56–65. See also Newton, '"Expolitio" per l'Umanesimo'.

Radding and Antonio Ciaralli argue that a manuscript fragment of Justinian's Code (Rome, Biblioteca Vallicelliana, Carte vallicelliane, XII, 3) was probably a product of Monte Cassino, and it can be assigned to the early Desiderian period (roughly 1058–71).[38] More specifically devoted to the *artes* are texts in grammar (Monte Cassino, MS 580) and grammatical reading (Eton, College Library, MS 150), dialectic (Monte Cassino, MS 191 and BAV, Ottob. lat. 1406), arithmetic (Monte Cassino, MS 189), and music (Monte Cassino, MS 318).

Lawrence furthermore makes it clear that in his day the traditional Quadrivium in Monte Cassino was expanded: in his time it included astronomy and medicine, in addition to the usual subjects of music, geometry, and arithmetic. This does not surprise us, because as Chapter 4 showed, medicine was included among the Liberal Arts, not just in Isidore and Vincent's works, but also graphically in a mid-twelfth-century depiction of the Liberal Arts (New York, Morgan Library and Museum, MS 982, from Salzburg *c.* 1150–*c.* 1160), where it forms the Quadrivium together with arithmetic, astronomy, and music. Medical learning is present in such eleventh-century manuscripts as Copenhagen, KB, GKS 1653 4° (medical texts copied jointly by Geraldus, the Bodleian Juvenal Scribe, and the Apuleius Rubricator), Monte Cassino, MS 225 (various medical works including the *Isagoge*), Monte Cassino, MS 351 (Paul of Aegina, copied by the Bodleian Juvenal Scribe), Paris, BnF, NAL 1628, a modest booklet consisting of fols 19–26 (the *Isagoge* copied by the Bodleian Juvenal Scribe with suppletions by Geraldus), and The Hague, KB, MS 73 J 6 (the *Pantegni*, copied by Geraldus and the Hague Rubricator).

The presence of *artes*-inspired manuscripts in the library of Monte Cassino cannot by itself be taken as sufficient evidence that these subjects were also taught in the monastery school. However, there are manuscripts that not only hold texts with an educational signature, but whose physical features also suggest that they themselves were used in education. These are, of course, the holster books discussed in Chapter 4. There are a number of holster books that survive from Monte Cassino. Particularly notable is BAV, Ottob. lat. 1354 of *c.* 1100, containing grammatical texts, including work by Alberic of Monte Cassino, because it is known to have been used in the classroom at Monte Cassino (see Chapter 4). As Gehl suggests, it reflects the 'novel, eclectic, compositional pedagogy pioneered by Alberic and the literary flowering at Monte Cassino'.[39] With a size of 180 × 100 mm, the relative width of the page is 0.56

[38] See Radding and Ciaralli, *The 'Corpus iuris civilis' in the Middle Ages*, pp. 85–86.

[39] Gehl, 'Vat. Ottobonianus lat. 1354', p. 307. On the mathematical treatise found here,

Table 5.1. Holster books produced at Monte Cassino.

	Manuscript	Contents	Height (mm)	Width (mm)	Relative width	1 line (mm)
1	BAV, Vat. lat. 3262	Ovid, *Fasti*	270	125	0.46	7
2	Milan, Biblioteca Ambrosiana, MS C 90 inf.	Seneca, *Dialogi*	350	185	0.53	10
3	BAV, Ottob. lat. 1354	*Grammatica*	180	100	0.55	3
4	The Hague, KB, MS 73 J 6	Constantine the African, *Theorica Pantegni*	235	128	0.55	3
5	BAV, Vat. lat. 3253	Virgil, *Georgica*	335	190	0.57	7
6	Monte Cassino, MS 105	*Homiliarium*	465	265	0.57	16
7	Monte Cassino, MS 451	*Ordo Romanus*	305	175	0.57	9
8	Florence, Laurenziana, MS Plut. 66.21	Justinus, *Epitome historiarum Pompei Trogi*	235	135	0.57	9
9	Oxford, Bodleian, MS Canon. Class. Lat. 41	Juvenal, *Satirae*	235	135	0.58	6
10	Monte Cassino, MS 520	Octateuchus	460	265	0.58	16
11	Monte Cassino, MS 571	*Prophetae maiores et minores*	485	280	0.58	16
12	Monte Cassino, MS 108	*Homiliarium*	455	270	0.59	15
13	Wolfenbüttel, Herzog-August Bibliothek, Cod. Guelf. 52.5 Aug 4°	Lucan, *Bellum civile*	185	110	0.59	6
14	Monte Cassino, MS 351	Paul of Aegina, *De curatione totius corporis*	285	170	0.60	7
15	Monte Cassino, MS 170	Augustine, *De disciplina Christiana*	265	160	0.60	8

(indeed the same as the Hague manuscript). As in the Hague manuscript, the writing space in the Ottoboni manuscript contains many lines (here fifty-two lines to the page) in tiny script.

see Gibson and Newton, 'Pandulf of Capua's *De calculatione*', with a miniature of the abacus teacher on p. 333.

What other books were likely made for such a classroom purpose, given their narrow dimensions? The holster book is not defined by a precise proportion, but 0.60 would be a safe cut-off point for this purpose. After all, this is much narrower than the norm, which puts the width between 0.68–0.72 of the folium's height.[40] Among the manuscripts certainly made in Monte Cassino during the abbacies of Desiderius and Oderisius, are fifteen holster books with a relative width of 0.60 or less (table 5.1).[41]

There were two main reasons for producing a manuscript with this seemingly puzzling tall appearance: it would either be fitted with a binding decorated with repurposed ivory plaques, or the manuscript was designed to be held in one hand.[42] The list above probably does not contain any manuscripts that would originally have had ivory boards, because these are too large in size, even though ivory would have been appropriate in the setting in which they were used, that is, the liturgy (e.g. nos 6, 10, 11, and 12). The table also holds a number of thinner codices that were almost certainly not bound with ivory plaques; these were likely made narrow so they could be held in one hand. Each of them has a clear connection to education as far as their contents are concerned, and the hand-held nature of these objects further suggests that they were used in such a setting.

The narrow format allowed teachers in an oral setting to hold the book in one hand, leaving one hand available for other tasks, such as pointing at passages or gesturing. The key benefit, of course, is that the holster format provided mobility: teachers could walk around as they were teaching. The largest group comprises classical manuscripts: nos 1, 2, 5, 8, 9, and 13. The Latin classics were popular texts for teaching novices grammar, rhetoric, and dialectic, together with other works from antiquity, alongside such purely grammatical texts as Donatus.[43]

Four additional holster books are included in table 5.1. One holds Augustine's *De disciplina Christiana* (no. 15). This was fundamental to Christian book culture and as such, unsurprisingly, is found in the same format, suit-

[40] See the discussion at pp. 122–23.

[41] The starting point for this investigation is the manuscript descriptions found in the back of Newton, *Scriptorium and Library*. In 2012 Julie Anne Somers, then research assistant at Leiden University, entered the dimensions from these descriptions into a database, from which table 5.1 was subsequently made.

[42] See Chapter 4, and Kwakkel, '"Dit boek"'.

[43] Kwakkel, 'Manuscripts of the Latin Classics'.

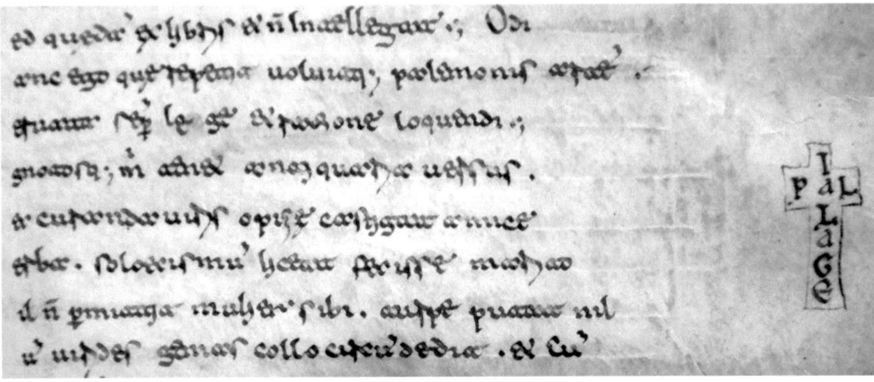

Figure 5.3. Hand of the Bodleian Juvenal Scribe, entering in alternating red and black and in a cross-shape, the rhetorical figure 'IPALLAGE' (= HYPALLAGE) in the margin of Juvenal's *Satires*, Oxford, Bodleian Library, MS Canon. Class. Lat. 41, fol. 23[r]. *c.* 1075–*c.* 1100. Reproduced with the permission of the Bodleian Library.

able for lecturing in the classroom. Its teaching function is also demonstrated by its beautiful marginal diagrams. Two other volumes have already been introduced: BAV, Ottob. lat. 1354, produced for use by a teacher at Monte Cassino (no. 3); and The Hague, KB, MS 73 J 6, our *Pantegni* copy (no. 4). The final holster book, Monte Cassino, MS 351 (no. 14), is also medical in nature. It contains Paul of Aegina's *De curatione totius corporis* (*Pragmateia*), the Latin translation of a Greek technical treatise. The codex, according to our new identification in Chapter 1, is copied by one of Constantine's team members, the Bodleian Juvenal Scribe, who executed both the main text and the rubrics. The margins hold Greek terms highlighted with yellow wash, also used for the rubrics, which would make it possible to easily locate and point out these terms in a classroom situation. This is the Bodleian Juvenal Scribe at his most formal, unlike his work in the Copenhagen medical manuscript. His hand is also somewhat less formal in his 'name manuscript', Bodleian, MS Canon. Class. Lat. 41 (fig. 5.3).

Given that smaller holster books were popularly used in the classroom, which is shown by both their physical appearance and contents, these items reveal something about the nature of education in Monte Cassino. While we would expect to find the classics, other works are more surprising to see in the abbey's classroom. For the present study, the medical works in table 5.1 are most important. After all, they can be taken as evidence that medical teaching was part of the curriculum at Monte Cassino. While this is the first time it has been suggested that medical teaching was conducted at Monte Cassino, the codicological evidence is straightforward, inasmuch as these books are format-

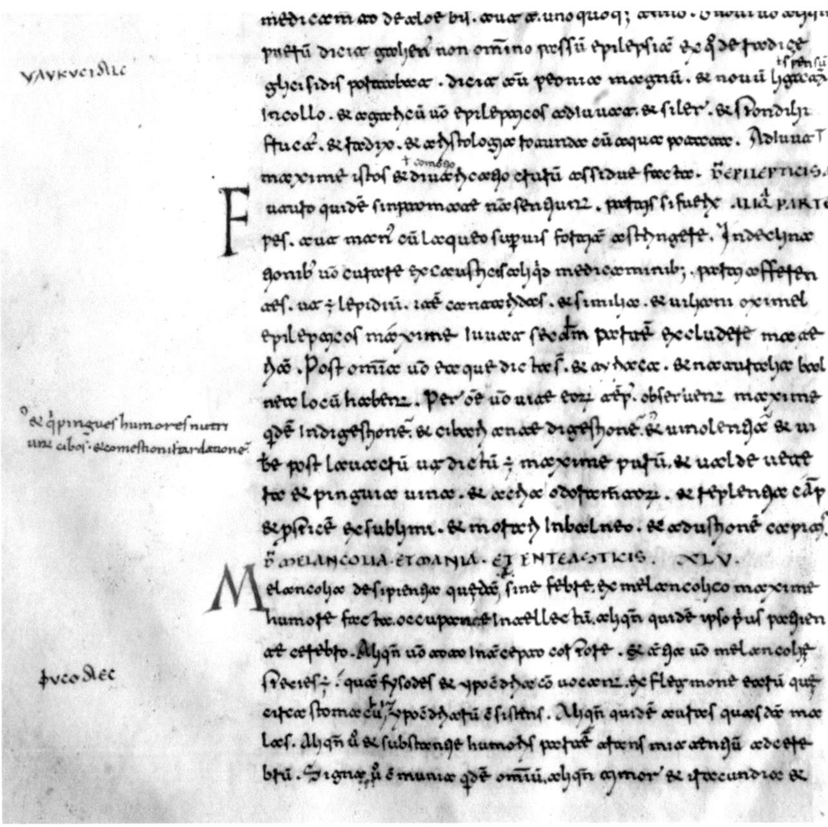

Figure 5.4. Hand of the Bodleian Juvenal Scribe writing in Greek (upper and lower marginal gloss), the main text (Paul of Aegina) in Latin, and the Latin correction (left margin, centre), Monte Cassino, Archivio della Badia, MS 351, p. 19. *c.* 1075–*c.* 1100.

ted for classroom use. That is, these books were suitable for teaching novices, Constantine's *introducendi*, in the central part of his Prologue. Perhaps we may even add that the teaching might have been overseen by Constantine, by his student 'Ioannes Medicus' (as he is called in Leo Marsicanus's calendar), or perhaps even by Geraldus or Atto/Theodemar, called Constantine's 'auditor' by Peter the Deacon.

There is, moreover, a fascinating parallel between two manuscripts, one classical (Juvenal) and the other medical (Paul of Aegina), in table 5.1. Both, as noted, are by the Bodleian Juvenal Scribe. Scholars have never observed that the Juvenal manuscript is fundamentally pedagogical in nature. The scribe marks rhetorical figures in the text by placing Greek terms in the margin beside the apposite passage. These marginalia are part of the original structure of the book, not only written in the hand of the text scribe but also decorated with colours by the original rubricator (fig. 5.3 and pl. XIII). This practice is precisely duplicated in Monte Cassino, MS 351, where Greek medical terms appear in the margin (fig. 5.4 and pl. XIV). Again, they are by the same hand as the text (in Greek characters rather than the Latin *capitalis* of the Juvenal manuscript), and are also decorated, although in a yellow wash in the Greek style, which is not present in the Juvenal manuscript. As with several other items in table 5.1, these two manuscripts created by the Bodleian Juvenal Scribe were produced for teachers for study and preparation, and equally for classroom use.

These specifics underlie the picture that Alfanus draws in his poems, of intense intellectual activity in the monastery during its golden age, specifically the 'expolitio' (polishing) of young minds that Desiderius so brilliantly fostered.[44] As Alfanus praised the qualities to be encouraged in inquiring young minds by their leaders, above all by Desiderius, so Constantine's *Pantegni* turned, in the chapter after his Prologue, to the ethical and moral qualities to be fostered (deontology) in those who pursued medical learning and practice. In placing the Hippocratic ethics immediately after the opening preface to the *Pantegni*, Constantine was following al-Maǧūsī's text, and indeed, endorsing yet again the Hippocratic-Galenic values upon which the new medicine of the late eleventh century was to be founded, as indicated by every aspect of Constantine's translation programme. The intellectual and ethical standards expressed here in the *Pantegni* mark an altogether new high-point.[45] The manuscripts that we have just examined were the tools used to make this kind of transformation happen.

Genesis and Diffusion of the Pantegni

According to the narrative of scholars until now, the history of the *Pantegni* as a school text began only at Salerno in the twelfth century; it was certainly used by a group of famous medical teachers by *c.* 1150. However, this study has shown that the roots of this educational history go back all the way to eleventh-century Monte Cassino itself, where the *Pantegni* and other medical

[44] See p. 164 in the present volume.

[45] Snippets of deontological values had been expressed rather tersely in early medieval medical texts known at Monte Cassino and elsewhere, but none of these approached the thoroughness of the *Pantegni*'s presentation. See MacKinney, 'Medical Ethics and Etiquette'; McVaugh, 'Bedside Manners'.

treatises were used in a school setting even during Constantine's lifetime. Now we add that the manuscript in The Hague is a key witness for yet another shift in our perception of the *Pantegni*: there is evidence to suggest that Constantine had started translating al-Maǧūsī's text even before he entered the Abbey of Monte Cassino. This claim is based on observations from other early *Pantegni* manuscripts and it hinges on three elements encountered on the first page of MS 73 J 6: the address to Abbot Desiderius by Atto/Theodemar, starting with 'Domino suo montis' (Part A); the part starting 'Cum totius', which was largely derived from al-Maǧūsī's text, though the latter's Prologue was not translated by Constantine in its entirety (Part B); and the concluding 'Vobis autem pater' section (Part C), also by Atto/Theodemar.

Our story of an attestation to the text before Monte Cassino begins with a manuscript that, paradoxically, was produced over fifty years after the Hague volume. The manuscript in question is Erfurt, Universitätsbibliothek, Bibliotheca Amploniana, Cod. Amplon. 4° 184, which has a colophon dating it to 1147. (The script shows it originated in Italy.)[46] Though copied later than the Hague manuscript, the Erfurt manuscript has important features that demonstrate that certain aspects of its text are earlier. It is precisely because we have the Hague *Pantegni*, with its clear demonstration of the work's production stages, that we are enabled to identify these earlier, pre-Hague stages.

There are three features that make the Erfurt codex stand out in the broader manuscript tradition. The first relates to the text of the Prologue. The Erfurt manuscript has neither Part A nor Part C; therefore the text in the codex represents the stage before those two framing parts, addressed to Abbot Desiderius, were added by Atto/Theodemar at Monte Cassino. In keeping with that absence, the part of the Prologue that the Erfurt manuscript does have (Part B) begins, 'Cum totius scientie generalitas', whereas the Hague manuscript has, 'Cum totius, Pater, scientiae generalitas'; the Erfurt manuscript lacks 'Pater', the resumptive naming of the addressee Desiderius. In other words, the Hague manuscript has all three elements — Part A, the resumptive 'Pater' in Part B, and Part C — that make up the full paraphernalia of dedication. Thus, the Prologue in the Erfurt manuscript appears to antedate the work of Atto/Theodemar.

Moreover, in the Erfurt manuscript, when the rubricator enters the incipit at the top of fol. 2^{r}, he writes 'Incipit liber pantegni a domno con-

[46] The Erfurt manuscript catalogue also identifies its origins in Italy. See Schum, *Beschreibendes Verzeichnis*, p. 441.

stantino translatus' (Here begins the book of the *Pantegni* translated by lord Constantine). Constantine is not given his full name. That full name 'Constantinus Africanus' appears in Part A of the Prologue, which is, as noted, omitted on this page of the *Erfurtensis*. Additionally, Constantine is not identified as a monk in the incipit. Furthermore, no connection with Monte Cassino is mentioned. Perhaps most surprisingly of all, he is called 'domnus Constantinus', a term that suggests a layman. These elements are strange indeed.

Just beneath the incipit stand the *capitula*, and these lack the mention of the 'Prologus' found in the Hague manuscript. Furthermore, the *capitula* that are present are not yet numbered, as they are in the Hague manuscript. In this respect, there are divergences; while some twelfth-century *Pantegni* manuscripts lack those numbers, most of the manuscripts from that century do contain them in the hand of the scribe or rubricator, though the exact numbering may vary. There are several copies made before 1150: Hildesheim, Dombibliothek, Hs 748 (*c.* 1125); Paris, BnF, Latin 6887 (*c.* 1100); Cambridge, Trinity College, MS R.14.34 (*c.* 1100–*c.* 1150); London, BL, MS Additional 22719 (*c.* 1100– *c.* 1150); and Oxford, Magdalen College, MS 51 (*c.* 1125–*c.* 1150).[47]

Beyond this, in Erfurt, Universitätsbibliothek, Bibliotheca Amploniana, Cod. Amplon. 4° 184, beneath the *capitula*, the initial **C** ('Cum totius') of the Prologue holds a stunning portrait of Constantine (or conceivably of his source, the author of the Arabic original). He is not dressed as a monk. He is a layman; in fact, dress and complexion are those of an African (cover image).

These elements paint a consistent and strikingly different picture: the Constantine of incipit, Prologue, and portrait is no monk. He is a layman. He has no connection with Monte Cassino. In fact, he is depicted in his native North-African gown, even though he does not have the name, 'Africanus', in the incipit. The stage represented by the text and the *capitula*, a stage of incompleteness *vis-à-vis* the forms found in the Hague manuscript, corresponds to an earlier stage in Constantine's career and work as we know it. Notably, if

[47] There are additional copies from the twelfth century containing *capitula* numbers: Hamburg, Staats- und Universitätsbibliothek, Cod. med. 228 (*c.* 1150–*c.* 1200); Florence, Laurenziana, MS Antinori 20 (late twelfth century); and Munich, Staatsbibliothek, Clm 9561 (late twelfth century). There are no numbered *capitula* in Basel, Universitätsbibliothek, MS D. III. 17 (*c.* 1100–*c.* 1150) which is perhaps incomplete, as it appears to lack rubrication, nor in Berlin, SBPK, MS lat. fol. 74 (1150–1200); nor Turin, Biblioteca Nazionale Universitaria, I.VI.24 (twelfth century).

Constantine was not at this time at Monte Cassino, he was still a layman and still in Salerno. This opens a completely new perspective on the genesis of this text. Without our understanding of the Hague manuscript and its manifest stages of production, it would be impossible to grasp this earlier, pre-Cassinese (and pre-Hague) stage of production in the Erfurt manuscript.

It is also curious that in the same Erfurt manuscript the scribe of the main text has added a note on an empty flyleaf (fol. 1^{v}), in the front of the codex and facing the beginning of the text on fol. 2^{r}. It is plain that the several matters of the note had not been available to the Erfurt scribe when he was initially copying the *Theorica*. Indeed, it seems probable that these notes were gleaned from some other manuscript, where they were probably jotted in the margins of the main text, but were combined into one collapsed notation by the Erfurt scribe.[48] It is not unlikely that either Constantine or a member of his circle in Salerno had jotted just such a note into the margin of Prologue Part B, that is, the section where the obscurity of Hippocrates and the confusing sophistic of Galen are detailed.[49] The texts of neither one ancient authority nor the other was sufficient to provide the best, clearest, and most thorough training for physicians. Nor did the Byzantine encyclopaedists do better; as Constantine perceived it, it was the *Pantegni* that would help fill that niche, even though translation of Arabic guides to understanding Galen's *Tegni* were also considered fundamental.[50] Moreover, the acknowledgement of Arabic authors present in the Erfurt note was something Constantine sometimes undertook while in Salerno, but appears to have abandoned altogether upon his arrival at Monte Cassino. These aspects point to the general contents of the Erfurt note as having originated in Salerno.

For our purposes, the most interesting aspect of the Erfurt note is that it addresses the absence of the *Pantegni* Prologue Parts A and C in the text that follows, as well as the role of the archbishop of Salerno as an early patron of

48 It may be significant that this scribe produced more than one copy of medical texts from Salerno; the same scribe is thought to have copied another surviving Salernitan text, the *Passionarius* of Gariopontus of Salerno, extant in Erfurt, Universitätsbibliothek, Bibliotheca Amploniana, Cod. Amplon. 4° 202. See Schum, *Beschreibendes Verzeichniss*, p. 460, and Glaze, 'Gariopontus and the Salernitans', p. 186. Might this scribe also have had access to a copy of the *Isagoge* with this brief introduction to the *Isagoge* in it?

49 On Prologue Part B, see Chapter 3 at p. 106 and Appendix C.

50 Both Cassinese accounts of Constantine's translations include the *Tegni*. The oldest manuscript of the *Tegni* in Latin, which dates from the last quarter of the eleventh century, will be examined in a future study.

Constantine's.[51] For example, the note calls attention to the absence of Part A and Part C of the Prologue and gives this explanation: 'Hic prologus debet esse in principio et est secundum Constantinum' (This Prologue should stand at the beginning, and it is according to Constantine). After this follows the address of Constantine to Abbot Desiderius (Prologue Part A), albeit in an abbreviated form. What is even more surprising is what then follows: a brief discussion that appears to concern the origins of the *Isagoge* or *Tegni* commentary (rather than the origins of the *Pantegni*), which is said to be the Prologue of none other than Archbishop Alfanus.[52]

> Gallienus locuturus de medicina libellum suum composuit quem intitulavit *Tegni.* Ad quem Iohannicius quidam, utraque lingua peritus videlicet greca et arabica, *Librum Ysagogarum* conposuit [...] [*lacunam indicav. F. Newton*] per quendam philosophum *Tegni* exponentem [exponente *E*] arabice, nomine Razis. A quo

[51] Burnett, 'Encounters with Rāzī the Philosopher', pp. 973–92.

[52] The same brief text appears in two thirteenth-century manuscripts: Gloucester, Cathedral Library, MS 17 (G), like the twelfth-century Erfurt, Universitätsbibliothek, Bibliotheca Amploniana, Cod. Amplon. 4° 184 (E) containing the *Theorica* alone; and Paris, BnF, Latin 6886 (P), containing both the *Theorica* and the *Practica*. The Gloucester manuscript is very similar to the Erfurt one in presenting a text that is earlier than that found in the Hague volume; (a) it lacks Prologues A and C; (b) Prologue B begins 'Cum totius scientie generalitas' (not including the address, 'pater'); (c) Prologue B ends, 'Gallienus et alii quidam in acuta egritudine mellitam dant aquam', not including the last three sentences of Prologue B as found in the Hague manuscript (see Appendix C for the text and translation of the Prologue in the Hague manuscript); (d) the list of capitula, which follows Prologue B has only twenty-four chapters, not including therefore the first chapter 'Prologus', listed in the Hague manuscript. We are greatly indebted to the study of this passage in Burnett, 'Encounters with Rāzī the Philosopher', especially pp. 976–79. See also the reading of Jordan, 'The Fortune of Constantine's *Pantegni*', p. 294 n. 28. As will be clear, we do not however concur with Burnett in understanding the 'Razis' treatise to have been the Latin *Pantegni*; we understand it to have been a brief exposition of the *Tegni*, with a prologue by Alfanus. This work of Rāzī's is not otherwise mentioned in Europe in the eleventh and twelfth centuries (a modern edition and translation of the work from Arabic into Spanish is available in Vázquez de Benito, *Libro de la introduccion*; we thank Grigory Kessel for the reference). The presence of this reference lends credibility and importance to the entire 'Gallienus locuturus' passage. This passage was certainly not a letter of introduction for Constantine; this misinterpretation of Creutz's is laid out by Bloch, *Monte Cassino in the Middle Ages*, p. 101 and n. 1. Nevertheless, the instinct to attribute it to Alfanus is sound; it is compatible with his style (note the paronomasia in *legi*/ *intellegi*). The following edition of the 'Gallienus locuturus' passage presents significant readings from all three manuscripts, and includes emendations by the editor; the punctuation and capitalization are modernized. For Creutz's erroneous interpretation, see Creutz, 'Additamenta zu Konstantinus Africanus', pp. 420–42.

brevitate comitante [comitante *G*, communicante *P*, *om. E*] sententias quasdam accepit, ex quibus *Libellum Ysagogarum* instituit. Cuius libellus sine *Ysagogys* [Ysagoys *E*] legi quidem poterat, sed intelligi nullatenus. Liber Razis nec uno momento [nec unmomento *E*, nec in momento *G*, vero immomento *P*, *em. F. N.*] prolixus. Arabice quidem institutus et in Latinitate quoque [in Latinum utcumque *E*, in Latinitate cumque *G*, in Latinitate quod *P*, *em. F.N.*] translatus, sic incipit. 'Hic est prologus archiepiscopi Salernitani' [Hic –Salernitani *E*, *om. GP*] (fol. 1^{v}).

(When Galen was preparing to speak of medicine, he composed his little book, to which he gave the title *Tegni*. For this a certain Johannicius, skilled in both languages, namely Greek and Arabic, composed a *Book of Introductions* [...] through [?] a certain philosopher who was expounding the *Tegni* in Arabic, by name Rāzī. From it he [Rāzī] took certain passages with a brevity to match, out of which he made up the *Little Book of Introductions*. His [Galen's] little book could be *read* without the *Introductions*, but it could certainly not be *understood*. The book of Rāzī is not even for a single moment wordy. Being produced in Arabic and also translated into Latin, it begins this way. 'This is the prologue of the archbishop of Salerno.')

After this, the note ends with Part C of the *Pantegni* Prologue. This passage added to the Erfurt manuscript as a discussion of various texts underscores the truth that Galen's *Tegni*, though a much briefer work than the *Pantegni*, was considered a difficult text to understand; the best guide to grasping Galen's meanings, both in the Islamic world and in the Latin West, was to study first the introductory book produced in the ninth century by Ḥunayn ibn Isḥāq.[53] The difficulties Constantine faced in producing a final, complete translation of

[53] Pormann and Savage-Smith, *Medieval Islamic Medicine*, p. 68, note that Ḥunayn had originally produced two versions of his introductory text to help students better comprehend the *Tegni*; the first was discursive, an *Introduction to Medicine*, while the second was erotematic, a *Questions on Medicine for Beginners*. The former, discursive version, they say, and not the question-and-answers version, provided the source from which the Latin *Isagoge* was produced. In the Arabic tradition, already by *c.* 1050 CE, Ḥunayn's text had become the subject of pedagogical commentary. The Latin *Isagoge* consequently became the first text in the Salernitan canon known as the *Ars medica* or *Articella*, and was soon being commented upon by Salernitan masters in the twelfth century. Elsewhere, it is noted that Ḥunayn's Arabic text had undergone abridgement already in the early eleventh century CE in North Africa; see the World Digital Library, 'Medical Questions', describing London, Wellcome Library, Arabic MS 258. In twelfth-century Salerno, the relationship between the *Isagoge*, the *Tegni*, the *Pantegni*, the *Megategni*, and the *Microtegni*, and the meanings of the titles of each, was explained by Master Bartholomaeus; see *Medieval Medicine*, ed. and trans. by Wallis, p. 157. We are grateful to Professor Wallis for sharing with us a plate of the Winchester manuscript preserving Bartholomaeus's commentary on the *Isagoge*.

Ḥunayn's text are manifest, as we have seen, in the two surviving, early-stage, and incomplete versions produced by scribes at Monte Cassino, now Monte Cassino, MS 225 and Paris, BnF, NAL 1628 (discussed above). Monte Cassino, MS 225, though the main text is not copied by a scribe trained at the abbey, nonetheless has the title *Liber isagogarum*, 'The Book of Introductions', written in a Cassinese hand.[54] In this, it echoes and validates the Erfurt note's use of that title. More notable still, this 'Gallienus locuturus' text added to the Erfurt manuscript bears a reference to Salerno and to Constantine's patron there, which is yet again a pointer to that city: like the pre-monastic, Salernitan status of Constantinus adumbrated in the incipit and portrait of the Erfurt manuscript. Significantly, another Erfurt manuscript (Erfurt, Universitätsbibliothek, Bibliotheca Amploniana, Cod. Amplon. 8° 62, early fourteenth century), contains a brief account of Constantine and Alfanus in a commentary on his *Dietae universales* by Master Mattheus F[errarius] of Salerno. In this account it is stated that Archbishop Alfanus wished to cover the cost of Constantine's completing the *Pantegni*.[55] It has never been explained why Alfanus (in Salerno) wished to provide funds for the completion of the *Pantegni* (at Monte Cassino). This is a third link between Constantine's early work on the *Pantegni* and the city of Salerno.

What does all this mean? To sum up, every aspect of the first text page of Erfurt, Cod. Amplon. 4° 184 points to a stage in Constantine's life when he was neither monk nor at Monte Cassino. In fact, this layman with the African dress and countenance would have then been working on his translation of the *Pantegni* in Salerno. This fits with the reference in the same manuscript, in the flyleaf addition, to 'the archbishop of Salerno', who could be none other than Alfanus. In another source, Erfurt, Cod. Amplon. 8° 62, Alfanus took an interest in the completion of that work. There is, moreover, another striking parallel between the text in the Hague manuscript and Erfurt, Cod. Amplon. 4° 184. As has been noted in Chapter 3, *Theorica* book III is missing a rubric for the chapter on sperm, 'De spermate', while this chapter is also missing from the *capitula* list of book III. In the Hague manuscript at fol. 19^{v} a space is reserved for a rubric, but it was never entered. The same is seen in the Erfurt manuscript, where at fol. 37^{r} a space is left for the rubric, but the rubric itself is not filled in. This final observation draws the Erfurt manuscript close to the lost Ur-text

[54] Plates of the opening leaves of both copies produced at Monte Cassino can be found in Newton, 'Constantine the African', figs 1 and 2, pp. 43–44.

[55] See pp. 183–84 in the present volume.

of the *Pantegni*, the early-stage exemplar also used to produce the Hague manuscript. In some other early manuscripts of the *Theorica*, like Hildesheim, Dombibliothek, Hs 748, the rubric *has* been filled in by the original rubricator ('De spermate et formatione pueri', fol. 22^v^). In other words, the missing rubric in Erfurt, Cod. Amplon. 4° 184, supports the view that this text is an early version, thereby legitimizing the information on its flyleaf pertaining to Constantine working in Salerno with his patron, the archbishop.

All this makes it highly probable that the translation of the *Pantegni* was advanced in Salerno to a large extent, with remaining problems ultimately resolved at Monte Cassino. This conclusion could only be reached because, as we have shown, the Hague manuscript sheds light on an early, but final stage of the text of the *Theorica*, as it was completed at Monte Cassino. The fact that the same Hague manuscript shows how two key additions to the Prologue were added during Constantine's stay at Monte Cassino (Parts A and C), among the enigmas with which this study began, and copied by known Cassinese scribes, opens the door to the explanation as to why the earlier stage of the text, attested by Erfurt, Cod. Amplon. 4° 184, will not have contained these components, and will therefore have been undertaken elsewhere: namely in Salerno.

Such is the Salernitan stage in the genesis of the *Theorica Pantegni*. The subsequent phase occurred at Monte Cassino. If our reconstruction above is correct, our newly gained view of the very earliest version of the *Pantegni* (that is, from the time before it became a Monte Cassino project) allows us to assess what precisely was done with the text in the abbey. First, the eloquent address to Abbot Desiderius (Part A) was added by Atto/Theodemar, identifying the translator from the start by his full name, Constantinus Africanus.[56] Moreover, it was only at Monte Cassino that a chapter heading was added to the *capitula* of book I ('Prologus') and the Hague Rubricator added chapter numbers (now twenty-five of them), as well as in all other books of the *Theorica*. The same rubricator also added the tailpiece to the Prologue (Part C) beginning 'Vobis autem', but did not put a title or *incipit* at the head of the text. Even though in Salerno the text was already named *Pantegni* (for this is what the work is called in the heading at the top of fol. 2^r^ in Erfurt, Cod. Amplon. 4° 184), it was nameless in Monte Cassino. Interestingly, with the disappearance of the title also vanished the qualifier 'translator', mentioned in the same Erfurt manuscript with its pre-Cassinese heading. This is the problem to which we now turn.

[56] In the Erfurt manuscript, Constantine identified himself within the *accessus* at fol. 3^v^: 'Est ergo constantinus africanus auctor quia ex multorum libris coadunator'.

Attribution and Misattribution

The incipit of the Erfurt manuscript of the *Pantegni* is not the only incipit that specifies that Constantine was a translator. Several other *Pantegni* manuscripts are similar in this respect:

1. Erfurt, Universitätsbibliothek, Bibliotheca Amploniana, Cod. Amplon. 4° 184, fol. 2r: 'Incipit liber Pantegni a domno Constantino translatus'.
2. Hildesheim, Dombibliothek, Hs 748, fol. 1r: 'Incipit liber Pantegni a Constantino Affricano translatus'.
3. BAV, Vat. Lat. 2356, fol. 1r: 'Incipit liber Panthegni a Constantino montis cassinensis monacho translatus'.
4. BAV, Vat. lat. 2457, fol. 1r: 'In Christi nominee incipit liber Pantegni, id est, tota ars. Nomen auctoris est Rasis. Nomen translatoris est Constantinus'.[57]

These forms of the incipit belong together, with the Erfurt manuscript having the Ur-form. As argued above, the Erfurt text represents the translation as far as it was completed at Salerno. It was only as the text was read aloud and copied out at Monte Cassino that Constantine and his team became aware of potential problems in the grammar and terminology that made lacunae necessary in the ongoing finalization of the text. As noted, the incipit openly proclaims that Constantine was the translator, whereas in the majority of *Pantegni* manuscripts, Constantine is named as author, or his authorship was at least implied.[58] What is particularly interesting is that the same incipit formula appears in at least two other manuscripts of Constantine's works:

1. BAV, Urb. lat. 1415, fol. 1v: 'In Christi nomine. Incipit liber de urina translatus a Constantino Africano in Latinam linguam ab Arabica'.
2. Padua, Biblioteca Universitaria, lat. 892, fol. 1v: 'Incipit liber Febrium a domno Constantino Africano translatus'.

Unlike the Erfurt *Pantegni*, these manuscripts of the *De urina* and *De febribus* were copied in the eleventh century, and both are closely tied to South Italy.

[57] For these manuscripts, see Jordan, 'The Fortune of Constantine's *Pantegni*', pp. 293–94.

[58] See Jordan, 'The Fortune of Constantine's *Pantegni*', p. 293. It is noteworthy that in the Erfurt manuscript, the Hague manuscript, and others, Constantine identified himself by name — Constantinus Africanus — in the *accessus*, which appears several folios into the text.

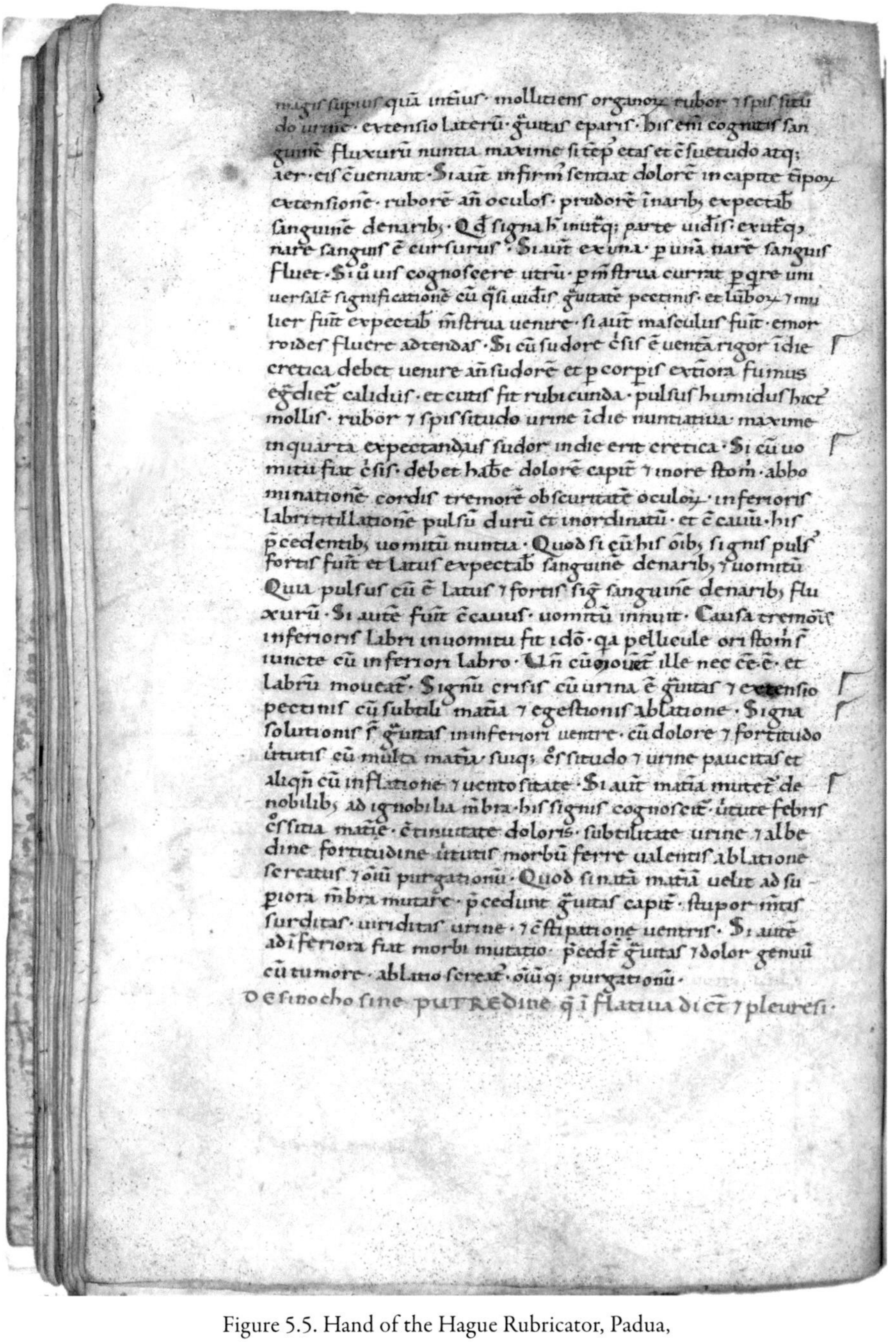

Figure 5.5. Hand of the Hague Rubricator, Padua, Biblioteca Universitaria, lat. 892, fol. 32[v]. *c.* 1075–*c.* 1100. *De febribus*.

The Vatican manuscript has headings (as, for example, this incipit) in eleventh-century Beneventan, as Henry W. Willard first observed, though the text itself is in Caroline minuscule.[59] The Padua manuscript was written by the first scribe of Aberdeen, UL, MS 106 (figs 5.2 and 5.5, and pls XII and XV), who has been identified as the Hague Rubricator, which would make it a product of the Cassinese scriptorium.[60]

As we have already seen, Constantine undertook considerable translation work while still in Salerno, and there are several reasons for considering that *De urina* dates from this same early period. The Salernitan account of Constantine's arrival in that city explicitly attests that it was Constantine's expertise in urinalysis that brought him to the attention of the famous Abbot Johannes de Curte;[61] the same Salernitan source appears to be based in part on the opening of *De urina*. Additionally, the literary style of the preface of this work is so rough that it cannot have been provided at Monte Cassino (as a prologue was for others of his works) by Atto/Theodemar.[62] All this fits with the Vatican manuscript's incipit 'translatus a Constantino' formula, which, as we have seen, is found in the Erfurt manuscript of the *Pantegni*, a form of that text which, we have concluded, dates from Constantine's stay in Salerno. A further anomaly that seems to point to a very early date is that, alone of Constantine's prologues, the Prologue of *De urina* specifically names the author of the Arabic original, 'Isaac son of Solomon, created this in the Arabic language'.[63] In this case, Constantine forthrightly credited his Arabic source.[64]

[59] In the first expansion of Lowe's original list of Beneventan manuscripts (1914), 'A New List of Beneventan Manuscripts', he cites Willard as having called his attention to the volume on p. 241.

[60] See p. 159. It must be emphasized that the ductus of the Aberdeen hand and that of the Padua manuscript do not match precisely. The script in the Aberdeen manuscript is more softly stroked and still has uncial **d**, while that of the Padua manuscript is more brittle and angular. The Tironian note for 'et' is also slightly different. Yet, it remains likely that the two manuscripts were executed by the same scribe, the Hague Rubricator. A different pen will account for some of these differences, but they may also be partly due to a later stage in the scribe's style.

[61] See the Introduction.

[62] See on this 'high-buskined style', pp. 98, 100–05.

[63] 'Fecit eum autem in Arabica lingua filius Salomonis Isaac'. We cannot agree with Bloch's observation, 'he admits that the book depended on a treatise of Isaac' (Bloch, *Monte Cassino in the Middle Ages*, p. 103); in this one treatise, probably his first translation, Constantine boldly and openly asserts (not 'admits') that Isaac was the author.

[64] Compare the opening of the *Pantegni*, where Constantine leaves out the passages from al-Mağūsī's original that named his Arabic sources. See Jacquart, 'Le sens donné par Constan-

On the other hand, in the case of the Padua *De febribus* or *Liber febrium*, the text is preceded by an artistic, elaborate preface addressed to Constantine's student, Johannes. This must be the work of Atto/Theodemar, and thus it was certainly added at Monte Cassino. But that is no bar to *De febribus* being considered an early work from Constantine's stay in Salerno. It is telling that in the Padua manuscript the Prologue precedes the incipit that we have cited above; it seems most likely that the Prologue was composed and added, at the beginning of the whole, without modifying the following 'Salernitan' incipit-formula, which like the Erfurt incipit retains the translator's name as 'domnus Constantinus'. These are the only two cases known to us that identify Constantine the translator as 'domnus'. This mode reflects the fact that at the time of this translation (as with the Erfurt draft of the *Pantegni*) Constantine was still a layman.

By a curious reflex, Constantine's honest, open, formulaic avowal of his work as a translation gave rise to a seriously false attribution.[65] This, we believe, is how it occurred. It seems that in a branch of manuscripts of the *Pantegni* in which the early formula 'translatus a Constantino' was found, this formula elicited from a reader a query, which we reconstruct in this fashion: 'If Constantine was only the translator of this masterly treatise, the *Pantegni*, who then was the original author?' Now in Erfurt, Cod. Amplon. 4° 184, where the simplest, probably Ur-form of this incipit-formula occurs, and which shows the earliest currently known form of the text of the *Pantegni*, on the flyleaf facing the opening text page is the brief text beginning 'Gallienus locuturus'. This obscure little paragraph, the text of which we have just given, discusses the origins of the *Isagoge* and *Tegni*, and speaks of the teacher Rāzī as having had a role in adapted versions of its transmission. The probability is that our hypothetical reader, pondering the above hypothetical question, plucked the name of Rāzī out of the facing curious little passage (it is the only Arabic name visible anywhere in the manuscript) and added it to the incipit.[66] This combination, of the

tin l'Africain', pp. 71–89. For the *Isagoge*, the author is called 'Iohannitius', a Graeco-Latinized adaptation of Ḥunayn ibn Isḥāq, meaning 'John, son of Isaac'. See the Cassinese accounts of the texts Constantine is said to have translated in Appendix B.

[65] On the early manuscripts and Constantine as translator, see Jordan 'The Fortune of Constantine's *Pantegni*', pp. 293–94; on p. 293, Jordan says, 'Many copies say nothing, but some of the earliest are quite careful in noting that Constantine is only a translator'.

[66] On titles subsequently added to Monte Cassino texts in manuscripts in which the original scribe/rubricator did not supply an author or title, see Radding and Newton, *Theology, Rhetoric, and Politics in the Eucharistic Controversy*, pp. 34–40. The subject of that book, the

challenging, question-raising incipit and the small paragraph containing the name of an Arabic medical writer, will, we believe, explain the presence of such incipits as these:

1. Hildesheim, Dombibliothek, Hs 748, fol. 1^{r}: 'Incipit Liber Pantegni. a Constantino Affricano translatus. Nomen auctoris fuit Rasis'.
2. BAV, Vat. lat 2457, fol. 1^{r}: 'In Christi nomine incipit Liber Pantegni, id est, tota ars, nomen auctoris est Rasis. Nomen translatoris est Constantinus'.
3. London, BL, MS Additional 22719, fol. 2^{v}: 'Incipit liber cuius nomen Pan Tegnae, vel Pasa Tegnae, id est tota ars dicitur. Nomen auctoris est Rasis apud grecos'.
4. Paris, BnF, Latin 6887, fol. 1^{r}: 'In Christi nomine incipit liber cuius nomen Pantegne vel Pasategne id est tota ars dicitur. Nomen auctoris est Rasis apud grecos'.[67]

Rāzī, of course, had nothing to do with the *Pantegni*, nor its source-text, al-Mağūsī's *Kitāb Kāmil aṣ-ṣinā'a aṭ-ṭībbiya*. The error arises from the little note attested in the Erfurt manuscript, and occasionally elsewhere. In this connection, it has been suggested that the phrase 'apud grecos' found in the above-listed London and Paris manuscripts might refer to Rāzī's reputation in Greek lands.[68] It seems more likely, inasmuch as the phrase occurs in two incipits in which the title 'Pantegni' is explained as 'Pasa Tegni', that the expression 'apud grecos' in the text of the incipit has been accidentally displaced from its original location beside the Greek words by the insertion of the phrase 'Nomen auctoris est Rasis' at the wrong point in the text. The original order would therefore have been, 'Pasa Tegni apud Graecos' (The Whole Art, according to the Greeks).

Conclusion: The Campaign and its Expense

In the narrative that we have presented, the story of Constantine's historic achievement has two parts and two geographical contexts. The work began at

treatise found only in Aberdeen, UL, MS 106, provides a precise parallel to a later scribe's hastily reading the opening sentences of an unattributed text and drastically misunderstanding the facts; the treatise is an attack upon the teachings of Berengar, but the writer of the heading ascribes the treatise to Berengar!

67 Jordan, 'The Fortune of Constantine's *Pantegni*', pp. 293–94.

68 See the useful discussion of Burnett, 'Encounters with Rāzī the Philosopher', pp. 973–92.

Salerno, the powerful, rich, and charming city described in all the sources as Constantine's first home in Italy. It is now clear that Constantine must have begun his great translation work there; in addition to *De urina* and *De febribus*, he would also have completed all, or a great part of, the *Theorica* of the *Pantegni* there. The rest of the tale takes place at Monte Cassino. It is here in St Benedict's own foundation, incredibly enlarged and enriched by its brilliant Abbot Desiderius, that Constantine revised his *Pantegni*, dedicating it to the 'Pater' who had received him so warmly.

What is curious is that, in the most reliable sources for the conditions in both seats of learning, one finds a striking detail that has never received sufficient attention. In the case of Salerno, the source is the account of Constantine's arrival in Salerno in the valuable and interesting passage of Mattheus F[errarius] in Erfurt, Cod. Amplon. 8° 62. This, the most reliable Salernitan source that we have about Constantine, ends with the sentence: 'Archiepiscopus Alfanus pro integratione Practica Pantegni expensas ei erogare voluit' (Archbishop Alfanus wished to pay his costs for completing the *Practica* of the *Pantegni*). It has been suggested that Alfanus wished to pay for procuring a copy of the full text of the *Practica* from Africa or from another source in the Islamic world.[69] The sentence is among the most enigmatic in all of our Constantine narratives.

The most trustworthy source for our knowledge of Constantine at Monte Cassino, the account of Leo Marsicanus or his successor Guido,[70] begins in this way: 'Istius porro abbatis tempore Constantinus Africanus ad hunc locum perveniens, sanctaeque habitum religionis induens, ecclesiam S. Agathae in Aversa a Richardo principe sibi concessam in hoc sancto loco devotissimus optulit' (In the time of this abbot, Constantine the African, coming to this place and donning the habit of a holy religious life, with deep devotion offered [to St Benedict] in this holy place the church of St Agatha in Aversa turned over to him by Prince Richard [of Capua]). This statement too is enigmatic, and strange. It has been suggested that the 'endowment' was an act of honour to Constantine, probably from a grateful patient (Richard of Capua) for a medical intervention by Constantine,[71] and this continues to seem a highly probable interpretation. But it remains incongruous. Constantine is the only intellectual among the distinguished figures described in the *Chronicle of Monte Cassino*

[69] See the Introduction of the present volume.

[70] On the reliability of this account, and its near-contemporary character, see pp. 103–04.

[71] Newton, 'Arabic Medicine and Other Arabic Cultural Influences in Southern Italy in the Time of Constantinus Africanus', pp. 40–43.

who is so endowed.[72] The statement, thrust forward to the very beginning of the Constantine section, is a stunning anomaly.

Two anomalies, then, are found: one in Salerno and one in Monte Cassino, in the two chapters of Constantine's life in Italy. As far as we know, the parallel has never been noticed, much less explained. But, viewed as a pair, the anomalies share an essential feature, which was economic: who was paying for the costs, the *expensae*, of these undertakings? In both phases it was remembered, in the most reliable source for Constantine's sojourn at Salerno and that at Monte Cassino, that Constantine's larger translation programme was a costly operation. In both places, a subvention was needed, that contemplated by Archbishop Alfanus in Salerno, and that actually provided by Prince Richard to Monte Cassino.[73]

In the present study, it has become abundantly clear that the work of producing translations of the *Pantegni* and the twenty-three (or more) other works was a task of multiple stages. Each work required a number of separate operations: copying the new translations, perhaps in various stages of completion, from wax tablets to *schedulae*, then from *schedulae* to parchment quires, and finally from these to a dedication copy. Many of these stages were never completed, as in the Paris *Isagoge* or indeed the Hague *Pantegni*. They required fresh supplies of parchment for a single work; parchment was a valuable resource,[74] as were ink, pens, and bindings.[75] And some of these separate works were long texts; just the *Theorica* of the *Pantegni* itself consisted of ten books. The whole was a vast undertaking. The two sentences, in the Salerno source and in the Monte Cassino one, reflect each community's memory of the enormous effort of it all.

With the economic factor in mind, one may summarize the narrative baldly in some such fashion as this: (a) at Salerno Constantine found as sponsors Abbot Johannes de Curte and Archbishop Alfanus, and began his translation

[72] *Chronica monasterii Casinensis*, ed. by Hoffmann, III.35, pp. 410–12. On a different case of Prince Richard of Capua's donation to Abbot Desiderius and Monte Cassino, all of it recorded by a secular scribe, see fig. 5.6, pl. XVI, and p. 189.

[73] In the case of individual manuscripts, we have been informed of an individual person who was the financial backer; for Monte Cassino, MS 99, see our discussion of Johannes Marsicanus above, p. 152.

[74] It may be estimated from commercially-made books in the Later Middle Ages that parchment constituted between 15 and 20 per cent of the cost. See Kwakkel, 'Commercial Organization and Economic Innovation', p. 183.

[75] On these expenses, see Clanchy, *From Memory to Written Record*, pp. 122–25.

project with such works as the *De urina* and the greatest part of the *Pantegni*, but Salernitan resources, both in money and in availability of a well-trained pool of scribes, proved inadequate for such an enormous job; (b) Prince Richard of Capua, perhaps moved by some medical intervention of Constantine's that benefitted his family or household, provided a subvention in the form of the gift of the church of St Agatha at Aversa; and, (c) with this gift in hand Constantine assumed the habit and entered the monastery of Monte Cassino, where he was warmly welcomed by Abbot Desiderius and where he found a strong support system, indeed a whole team of able scribes and also at least one eloquent advisor in Latin style, and pursued his grand undertaking for the remainder of his life.

The blunt sentences about financial matters stand out like a sore thumb in the medieval narratives of Constantine the African's arrival in Italy. It is true that the body of his work was huge. It was also unprecedented in medieval Europe. For centuries before this, from virtually the beginning of the Middle Ages, learning had been in the hands of monastic communities, and one can trace great copying projects or campaigns in such communities over those centuries. But nowhere before this is it recorded that a single centre, in the space of a single generation, deliberately embarked upon an undertaking so vast, and so new in kind. What is new is the production of a great body of secular texts in a single discipline within the *artes*. Down to this point we have seen this effort only in the case of religious texts, for example, in the campaign of monks of Monte Cassino, in Desiderius's time, to assemble a very large corpus of texts by Augustine.[76] (Many of these texts also go back to North Africa!)[77] With Constantine's medical translations, studied in this book, we see a similar campaign to produce copies of a single author. Yet there are a number of important differences: this campaign is focused upon a house author; the house author was a specialist and concentrated upon a secular, rather than religious, genre; in fact, among the secular *artes*, his specialty was medicine alone, and not just the copying of medicine, but the translating of it. Constantine's work went through the complex, multi-stage process that was the very difficult work of translation; this complex process required backing on a scale that seems to have been unprecedented.

If we return to read once again our main Monte Cassino source for the Desiderian age, the abbey's *Chronicle*, which has been repeatedly invoked in this study, the singularity of Constantine and his achievement stands out. In

[76] Newton, *Scriptorium and Library*, pp. 80–85, 251–52.

[77] Newton, *Scriptorium and Library*, pp. 319–23.

the chapter that describes the four great writers of that age, Alberic, Alfanus, Amatus, and Constantine,[78] the last is not only the climactic figure, but his notice is longer than the other three notices put together. He also stands out in another way: whereas the first three were generalists writing in a wide range of genres — prose and poetry, sacred and secular — Constantine, in contrast, focused upon a single *ars*: he was a specialist. His immense accomplishment was concentrated upon the great tradition that goes back to Hippocrates and Galen.

What the present study illuminates most of all, however, is the effort of Desiderian scribes. The present study has sought to show, in concrete ways, a side of the Monte Cassino scriptorium scarcely investigated before: Constantine's achievement could not have occurred without the team of scribes that carried out the work. More importantly, at Monte Cassino, alongside the well-known and studied team of scribes that produced the glorious liturgical books such as Monte Cassino, MS 99 (Leo's Homiliary of 1072) and BAV, Vat. lat. 1202 (the lectionary that celebrated the completion of the basilica and atrium complex in 1075) in the beautiful new Desiderian form of Beneventan script, there existed a second team of scribes engaged in creating volumes of learning in the *artes*, and this latter team can be observed at work in Constantine's service. Some of the scribes on whom these medical book projects depended wrote an unorthodox, non-Cassinese form of Beneventan, while others wrote the alien Caroline minuscule; most surprising of all, some wrote both, even on the same page.[79] Despite their palaeographical anomalies, the latter group of scribes produced books that would ultimately help transform the study of medicine in twelfth- and thirteenth-century Europe. These hitherto unsung, humble scribes, working under the auspices of the elite of church or state, are the heroes of this revolution.

As this book has shown, it is at Monte Cassino that, for the first time, we can identify and give names, or at least titles, of these men. Their *labor* (the Latin word expressing the toil of copying) made possible the fulfilment of Constantine's vast project. Our roll-call of Cassinese scribes enlisted in this

[78] *Chronica monasterii Casinensis*, ed. by Hoffmann, III.35, pp. 410–12.

[79] On Caroline minuscule in the Beneventan zone, see Brown, '"Where Have All the Grammars Gone?"', pp. 404–09, and in her valuable appendix, a list of grammatical manuscripts (pp. 410–14), with a separate list of grammatical texts 'in Caroline minuscule with Beneventan associations' on p. 414. For earlier bibliography on the subject, see her n. 37 on p. 407. It is Brown's conclusion that 'towards the end of the eleventh century, Caroline minuscule came to be regarded at Montecassino as a more suitable vehicle for grammatical texts' (p. 409).

cause includes Geraldus, the Hague Rubricator, the Bodleian Juvenal Scribe, and the Apuleius Rubricator. Alongside these scribes stands the skilled Atto/Theodemar, who adorned Constantine's works with prose prefaces in the 'high-buskined style'.

Behind Constantine and the assembled team that helped him in his endeavour, stood the towering figures of their secular backers. They were, above all, Normans. According to the *Chronicle of Monte Cassino*, the greatest of the Norman magnates, Duke Robert Guiscard, held Constantine 'in great honour'.[80] The two would have met, in the estimation of Hoffmann, upon Guiscard's capture of Salerno in 1076.[81] Given the dynastic complexities, he would also have known Guiscard's wife, Sikelgaita, who was the sister of the last Lombard ruler of Salerno, Gisulf II, and also of Johannes, 'Abbas de Curte'.[82] And this is only the beginning of the nexus. These were some of the *committenti*, the visionaries whose *studium* (the Latin word that summed up their interest and active support)[83] made possible this great leap forward in the intellectual history of Europe.

It was another prince of the new Norman hegemony who took the critical step. Before his death in 1078, Prince Richard of Capua endowed Constantine with the church of St Agatha in Aversa which, upon his entry into Monte Cassino, Constantine turned over to the abbey; this provided the solution to the financial problem that looms so large in both the Salerno and Monte Cassino accounts of his coming. In turn, Richard's son, Prince Jordan, confirmed the gift in a document of 22 February 1086 that is still preserved at Monte Cassino (Archivio, Aula III, Caps. XI.26).[84] The document states expressly that Jordan acted 'at the intervention of my wife, the Princess Gaitelgrima'. As stated earlier, Gaitelgrima was a Lombard, another sister of Gisulf II, of Abbot Johannes de Curte, and of Robert Guiscard's wife Sikelgaita. In this close-knit web of relationships, it is easy to reconstruct a scenario: if Constantine had carried out a medical intervention for one member of the clan, perhaps for Guiscard (he did hold Constantine 'in great honour') or Sikelgaita, the renown of his skill would

[80] *Chronica monasterii Casinensis*, ed. by Hoffmann, III.35, p. 412.

[81] Hoffmann, 'Der Kalender des Leo Marsicanus', p. 133 n. 36.

[82] Glaze, 'Salerno's Lombard Prince'.

[83] On 'labor' and 'studium' see Newton, 'Leo Marsicanus and the Dedicatory Text and Drawing in Monte Cassino 99', pp. 190–93.

[84] This donation is discussed by Newton, 'Arabic Medicine and Other Arabic Cultural Influences in Southern Italy in the Time of Constantinus Africanus', pp. 40–43.

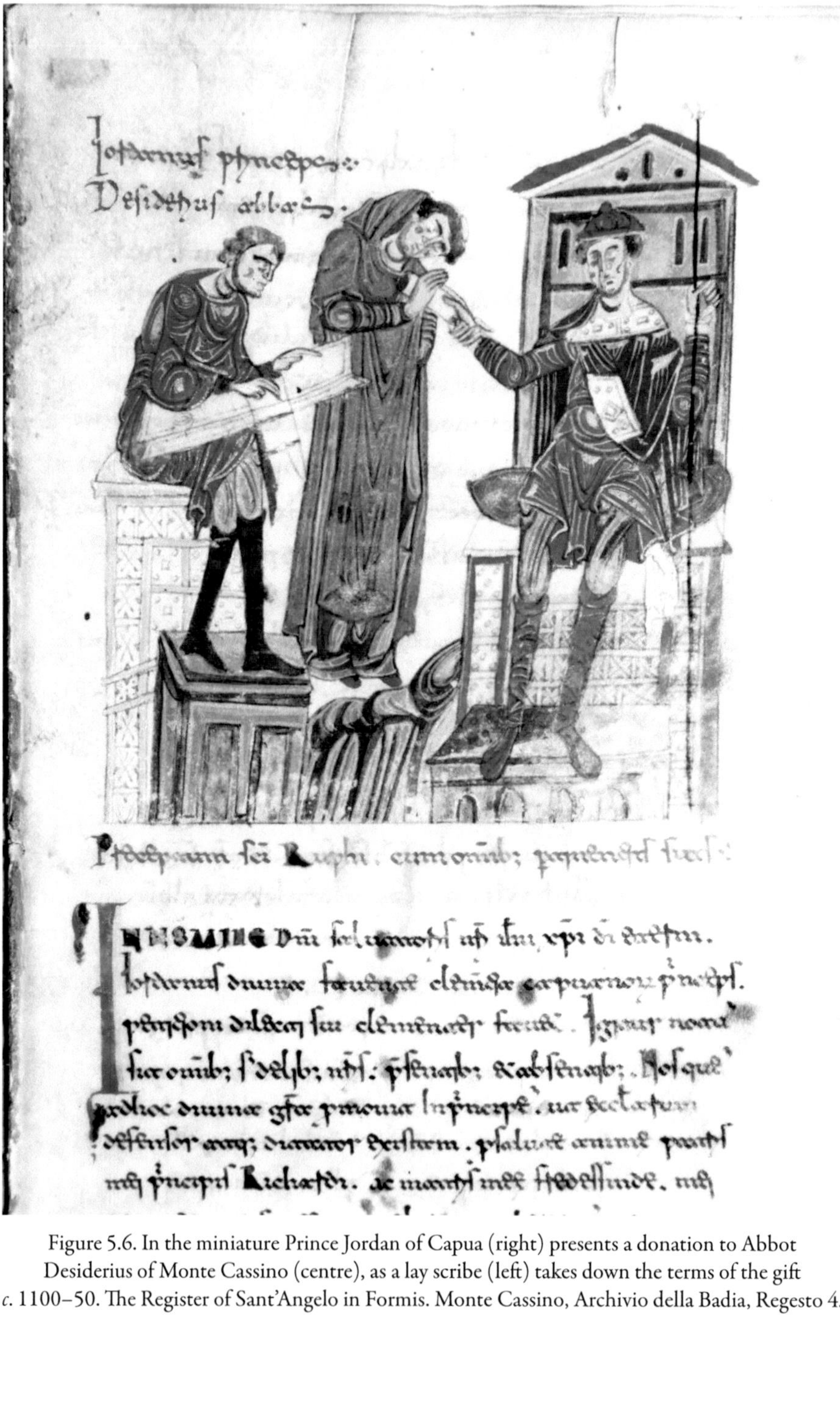

Figure 5.6. In the miniature Prince Jordan of Capua (right) presents a donation to Abbot Desiderius of Monte Cassino (centre), as a lay scribe (left) takes down the terms of the gift *c.* 1100–50. The Register of Sant'Angelo in Formis. Monte Cassino, Archivio della Badia, Regesto 4.

have inevitably spread from palace to palace and would explain Gaitelgrima's 'intervention'.

An image of Jordan's resultant generosity is preserved for posterity in a miniature found in the *Register* of Sant'Angelo in Formis (near Capua), a *c.* 1100–50 manuscript kept, like so much of this monograph's evidence, at Monte Cassino itself (Regesto 4) (fig. 5.6 and pl. XVI).

The miniature depicts, on the right, Prince Jordan of Capua granting a donation (but not the Prince Jordan document that has been linked with Constantine in our study) to Abbot Desiderius of Monte Cassino (centre), while the scribe bends over his writing-board — observe the scribe's bent shoulders, his hand at the ready, and his attentive gaze, as *auditor*, fixed here on the prince's face and his every utterance. Though the miniature stands above the gift of a church of St Ruphus rather than that of St Agatha, the scene is fundamentally important as a paradigm of that Norman's largesse towards the Abbey of Monte Cassino. Jordan, in princely costume, places the document directly in the hands of Desiderius, abbot of Monte Cassino, in modest dress and mien.

It was in the person of Desiderius, of course, that Constantine found the greatest of patrons and *committenti*, Desiderius, the 'bibliophile abbot', who welcomed him warmly into the abbey. In response, Constantine, calling himself 'his [Desiderius's] monk', dedicated the *Pantegni* to his patron, whom he called on the first page of the Hague manuscript 'the preeminent shining jewel of the entire ecclesiastical order'. Alfanus, in Poem 39 quoted earlier in this chapter, described Desiderius as having created a school at Monte Cassino where the teaching of monks could be likened to the polishing of gems. For Constantine and his team, their teacher and model Desiderius, depicted here in his role of humility, was the most polished gem of all.

Appendix A

Description of The Hague, Koninklijke Bibliotheek, MS 73 J 6

Pantegni (Theorica) • Medical Excerpts

Parchment • 89 fols • 235 × 128 mm • 463 grams • Monte Cassino and Southern France • c. 1075–c. 1085 (main text) and c. 1150–c. 1200 (added excerpts)

Genesis and Provenance

MS 73 J 6 is the oldest surviving manuscript of the *Theorica Pantegni*, part of Constantine the African's Latin translation and adaptation of the Arabic *Kitāb Kāmil aṣ-ṣināʿa aṭ-ṭibbīya* (*Complete Book of the Medical Art*) written by the Persian physician ʿAli ibn al-ʿAbbās al-Maǧūsī (d. 982). The codex consists of two codicological units, the second of which contains the *Pantegni*. This unit was produced by Geraldus, a known scribe at Monte Cassino (see Chapter 1), probably under supervision of, or in consultation with Constantine himself (see Chapter 5). After almost a century of use, a second codicological unit was added (now part I). The addition is modest in scope and encompasses a bifolium (fols i–ii) and a singleton attached with glue (fol. iii), both filled with excerpts of a medical nature. The leaves were probably added early in the second half of the twelfth century (*c.* 1150–*c.* 1175), given the date of the earliest writing it contains; Scribe E was likely responsible for the addition. Two scribes in part I present palaeographical features attributable to Southern France, suggesting that the leaves were probably added and filled there (see Chapter 2). Parts I and II remained in use as a single entity through to the present day.

In the thirteenth century the manuscript relocated to Northern France, in or near Arras, given the following note at fol. 89^{r}: 'le samedi deuant le nuit de noel la furent huies mes garsons, wautiers mes wallers. jehans de hersin freres mon segneur Rogier. miles li freres [...]n le blannc le dame de maison. en m[...] aaras. Hues li blains me doit [...] men doit i de goi[s..].' (The Saturday before Christmas night were present: Huies, my servant; Wautier, my friend; John of Hersin, the brother of my lord Rogier; Miles, the brother of [...] le Blanc, the lady of the house; and [...]. Hues le Blanc owes me [...], [...] owes me a [...].)[1] A fifteenth-century hand wrote an ownership description at fol. iii^{v}: 'Iste liber est pro petro de [la ... erased]'. The present binding (red velvet over cardboard) probably dates from the nineteenth century. The manuscript was owned by Joseph Désiré Lupus (d. 1822) of Brussels and was acquired with the rest of his collection in 1819 by King William I of the Netherlands. It was transferred to the Royal Library in 1823.

Part I (fols i–iii): Southern France, *c.* 1150–*c.* 1175

Codicology: Parchment of good quality with horizontal cuts, which were present before Scribe E wrote his text • Quires: Post-medieval flyleaf (unfoliated); 1^{I+1} (fol. iii) (bifolium with a singleton attached to the back, glued) • Page dimensions: 235 × 128 mm (relative dimensions: 0.54) with textblock dimensions of 179 × 105 mm (fol. i^{r}), 200 × 100 mm (fol. i^{v}–ii^{r}) and 180 × 100 mm (fol. ii^{v}) • No pricking or ruling visible, 1 col., 39 (fol. i^{r}) to 44 (fol. ii^{r}) lines • No quire or leaf signatures.

Palaeography: Scribe E (Pregothic script with traits from Southern France (e.g. shape Tironian note and *con* abbreviation), *c.* 1150–*c.* 1175, see pl. IX): main text fols i^{v}–ii^{v}; Scribe F (Pregothic script with the same Southern-French peculiarities as Scribe E, *c.* 1150–*c.* 1175, see fig. 2.15): fol. i^{r}, lines 1–10; Scribe G (Pregothic script, *c.* 1150–*c.* 1175, see fig. 2.15): fol. i^{r}, lines 10–24; Scribe H (Pregothic script, *c.* 1150–*c.* 1175): fol. i^{r}, lines 24–end of page; Scribe I (Pregothic script, *c.* 1200–*c.* 1225, see fig. 2.16): notes in lead point at fol. iii^{r+v}.

Decoration: not present.

[1] Transcription by Ed van der Vlist (The Hague, Koninklijke Bibliotheek), translation by Julia Szirmai (Leiden).

Contents:[2] Excerpt from *Viaticum*, book VII, chapter 21 ('De carbunculis') (fol. i^{r}, lines 1–10); Excerpt from *Viaticum*, book II, chapter 22 ('De gingivis') (fol. i^{r}, lines 10–12); Excerpt from *Viaticum*, book II, chapter 23 ('De fetore oris') (fol. i^{r}, lines 12–22); Extracts from unknown texts on laxative food and drink (fol. i^{r}, line 22 to end of page); *Viaticum*, book III, chapter 6 ('De tussi') (fol. i^{v}, line 1–fol. ii^{v}, line 7); *Viaticum*, book IV, chapter 9 ('De fastidio') (fol. ii^{v}, line 7–fol. ii^{v}, end); Medical notes (fol. iii^{r+v})

Part II (fols 1–89): Monte Cassino, *c.* 1075–*c.* 1085

Codicology: Parchment of medium quality, with some minor holes (e.g. fol. 25), small unrepaired cuts (e.g. fol. 15), translucent patches, some pronounced follicle patterns (so bad at fol. 37^{r} that the scribe avoided the lower part of that page), many pages with visible streaks from the parchmenter's *lunellum*, and with (pre-copying) knife cuts in the parchment (fols 15, 16, 41, 44, 47, 75, and 76) • Quires: 2–11^{IV} (80), 12^{IV+1} (89) • Dimensions: 235 × 128 (189 × 98) mm (relative dimensions: 0.54) • Pricking visible, blind ruling (runs through the gutter), 2 cols, 62 lines (10 lines measure 30 mm in height) • Contemporary bookmark (parchment strip stitched in corner of page) at fol. 29, probably attached to mark the diagram found on fol. 29^{r}; another bookmark was once attached to fol. 82 (imprint remains).

Palaeography: Scribe A [= Geraldus] (Caroline minuscule with Beneventan features (*ri* ligature), *c.* 1075–*c.* 1085, see pl. I): main text fols 1^{r}–85^{r}, including the chapter tables (the main text includes nine lacunae as outlined in Chapter 2); Scribe B [= Hague Rubricator] (Caroline minuscule, *c.* 1075–*c.* 1085, see pl. IX), rubrication in bright red ink at fols 1^{r}–77^{v}; Scribe C (Pregothic script with Beneventan abbreviation for *autem*, *c.* 1150, see pl. VII): main text fols 85^{v}–87^{v}, including text colophon at the end, omitted lines in part of Scribe A (fol. 21^{r}, inner margin; fol. 26^{r}, inner and lower margin; fol. 68^{r}, inner margin), in dark red ink nine rubrics that were not executed by Scribe B (fols 78^{r}–85^{r}), as well as, in brown ink, the text of the rubric at fol. 19^{v} (upper margin, partly cut); Scribe D (Pregothic script, *c.* 1150–*c.* 1200, see pl. VIII): excerpts at fols 87^{v}–88^{r} and at 89^{r}, written down intermittently (duct and ink variation). In addition to these main hands, there are some incidental marginal words throughout main

[2] The identifications from *Viaticum* books III and IV were made by Eliza Glaze, all other by Ed van der Vlist (The Hague, Koninklijke Bibliotheek).

text by other individuals, as well as several pen trials at fol. 89^{r}, the largest one dating to *c.* 1100–*c.* 1125 ('In flumine Jordanis centum scaturigines habentur. | Unus quisque homo centum venas habet. | ita sanguis perficere quod dominus iubet.').

Decoration: initial C at fol. 1^{r} in red and light blue, and with yellow wash, 8 lines in height, in the style of the Beneventan Zone (figure 1.10 and plate V). At various locations in the text tiny drawings of bones are provided within the running text, never taller than a single text line (fol. 7^{v}, col. B, lines 32, 33, 34, and 35; fol. 14^{r}, col. A, line 16, col. B, line 38 and 41; and fol. 17^{r}, col. A, line 35).

Contents: Constantine the African, *Theorica Pantegni* (fols 1^{r}–86^{v}); Excerpts of mostly medical nature (fols 87^{v}–88^{r} and 89^{r})

Appendix B

The Biographies of Constantine the African

Although these biographies have certain elements of the fantastical about them, they share three points between them:

1. Constantine was trained in the medical literature of experts from across the Islamic world, who had composed their texts originally in multiple linguistic traditions;
2. After his arrival in Salerno, Constantine earned the respect and patronage of the local elite;
3. By returning repeatedly to the Arabic sources from which he worked, he effectively transmitted into Latin a vast and varied corpus of both general and highly specialized texts with the overall goal of improving the corpus by which better medical knowledge and practice could be effected.

I. The Monte Cassino Tradition (in Two Forms)

Cas. 1: From Monte Cassino, MS 450 (*c.* 1140–50), pp. 278–79, by Leo Marsicanus or Guido, published in *Chronica monasterii Casinensis*, ed. by Hoffmann, III.35, pp. 411–12. Translated here by Francis Newton. The account of Constantine immediately follows upon the *Chronicle*'s description of the writings of Alberic, Alfanus of Salerno, and Amatus of Monte Cassino. The *Chronicle*'s description of Constantine and his work occupies as many lines by itself as the account of the previous three authors combined.

Istius porro abbatis tempore Constantinus Africanus ad hunc locum perveniens sancteque habitum religionis induens ecclesiam sancte Agathe in Aversa a Richardo principe sibi concessam in hoc sancto loco devotissimus optulit. Necessarium plane videtur ad posterorum memoriam, quantus hic vel qualis fuerit, litteris tradere. Hic igitur e Cartagine, de qua oriundus erat, egrediens Babiloniam petiit, in qua grammatica, dialectica, geometria, arithmetica, mathematica, astronomia nec non et phisica Chaldeorum, Arabum, Persarum, Saracenorum, Egiptiorum ac Indorum plenissime eruditus est. Completis autem in edisscendis istiusmodi studiis triginta et novem annorum curriculis ad Africam reversus est. Quem cum vidissent Afri ita ad plenum omnium gentium studiis eruditum, cogitaverunt occidere eum. Quod Constantinus agnoscens clam navem ingressus Salernum advenit ibique sub specie inopis aliquandiu latuit. Deinde a fratre regis Babiloniorum, qui tunc eo advenerat, agnitus ac in magna honorificentia apud Robbertum ducem habitus est. Exinde vero Constantinus egrediens ad hunc locum pervenit et ordine, quo supra retulimus, monachus factus est. In hoc vero cenobio positus transtulit de diversarum gentium linguis libros quamplurimos, in quibus sunt hi precipui: Pantegnum, quem divisit in libros duodecim, in quo exposuit, quid medicum scire oporteat. Practicam, in qua posuit, qualiter medicus custodiat sanitatem et curet infirmitatem. Librum graduum. Dietam ciborum. Librum febrium, quem de Arabica lingua transtulit. Librum de urina. De interioribus menbris. Viaticum, quem in septem partes divisit, videlicet de morbis in capite nascentibus, dehinc de morbo faciei, de instrumentis, de stomachi et intestinorum infirmatitbus, de languore epatis, renum, vesice, splenis et fellis, de his, que in exteriori cute nascuntur. Expositionem aforismi. Librum tegni, megategni, microtegni, Antidotarium. Disputationem Platonis et Ypocratis in sententiis. De simplici medicamine. De genecia. De pulsibus. De experimentis. Closas herbarum et specierum. De oculis.

In the time of this abbot [Desiderius, abbot 1058–87], Constantinus Africanus, coming to this place and donning the habit of the holy religious life, with deepest devotion presented in this holy place the church of St Agatha in Aversa, which had been granted to him by Prince Richard [of Capua]. It seems altogether necessary to hand down to the memory of future generations a written account of his nature and his greatness. He then, departing from Carthage, where he was born, made his way to Babylonia [Old Cairo], where he received a thorough education in grammar, dialectic, geometry, arithmetic, mathematics, [and] astronomy, as well as in the physic [healing art] of the Chaldaeans, Arabs, Persians, Saracens, Egyptians, and Indians. Now when he had completed thirty-nine years in scholarly studies of this kind, he returned to Africa. When the Africans saw that he was so deeply learned in the fields of study of all nations, they conceived the idea of killing him. Learning this, Constantine secretly embarked on a ship and came to Salerno, and for some time remained hidden there under the guise of a poor man. Thereafter, he was recognized by the brother of the king of the Babylonians, who had come there at the time, and [Constantine] was treated with great honour by Duke Robert

[Guiscard, the Norman conqueror of Salerno in the year 1077]. Then, leaving there, Constantine came to this place [i.e. Monte Cassino], and became a monk, as I have said. And, established in this monastery, he translated out of the languages of diverse peoples a great quantity of books. Among them were these in particular: the *Pantegni*, which he divided into twelve books, in which he set forth what a doctor ought to know; the *Practica*, in which he expounded the means by which a doctor preserves health and cures sickness; the *Book of Degrees*; the *Diet of Food*; the *Book of Fevers,* which he translated from Arabic; the *Book on Urine*; *On the Inner Organs*; the *Viaticum*, which he divided into seven parts, namely, *On Diseases Arising in the Head*, *On Facial Disease*, *On Utensils*, *On Infirmities of the Stomach and Intestines*, *On Affliction of the Liver, Kidneys, Bladder, and Spleen, and Gall-Bladder*; *On Things That Arise without on the Skin*; the *Exposition of the Aphorisms*; the *Book of the Tegni*; *Of the Megategni*; *Of the Microtegni*; the *Antidotarium*; the *Dispute of Plato and Hippocrates on the Sentences*; *On Simple Medicine*; *On Gynaecology*; *On Pulses*; *On Experiments*; *Glosses on Herbs and Spices*; *On Eyes.*

Cas. 2: From Monte Cassino, MS 361 (*c.* 1150), fols 69^{v}–70^{r}, Peter the Deacon, *De viris illustribus*, chap. 23, published in *Monte Cassino in the Middle Ages*, I, ed. by Bloch, pp. 127–28. Translated here by Francis Newton.

XXIIII [*sic*]. Constantinus Africanus eiusdem cenobii monachus omnibus philosoficis studiis plenissime eruditus, Orientis et Occidentis magister, novusque effulgens Hypocras, Cartagine, de qua oriundus erat, egrediens, Babiloniam petiit, in qua grammatica, dialectica, rethorica, geometria, arithmetica, mathematica, astronomia, necromantia, musica, phisicaque Chaldeorum, Arabum, Persarum, Saracenorum plenissime eruditus est. Indeque discendens, Indiam adiit eorumque se studiis erudiendum tradidit. Et dum ad plenum artes edoctus fuisset, Ethyopiam petiit, ibique rursus Ethiopicis disciplinis eruditur. Cumque eorum studiis affatim repletus fuisset, Egiptum profectus est, ibique omnibus Egiptiorum artibus ad plenum instruitur. Completis igitur in ediscendis istemodi studiis triginta et novem annorum curriculis, Africam reversus est. Quem cum vidissent Afri ita ad plenum omnibus gentium studiis eruditum, cogitaverunt occidere eum. Quod Constantinus agnoscens, clam navem ingressus Salernum advenit, ibique sub specie inopis aliquandiu latuit. Deinde a fratre regis Babiloniorum qui tunc ibidem advenerat agnitus, ac in magna honorificentia aput Robertum ducem habitus est. Exinde vero Constantinus egrediens, Casinense cenobium petiit, adque a Desiderio abbate libentissime susceptus, monachus factus est. In eodem vero cenobio positus, transtulit de diversis gentium linguis libros quamplurimos, in quibus precipui sunt hi: Pantegnus (quem divisit in libros XII), in quo exposuit quid medicum scire oporteat. Practicam, in qua posuit, qualiter medicus custodiat sanitatem et curet infirmitatem (quam divisit in libros XII). Librum graduum. Dietam ciborum. Librum febrium, quem de Arabica lingua transtulit. Librum urine. De interioribus membris. De coitu. Viaticum, quem in septem partes divisit: primo de morbis in capite nascentibus; dehinc de morbo faciei; de instrumentis; de stomachi et intestinorum infirmitatibus; de infirmitatibus epatis, renum, vesice, splenis, et fellis; de his que in genitivis membris nascuntur; de omnia que in exteriori cute nascuntur. Expositio Aforismi. Librum Tegni. Megategni. Microtegni. Antidotarium. Disputatio Platonis et Hypocratis in sententiis. De simplici medicamine. De genecia, idest de membris ac corporibus feminarum. De pulsibus. Pronostica. De experimentis. Close herbarum et specierum. Cyrurgia. Librum de medicamine oculorum. Hic vir quadraginta annis in ediscendis diversarum gentium studiis explevit. Novissime vero senex et plenus dierum in Casino obiit. Fuit autem temporibus supradictorum imperatorum.

XXIIII. Constantine the African, a monk of the same monastery [Monte Cassino], most fully educated in all the pursuits of philosophy, master of East and West, and a new brilliant Hippocrates, departing from Carthage, where he was born, made his way to Babylonia [Old Cairo], where he received a thorough education in grammar, dialectic, rhetoric, geometry, arithmetic, mathematics, astronomy, necromancy, music, and the physic [healing art] of the Chaldaeans, Arabs, Persians, [and] Saracens. And, turning south from there, he went to India and devoted himself to instruction in their studies. And when he had been fully trained in the arts, he betook himself to Ethiopia, and there in turn was instructed in the Ethiopian disciplines. And when he had been well filled with their studies, he set out for Egypt and there was fully instructed in all the arts of the Egyptians. Therefore when he had completed thirty-nine years in learning studies of this kind, he returned to Africa. When the Africans saw that he was so deeply learned in the fields of study of all nations, they conceived the idea of killing him. Learning this, Constantine secretly embarked on a ship and came to Salerno, and for some time remained hidden there under the guise of a poor man. Thereafter, he was recognized by the brother of the king of the Babylonians, who had come there at the time, and [Constantine] was treated with great honour by Duke Robert [Guiscard, the Norman conqueror of Salerno in the year 1077]. Then, leaving there, Constantine made for the Cassinese monastery, and was most heartily welcomed by Desiderius the abbot and became a monk. And established in this monastery, he translated out of the languages of diverse peoples a great quantity of books. Among them were these in particular: the *Pantegni*, which he divided into twelve books, in which he set forth what a doctor ought to know; the *Practica*, in which he expounded the means by which a doctor preserves health and cures sickness (which he divided into twelve books); the *Book of Degrees*; the *Diet of Food*; the *Book of Fevers*, which he translated from Arabic; the *Book of Urine*; *On the Inner Organs*; *On Sexual Intercourse*; the *Viaticum*, which he divided into seven parts, namely, *On Diseases Arising in the Head*, *On Facial Disease*, *On Utensils*, *On Infirmities of the Stomach and Intestines*, *On Affliction of the Liver, Kidneys, Bladder, Spleen, and Gall-Bladder*; *On Those That Arise in the Organs of Generation*; *On Those that Arise in the Exterior Skin*; the *Exposition of the Aphorisms*; the *Book of the Tegni*; *Of the Megategni*; *Of the Microtegni*; the *Antidotarium*; the *Dispute of Plato and Hippocrates on the Sentences*; *On Simple Medicine*; *On Gynaecology*, that is, the limbs and bodies of women; *On Pulses*; the *Prognostica*; *On Experiments*; *Glosses on Herbs and Spices*; the *Surgery*; the *Book on Healing of Eyes*. This man completed forty years in pursuing the learned studies of different nations. And finally as an old man and full of days he died in Monte Cassino. He lived in the times of the aforesaid emperors [that is, Michael VII, Constantine X, Alexius I, and Henry IV].

II. A Salernitan Tradition

Erf.: From Erfurt, Universitätsbibliothek, Bibliotheca Amploniana, Cod. Amplon. 8° 62 (early fourteenth century), fols 49^{v}–50^{r}. Transcribed and translated here by Francis Newton.

Sed notandum quod hoc opus non Constantinus sed Ysáác UT diximus composuit, Constantinus autem translatavit. Sed quoniam dictus Constantinus nusquam qualiter huc venerit, et libros translataverit diximus, ideo hic congruum duximus dicere. Constantinus autem Sarracenus exstitit, mercator tamen, quia mercationis causa huc venit, et multas mercationes secum attulit. Qui cum casu per plateam pergeret, ad curiam sancti Petri ascendit, in qua erat peroptimus medicus frater principis, qui 'abbas de curia' nuncupabatur. Constantinus ergo ipsum urinas iudicantem intuens, et nostram linguam penitus ignorans, servis Sarracenis precium tribuit, ut ei que iudicaret interpretarentur. Qui per interpretes cognoscens ipsum in medicina satis valere, per interpretes eius querebat de colore et substantia urinae, et in omnibus de urinis bene responderet [*sic*]. Eum per Sarracenos interrogavit, utrum multi in Latino haberentur libri de physica; qui respondit non haberi, sed modo studio et exercitio se ipsam comparasse. Constantinus ergo rediens in Africam tribus continuis annis physice diligenter adhibuit operam, et demum multos accipiens libros huc rediit. Qui dum Palinurum venisset, tempestate maris superveniente multa aqua in navem intravit et quandam *Pantegni* partem, scilicet 'Practicam' videlicet, dissipavit; sed dum huc venisset, et Romanam Latinam linguam didicit, et, Christianum se faciens, ad Sanctum Benedictum de Monte Cassino se monachum optulit, et libros illos in nostram linguam transstulit. A 'Practica' vero *Pantegni* non nisi tres libros translatavit. Erat namque ab aqua dissipata. Stephanon autem quidam Pisanus ad illas partes ivit et linguam illam addiscens eam ex toto transtulit, quae nunc 'Practica *Pantegni*' et Stephanonis dicitur. Sed Constantinus eius loco *Libros simplicium medicine* et *Librum graduum* edidit et Archiepiscopo Alfano ex sua parte *Librum stomachi* fecit, qui maximam eius contulit utilitatem. Archiepiscopus Alfanus pro integratione 'Practice *Pantegni*' expensas ei errogare voluit.

But it must be remarked that it was not Constantine but Isaac who composed this work [Isaac Iudaeus, *Liber diaetarum universalium*], and Constantine translated it. But since we have nowhere related how the aforesaid Constantine came here and translated the books, I have considered it for this reason appropriate to speak of it here. Now Constantine was a Saracen, but a merchant, for he came here for the sake of trade, and brought considerable trading goods with him. As he was by chance making his way through the public square, he climbed up to the Curia of St Peter, where there was an excellent physician [John], the brother of the prince [Gisulf II, the last Lombard prince of Salerno], who was called 'abbot of the Curia'. Therefore Constantine, observing him as he was passing judgement upon urine specimens, and being completely unacquainted with our language, gave a payment to the Saracen slaves to translate for him the judgements that he [the abbot] rendered. He [Abbot John], learning through the interpreters that the man himself [Constantine] had considerable competence in medicine, asked him through his interpreters about the colour and consistency of the urine; and in all respects he answered well regarding the urine specimens. He [Constantine] asked him through the Saracens whether many books on medicine were available in Latin. He answered that there were not, and that he himself had gained it [medical knowledge] only by dint of concentrated interest and practice. Constantine therefore, returning to Africa, for three straight years diligently directed his attention to medical science; and at last, taking many books, returned here. When he had reached Cape Palinurus, a sea storm broke out, and a great quantity of water came into the boat and destroyed a certain part of the *Pantegni*, namely the 'Practica'. But when he had come here, he both learned the Roman Latin tongue, and, making himself a Christian, offered himself as a monk at St Benedict of Monte Cassino. He also translated those books into our language. But of the 'Practica' of the *Pantegni* he translated only three books, for it had been destroyed by the water. Stephanon, however, a certain Pisan, went to those parts and, learning that language, translated it in its entirety, what is now known as the 'Practica' of the *Pantegni* of Stephanon as well. But Constantine, in place of it [the missing part] published the *Books of the Simple Medicine* and the *Book of Degrees*; and for Archbishop Alfanus he independently created the *Book of the Stomach*, which proved of the greatest usefulness to him. Archbishop Alfanus wished to reimburse him his costs for completing the 'Practica' of the *Pantegni*.

III. An Account from Cordoba and Montpellier

Sloane: From London, BL, MS Sloane 2426, fols 7^{v}–8^{v}, published by Singer, 'A Legend of Salerno'. Text collated and translated here by Francis Newton.

[In discussion of muscles and ligaments:] De partibus musculos seu lacertos componentibus disputabimus, qui sunt ligamenta, caro, nervi, atque panniculi, quibus musculi vestiuntur; etiam de aliis partibus corpus componentibus, ut sunt venae, et arteriae, ossa; et de quibusdam superfluitatibus corpus honestantibus et iuvantibus, ut sunt ungues et pili. Ut ratio anatomiae totius corporis sit evidentior, tractare non praetermittemus secundum auctoritatem Galeni et Albansoardi Cordubensis, qui *Pantegni* composuit, quamvis Constantinus ipsum composuissse mentiatur; tamen ipsum Constantinus et Stephanus nepos patriarche Antiochensis transtulerunt. Unde constat ipsos non fuisse auctores et inventores, sed tamen interpretes et expositores, ut Theophilus fuit expositor *Libri urinarum*, quod ipse indicat tituli impositione. Verumtamen, cum ipse Albonsoardus inter omnes medicos Cordubenses summus, qui erant numero mille CCCCti haberetur, plures discipulos habuisset, inter quos sapientiores erant Constantinus et Ali, filius tabernarii. Qui iussu et auxilio sui magistri *Viaticum*, *Dietas utrasque*, *Librum stomachi*, *Cirurgiae*, *Librum graduum*, et quamplures alios composuerunt. Accidit ut rex Cordubensis, qui lingua illa Almansor dicitur, longe a civitate infirmaretur. Qui cum ad Albasoardum legatos ut cito veniret misisset, tanquam dedignans venire quia sapientia et nobilitate pollebat, finxit se infirmari, et misit Constantinum et Ali. Qui cum circa regem evigilanter et multo studio plura ex ratione fecissent, purgato corpore ut quartanam omnino expellerent, ipsi in balneo posito opium in nimia quantitate Constantinus obtulit. Et bene fecit, quia opium dedit, sed male, quia quantitatem facta virium comparatione non consideravit. Tandem, cum ad ipsum venisset [Tandem-venisset *iteravit* S; *corr.* S2], prorsus humore congelato ne deinceps ad locum putrefactionis flueret, et spiritu frigiditate opii extincto, omnino curatum invenit, nil mali sentiens. Quod videns, timens usque in ultimum diem sibi sociari et in sepulcro poni, iniunxit circumstantibus ne streperent, et quieti essent, quia rex dormiebat et liberaretur in brevi. Quod minime suo indicans socio, qui causa spatiandi villam exierat, amotis sarcinis et omnibus libris — nemine socio iuncto — portum venit. Ubi casu navem remis et velo paratam, prospero succedente vento, littora relinquentem [*FN*, relinquente *Singer*] invenit. Et cum itinere unius diei nautae maria sulcassent, (ut credo) nutu Domini et eius providentia, qui hanc artem in Christianos transferre volebat ad medelam ipsorum, a Salernitanis nautis causa praedae maria solito transfretantibus sunt captivati et Salerni deducti, et, ut mos est captivorum, venales per villam ducti. De quorum numero Constantinus existens, a quodam coriario emptus est, qui Constantinum suo negotio destinavit. Quem cum contigisset iuxta littus maris coria reparare, transivit princeps Salerni, gravi morbo afflictus. Qui cum infinita in medicos expendisset — qui tunc temporis raritate cariores prophetis habebantur — a nullo curatus fuerat. Quem intuens Constantinus ait, 'Si me ab hoc coriorum periculo liberaveris, et ego a languore te liberabo.' Qui subridens, credens ipsum desipientem quia captivum et vili veste indutum videbat — nesciens quod in vili vase mirabile vinum contineatur, odore etiam cuius omnes sacientur, et in vili corpore magna scientia latere possit — inquit, 'Tu iminenti periculo quo torqueris, periculo iam factus medicus, liberari velles', non credens medicum esse ipsum; 'Tamen, si ita est ut testaris, prius facta in aliquo eadem infirmitate detento curatione, secundo in me transferas.' Et factum est sic. Curatur prior; curatur — gratia Dei qui hanc artem per Constantinum ad nos volebat transfundere — et princeps. Deinde ubique terrarum famosus, cum in multo honore a Christianis haberetur, factus est et Christianus, et postea Montis Cassinensis monachus. Inde Salernus primatum sibi et primum medicum est sortita. Ubi usque in hodiernum diem eius gesta referuntur; sed iam, senio dissoluta, a modernis ibi sub umbra scientiae possidentur. Sed inde huius scientiae propaginum extensis palmitibus usque ad Montem Pessulanum celeberrime ibidem renascitur. Iam tempus amonet promissa solvere, et primo de ligamentis qui sunt partes musculorum iam premissa nervorum disputatione.

I intend to discuss the parts that compose the muscles or *lacerti*, which are the ligaments, the flesh, the nerves, and the *fasciae* which cover the muscles; also the other parts that compose the body, such as the veins, the arteries, and the bones; and certain accessory adornments and aids to the body, such as the nails and the hair. In order that our general anatomical account may be clearer, I shall take care to treat it in accordance with the authority of Galen and Albansoardus of Cordoba, who composed the *Pantegni*, though Constantine lies; he says that *he* composed it; but really Constantine and Stephen, nephew of the patriarch of Antioch, translated it. So it is clear that they were not the authors and originators; they were its translators and interpreters, as Theophilus was the interpreter of the *Book of Urines*, as he himself shows by the title he gave it. But Albonsoardus himself was supreme among all the doctors of Cordoba, numbering about fourteen hundred, and he had many students; the wiser ones were Constantine and Ali, the son of the innkeeper. At the command of their teacher and with his help, they composed the *Viaticum*, the two *Diet Books*, the *Book of the Stomach*, the *Book of Surgery*, the *Book of Degrees*, and quite a number of others. It happened that the king of Cordoba, called Almansor in that language, fell sick far from his home city. When he sent messengers to Albasoardus asking him to come quickly, the latter, relying on his noble rank and his wisdom, thought it beneath him to go; he made up the excuse that he was unwell and sent Constantine and Ali. They carried out a full scientific treatment actively and attentively, purging the king to rid him completely of the quartan fever, and then Constantine had him placed in a bath and administered a dose of opium that was too large. Now it was good that he gave him opium, but bad that, in drawing up the dose, he did not pay attention to its relative strength. After some time, coming to him, he found that the humour had thoroughly solidified so that it could not any longer flow towards the diseased site, and that its essence was destroyed by the chilling effect of the opium; suspecting no problem, he considered him completely cured. When he saw that, the fear came upon him that he would be bound to the king until the last day of his life and until his burial. So he gave orders to those present not to make any noise and to remain quiet, because the king was asleep and would shortly be free of illness, and, without sharing his plan with his colleague, who had left the villa to take a walk, he had his bags and all his books carried out and — with no traveling-companion — reached the harbour. By chance he found a ship there already outfitted, oars, sails, and all, and on the point of leaving shore under a favourable wind.

And when the crew had ploughed through the sea a day's voyage — by (as I believe) the will of the Lord and his providence, who desired that this art be transferred to Christians, for their healing — they were captured by Salernitan sailors who made a practice of cruising the seas for booty; they were brought to Salerno and put on sale and led through the city, as captives are. Constantine, being one of them, was bought by a tanner, who assigned him to work in his business. And as he happened to be dressing skins by the sea shore, there passed by the prince of Salerno, who was suffering from a very serious illness. The prince had spent huge sums on doctors — being at that time so rare, they were considered more valuable than prophets — and had found no one to cure him. Constantine fixed his gaze on him and said, 'If you will free me from this dangerous tanning work, I will free *you* from your sickness'. The prince smiled, thinking that he was witless because he saw he was a captive and dressed in worthless clothes — not knowing that a worthless vessel can contain wine so marvellous that the mere bouquet of it by itself would be enough to give everyone great pleasure, and that a great amount of knowledge could lie hidden in a worthless body — said, 'You would like to turn into a doctor and free yourself from the dangerous burden that torments you!' not believing that he *was* a doctor: 'Still, if things are as you say, first cure someone afflicted with the same illness I suffer from, and then you may try the treatment on me'. And that is what they did. The first man was cured; then a cure — thanks to God, who wanted to transfer this skill to us, through the agency of Constantine — was worked upon the prince. After that, Constantine was renowned all over the world and, being held in high esteem by Christians, he became a Christian, and afterwards a monk of Monte Cassino. This is how Salerno won the first place of leadership for itself, and the first doctor too. They talk about his deeds there even today; but, in the hands of the moderns there, it all grows old and decrepit and a shadow falls upon their science. But, from there, fresh offshoots from the vine of this the most famous science have spread all the way to Montpellier, and there it is being reborn. But now time reminds me to fulfil my promise and first to talk about the ligaments that are part of the muscles, prefacing it with a discussion of the nerves.

Appendix C

Latin Text and English Translation of the Prologue of the *Pantegni*

This transcription of The Hague, KB, MS 73 J 6, fol. 1r (fig. 1.1 and pl. I) uses majuscules to represent the manuscript's *capitalis* incipits, employs modern punctuation to indicate pauses, and expands all abbreviations. Irregular abbreviations and corrections are remarked upon in footnotes. The late twelfth-century headings are ignored here, as are the thirteenth-century retracings.

DOMINO SUO MONTIS CASSINENSIS abbati, Desiderio, Reverentissimo patrum patri, immo totius ordinis aecclesiastici gemme praenitenti, Constantinus africanus, licet indignus (suus tamen monachus) oculatis[1] intus et exterius caeli ascribi animalibus.

CUM TOTIUS, Pater, scientiae generalitas tres principales partes habeat, omnes enim saeculares seu divinae litterae subiciuntur Logicae, aethice, seu phisicae, medicina tamen litteralis cui harum possit subici a compluribus solet dubitari. Soli enim logyce non supponitur, cum neque propria inventio, neque iudicium in ea dominentur. Phisicae soli non subicitur, cum non tantum necessariis, sive probabilia seu non probabilia sint, fulciatur argumentis. Aethice soli videtur absurdum subici, cum disputare de solis moribus non suae sit intentionis. Sed cum oporteat medicum esse rationabilem rerum naturalium et moralium tractatorem, constat quia in omnes incidit, diversis cogitationibus omnibus subici. Unde ego Constantinus[2] tantam huius artis utilitatem perpen-

[1] The abbreviated 'tius' is here corrected to 'tis'.

[2] The manuscript contains '.C.', which certainly names Constantine the African; the

dens, latinorumque volumina percurrens, cum licet multa essent, non tamen introducendis etiam sufficere viderem,[3] recurri ad nostros, veteres sive modernos. Revolvi enim ypocratem in hac arte maximum; revolvi et galienum, et de novis alexandrum. paulum quoque et oribasium.[4] Sed ypocratem in aphorismis gloriosissimum, et in aliis etiam huius artis tractatorem praecipuum, solum imitare[5] nolui, quia adeo obscurus atque brevis extitit, ut multos iam ab hac utilitate repulerit.[6] Galienus de rebus singulis singula volumina fecit. Assidua enim verborum iteratione, et cavillosa diversarum questionum argumentatione centum .LX. fecit volumina eademque maxima. Multiplicitate quorum multi tedio affecti sunt. Vix enim tantum .XVI. volumina leguntur. Quae sunt: Piriton hereseos [*sic*] medicorum. particula una. Microntegni .i. Pulsuum minores particule .ii. Epistole ad Glaucum .ii. De elementis .i. De complexione tres. De virtutibus naturalibus .iii. De anathomia .v. De morbo et accidentibus .vi. Mega pulsuum .xvi. De interioribus membris .vi. Criseos .iii. ymera criseos .iii. De febribus .ii. Megategni .xiiii. De regimento sanorum .xii. Auribasius in libro de re publica ad Unesum filium suum nichil tetigit naturalium, de aliis vero parum. Scribit quoque alterum ad quendam Stacium similiter suum filium in .viiii. particulas divisum, in quo parum profuit, quia nichil de naturalibus ibidem scripsit, id est, de elementis, complexione, humoribus, menbris, virtutibus, actione, spiritu. In alio vero volumine lxx. particulas continente, vix aliquid invenitur naturale, nisi in una particula invenitur interiorum membrorum anathomia. Paulus quicquid scripsit, bene dixit, set et naturalia omisit, et libros male ordinavit. Alexander similiter. Ego autem communi consulens utilitati, scribere tantum necessaria disposui, in sanitate sanorum custodientia[7] et infirmitate medicinanda. Dixi quoque morborum causas, et eorum naturas, significationes quoque, et accidentia. Infirma enim curare, his ignoratis, est impossibile. In multis tamen locis testimonia introduxi Ypocratis atque Galieni, ab ipsis experimento comprobata et rationibus de dieta et medicaminibus confirmata. In pluribus vero locis multa dicunt de medicinis quae nostro tempore sta-

abbreviation means that it was taken for granted that Constantine's name would have appeared in a heading at the beginning.

[3] The '-re' ending 'sufficere' and 'vi-' beginning 'viderem' have been conspicuously retraced by a later reader.

[4] 'Auribasium' is here corrected to Oribasium by the first hand, that of Geraldus.

[5] The original 'imitare' is here corrected by a later medieval hand to 'imitari'.

[6] Here 'repulerit' is here corrected from the manuscript's 'reppulerit'.

[7] The original 'custodientia' is here corrected by a late medieval hand to 'custodienda'.

tuimus non sequi, utpote in quarto climate constituti. Ypocras enim praecepit in peri ton oxeon nosomaton, in solutione ventris elleborum nigrum dari pleureticis. Galienus et alii quidam in acuta egritudine mellitam dant aquam. Nos vero pro mellicrate siropum iulab et siropum rosatum assuevimus dare, et solvimus ventrem in acuta egritudine cum cassia fistula, manna, oxifenicia, viola, et similibus. Auctoritatem tamen non fugimus cum precepta sequamur sed situs regionum consideramus. Est autem intentio libri huius, quomodo infirmitates cognoscantur, et ex ordine suo eis curationes adhibeantur.

Vobis autem, pater, hoc nostrum opusculum tribus ex causis destinavimus nos daturum, ut cum supradictis philosophie partibus inhianter vos insudare noverimus, hac eiusdem parte, utpote potiore, noluerimus vos carere; secundo etiam, quia ut philosophus ait quidam, cum omne bonum per se fit[8] iocundum, in commune tamen deductum et praesertim inter amicos ventilatum, fit iocumdissimum; tertio, ut cum in actibus humanis nichil ex omni parte perfectum sit, corrigenda corrigatis. auctorizanda vestra consideratione digna iudicetis.

English Translation

TO HIS LORD, ABBOT OF MONTE CASSINO Desiderius, most reverend father of fathers, nay rather, pre-eminently sparkling jewel of the whole ecclesiastical order, Constantine the African, although unworthy (yet still his monk) to be counted among creatures of heaven endowed with vision within and without.

WHILE FOR THE WHOLE of knowledge, O father, the general field has three major parts, since all letters, secular or divine, fall within the category of the logical, the ethical, or the physical; there is, however, doubt on the part of many men under which of these medicine as a written art can be subsumed. For it is not set under logic alone, since neither invention proper nor judgement is the ruling force in it. It is not set under the physical alone, since it does not rest upon necessary arguments, be they probable or improbable. It seems absurd for it to be set under the ethical alone, since it is not part of its purpose to dispute morals alone. But since a doctor must be a rational creature who treats things natural and things moral, it is well understood, since it falls under all of them, that it is set under all these varied thought-systems. Wherefore I, Constantine, pondering the great usefulness of this art, and skimming through the volumes

[8] The scribe wrote 'fit' in error for 'sit' (the '*cum* clause' requires a subjunctive), perhaps influenced by the 'fit' in the next line.

of the Latin writers (though they were many, I saw that they were not adequate for beginners), turned back to our people, whether ancient or modern ones. I leafed through the pages of Hippocrates, who was supreme in this art; I leafed also through Galen, and, among the new authors, Alexander, and also Paul and Oribasius. But Hippocrates who was most distinguished for his Aphorisms, and in his other works even the foremost expounder of this art, I did not choose to imitate alone, because he was so obscure and so brief that he has driven many men away already and discouraged them from pursuing this useful field. Galen created individual books on individual subjects. For by constant repetition of words, and carping discussion of diverse questions, he created one hundred sixty volumes, very large ones.[9] By reason of the large number of them, many [students] have been overwhelmed by weariness. For it is very difficult to read [even] the sixteen volumes, which are: *On the Sects*,[10] one segment; the *Microtegni*, one; *The Lesser Segments on Pulses*, two; the *Letters to Glaucus*, two; *On Elements*, one; *On Complexions* [temperaments], three; *On the Natural Virtues*, three; *On Anatomy*, five; *On Illness and Accidents*, six; *The Great Text on Pulses*, sixteen; *On Internal Organs*, six; *On Crisis*, three; *The Day of Crisis*, three; *On Fevers*, two; the *Megategni*, fourteen; *On the Regimen of Health*, twelve; Auribasius, in *The Book on the State to Unesus*, his son, did not touch on the Naturals at all, and hardly on other subjects. He writes also another book to a certain Statius, similarly his son, and divided it into nine segments; in this he accomplished little, for in it he wrote nothing about the Naturals, that is, the elements, the complexions [mixtures of qualities], the humours, the members [of the body], the powers [*virtutes*], the faculties [*actiones*], and the spirits. But in another volume, containing seventy segments, hardly any mention of the Naturals is found, except that in one segment the anatomy of the inner organs is found. Whatever Paulus wrote was well written, but he also omitted

[9] The number of works offered here, sixteen, follows the medical curriculum in Galen that was established at Alexandria in Late Antiquity, and which is reflected in Ḥunayn's *Isagoge*. The sixteen titles Constantine lists comprise the Alexandrian curriculum, here itemizing a total of eighty segments (*particulae*). On the curriculum advocating the study of sixteen of Galen's texts, see Iskandar, 'An Attempted Reconstruction of the Alexandrian Medical Curriculum', especially pp. 237–38. On the use of designations for *particulae* (sections) and *capitula* (chapters) in the Hague *Pantegni*, see the discussion in the Introduction of the present study.

[10] The standard summary of the Naturals is given in the *Isagoge*, the translation and adaption of which Constantine and his team were busy producing, revising, and improving at approximately the same time they were perfecting the *Theorica*. For a translation of the *Isagoge*, see Wallis, 'Medical Theory' in her *Medieval Medicine*, pp. 139–56.

the Naturals and organized the books in a poor way. Similarly with Alexander. But I, seeking to make it useful to all, have determined to write only what is necessary to protect the health of the healthy and to heal illness. I have also listed the causes of diseases, and their natures, their signs also, and the accidentals. For healing sickness without knowledge of these matters is impossible. Yet in many places I have brought in the witness of Hippocrates and Galen, demonstrated by them through experience and confirmed by their reasoning regarding diet and medicines. And in many places they say a great deal about medicines which I have decided in our circumstances not to follow, living as we do in the fourth climate. For Hippocrates in the treatise *On Severe Diseases* taught that for bowel movement black hellebore be given to pleurisy patients. Galen and some others in case of acute illness prescribe honey water. But I, instead of *mellicrates*, usually prescribe syrup of julep and rose-syrup; and in cases of acute illness we cause bowel movement by means of an enema using cassia, manna, oxyphoenicia, violet, and the like.[11] Yet we do not shun [their] authority when we follow their teachings, but take the geographical location into consideration. The goal of this book is the identification of diseases, and, thereafter, the application of cures for them.

And I determined to present this my little work to you, O father, for three reasons, so that since I know that you with panting zeal sweat over the three aforementioned parts of philosophy, I did not wish you to be deprived of this part of the same, the very best part. In the second place, besides, as a certain philosopher says, 'While every good thing in and of itself is pleasing, still that which is shared and especially that aired among friends becomes supremely pleasing'. In the third place, since in the doings of human creatures nothing is in every way perfect, so that you might correct what is in need of correction, and might judge worthy what is to be authorized by your consideration.

[11] On the early integration of pharmaceutical practices from the Byzantine and Islamic East into Salernitan practice immediately prior to Constantine's activities in Italy, see Glaze, 'Salerno's Lombard Prince'.

Appendix D

English Translation of the Theodemar Chapter of *Ortus et vita*

Peter the Deacon, Ortus et vita iustorum cenobii Casinensis, chap. 49 (ed. by Rodgers, pp. 71.8–73.23).[1]

XLVIIII. Theodemarius Alamannia prouincia ortus, Agnetisque imperatricis capellaneus fuit. Hic igitur dum relictis spretisque seculi pompis Casinum peteret, uenit ad fluuium Viride qui secus Ciperanium influit; quem dum transmeasset, famulum eius unda rapiens introrsum traere cepit. Quod ubi aduertid, se confestim ibidem in orationem dedit, moxque ut ab oratione surrexit, famulum eius unda foras proiecit. Cum autem Casinum uenisset, sancte conuersationis habitum prout obtabat accepit. Quante autem religionis quanteque perfectionis eius uita extitit, et in quantum Deo placuerit, in sequentibus declarabitur.

Quadam uero die dum sacrificium omnipotenti Deo offerret, quidam claudus elemosinam petens aduenit. Cuius cum uir Dei manus abpreendisset, confestim sanatus est. Nec hoc silendum uidetur, quod post misse consumationem aqua que de eius manibus effluebat in potum inerguminis data sanabantur. Eodem preterea tempore episcopus Tranensis | nepotem suum, Phocam nomine, quem immundus acriter uexabat spiritus ad eum midtere studuit, rogans ut ob eius liberationem omnipotenti Deo preces fundere dignaretur. Super quem cum orationem fudisset, ab eo diabolum effugauit.

[1] The Latin edition of this text (without editorial notes) is reproduced here with the kind permission of R. H. Rodgers.

Illis porro temporibus Berengarius diaconus Andecauensis sui nominis heresim condidit, dicens sacrificium quod omnipotenti Deo offertur esse figuram corporis Christi, non ueritatem. Hoc ubi Romano pontifici nuntiatum est, Dominum Iesum Christum precibus pulsare admonuit, ut populum suo sanguine redemptum ad uiam dignaretur reducere ueritatis. Igitur dum omnes ob hoc Domini flagitarent clementiam, supradictus Theodemarius redemptionis nostre hostiam Deo oblaturus accedit. Cumque ad consecrationem uentum fuisset, predictam oblationem in carnem repente mutatam conspicit. Quod dum Romano pontifici nuntiatum fuisset, omnium bonorum reseratori gratias retulit, Berengariumque cum suis sequacibus eandem heresim renuntiare coegit.

Stephanus Capuanus dum a ciuitate sancti Germani Casinum uenisset, ad altare beate Marie semper uirginis Deum rogaturus perrexit. Ad idem uero altarium uir Domini Theodemar diuina misteria celebraturus accesserat. Ab oratione igitur Stephanus dum surrexisset, ad Theodemarium fortuitu oculos uertens, uidit in capite eius coronam auream gemmis ac margaritis ornatam. Ad hanc uisionem stupefactus, Oderisium abbatem adiit eique cuncta que uiderat per ordinem pandit. Alio quoque tempore dum idem Theodemar sacris astaret altaribus, ac se in cordis contritione Domino Iesu Christo mactaret, hi qui ibidem astabant uiderunt super scapulam eius dextram columbam niuei coloris residentem.

Eo preterea tempore dum omnis tellus aresceret, Oderisius abbas fratres ad se euocans, Dominum Iesum Christum ac uirginem Mariam precibus pulsare admonuit, ut qui in deserto aquam de petra produxit, ipse arenti mundo pluuiam daret. Quod dum fratribus placuisset, statuerunt ad beate Marie ecciesiam in eodem monte constructam discalciatis pedibus pergere ibique Dei omnipotentis clementiam subplicare. Adueniente autem die, predicto Theodemario abbas precepit, ut cum fratribus pergeret ac pro terre siccitate sacrificium Deo offerret. Igitur dum ea que sibi iniuncta fuerant implere satageret, cogitare intra se cepit, nullum in Casino sui similem aut meliorem esse; ideoque sibi utpote meliori ac sanctiori hoc iniuncxisse. Peracta igitur letania, fratres rediere Casinum, set aer in ea qua fuerat serentiate[2] permansit. Vir autem Domini hoc cernens, se in precibus strincxit, triduoque sine intermissione Deum rogare adtentius cepit. Tertia autem nocte adueniente, assiduis Deum rogare precibus cepit. Mane uero facto surgens, expansis ante altare manibus ait, "Non deponam manus meas usquequo pluuiam nobis Dominus dare dignetur." Eodem uero die tanta inundatio pluuie erupit, ut tota affatim terra aqua repleretur.

[2] *Nos* serenitate *scripsimus*; serentiate *ed.*

Quodam preterea tempore dum Neapolim aduenisset, quidam uir magnis detentus febribus, oratione eius interueniente confestim sanatus est. In ciuitate Salernitana quidam rusticus filium claudum habebat, quem ad abbatem ferens de curte, exposcit ut aliquod remedium claudo impertiret. Abbas uero uirum Dei Theodemarium ad se uenientem aspiciens, puerum ante eum proiecit eumque rogare cepit ut puerum a terra leuaret. Vir autem Dei quid in re esset ignarus, extendens manum abpreendit puerum dicens, "Surge;" et confestim surrexit.

Alio quoque tempore cum idem uir Dei sacris astaret altaribus, uir sanctissimus Ebyzo cum eo stare consueuerat. Set sicut est natura humana segnis ad Dei seruitium, multotiens uocatus renuebat. Illo uero die quo sacram hostiam Deo ad <altare> beate Marie semper uirginis offerebat, supradictus Ebyzo sopore deprimitur uidetque angelum Domini iusta se stantem et dicentem, "Ebize, animaduerte et uide cui tu seruire contempnis, quomodo ei angeli seruiunt, et tuo ei seruitio denegato, Dominus ei angelos misit." Stabant autem iusta eum duo angeli, unus a dextris et unus a sinistris.

English Translation

49. Theodemar was born in the Alemannic province and was chaplain to the Empress Agnes. So when, forsaking and despising the pomp of the world, he was making his way to Monte Cassino, he came to the River Liri outside Ceprano; when he had crossed it, a wave seized his servant and began to drag him under. When he observed this, he at once fell to praying on the spot, and, as soon as he rose from prayer, a wave cast the servant out upon the bank. And when he had reached Monte Cassino, he put on the habit of a holy life. And what a perfect religious life his was, and how pleasing to God, will be made clear in what follows.

Now one day, as he was offering sacrifice to almighty God, a lame man came up to him, begging alms. And when the man of God had taken his hands, at once he was healed. And I should not, it seems, pass this over in silence, that after the completion of the Mass, the water that dripped from his hands was given to the sick to drink, and they were healed. Moreover, at this same time the bishop of Trani, whose nephew, Phocas by name, was tormented by an unclean spirit, decided to send him to him [Theodemar], asking him that he would deign to offer prayers to almighty God for his release. When he had poured forth a prayer over him, he drove the devil out of him.

In those times the deacon Berengar of Angers [that is, Berengar of Tours] initiated the heresy that bears his name, saying that the sacrifice that is offered to almighty God is only a figure and not truly the body of Christ. When this was reported to the pontiff in Rome, he advised them [Monte Cassino's congregation?] to importune our Lord Jesus Christ with prayers to bring the people that he had redeemed with his own blood back into the way of righteousness. Therefore, as they [the Cassinese congregation] were all beseeching the mercy of the Lord to this end, the aforementioned Theodemar came forward to offer to God the sacrifice of our redemption. And when they had reached the consecration [of the Host], he observed that the aforesaid offering had changed into flesh. Once that was reported to the pontiff in Rome, he offered up thanks to the Revealer of all good things, and compelled Berengar with his followers to renounce that same heresy.

When Stephen of Capua had come from the town of San Germano [medieval Cassino] to Monte Cassino, he directed his steps to the altar of the Blessed Mary Ever-Virgin, to ask God [God's help]. The man of the Lord, Theodemar, had come to the same altar to celebrate the divine mysteries. And so when Stephen had risen from prayer, by chance turning his eyes in Theodemar's direction, he saw on his head a crown of gold studded with jewels and pearls. Astounded at this vision, he went to Abbot Oderisius and poured forth to him all that he had seen from beginning to end. Besides, on another occasion, as the same Theodemar was standing at the holy altar, and offering himself in contrition of heart to our Lord Jesus Christ, those who were standing by in the same place saw a snow-coloured dove sitting on his right shoulder.

Moreover, at a time when the entire land was suffering from drought, Abbot Oderisius summoned all the brothers and admonished them to importune the Lord Jesus Christ and the Virgin Mary in their prayers, like him who in the desert brought forth water out of a rock, to grant rain to the drought-stricken world. As this pleased the brothers, they decided to go in procession barefoot to the church of the Blessed Mary built on the same mountain and there to beg the mercy of Omnipotent God. And when the day came, the abbot bade the aforementioned Theodemar to go with the brothers and offer sacrifice to God for the drought in the land. Therefore while endeavouring to carry out the commands that had been laid upon him, he began to think within himself that there was no one at Monte Cassino like himself or better, and therefore that he had laid the command upon him as being better and more holy. Therefore, when the litany was done, the brothers returned to Monte Cassino, but the sky still remained as clear as before. Now the man of God, seeing this, bound himself in his prayers and began a three-day course of intense prayer to God, without break. And when the third night arrived, he began to beseech God with continuous prayers. And, arising at morning and spreading his hands before the altar, he said, 'I shall not put down my hands until the Lord may deign to grant us rain'. That same day such an inundation of rain burst forth indeed that the entire land was filled.

Moreover, at a certain time when he had come to Naples, a great man who was afflicted with bouts of high fever, at his prayer of intercession, was immediately healed. In the city of Salerno a certain countryman had a son who was lame, and he took him to the Abbas de Curte [the abbot of the court] and asked him to confer some remedy upon him who was lame. But the abbot, seeing the man of God Theodemar approaching, threw the boy down in front of him and began to beg him to take the boy up from the ground. And the man of God, quite unaware what was going on, stretched out his hand and took the boy, saying, 'Arise'; and at once he stood up.

At another period, when the same man of God would stand at the holy altar, the most holy Ebyzo had formed the habit of standing with him. But such is human nature, sluggish in carrying out God's service, time and again when called on, he refused. But on that day when he was offering the sacred sacrifice to God at the altar of the Blessed Mary Ever-Virgin, the aforementioned Ebyzo was overcome by sleep and saw an angel of the Lord standing beside him and saying, 'Ebyzo, pay attention and observe who it is to whom you disdain to offer service as his angels serve him, and (as you have denied him your service), the Lord has sent him angels'. And there stood beside him two angels, one on the right and one on the left.

Appendix E

Holster Books Copied Prior to 1200

The following table presents eighty holster books selected from a variety of inventories and manuscript catalogues. The corpus is limited to books written before *c.* 1200 that have a relative width of 0.60 or less; these proportions ensure only books that were intentionally made differently are included, and exclude those that may have been accidentally made slightly narrower than usual, or trimmed considerably during binding.

	Manuscript	**Date**	**Verse or prose**
1	St Gall, SB, Cod. Sang. 360	*c.* 1100	Prose
2	Paris, BnF, Latin 8824	*c.* 1050	Prose
3	London, BL, MS Harley 5431 (fols 4^{r}–126^{v})	*c.* 975–*c.* 1025	Prose
4	Paris, BnF, Latin 6898	1094	Prose
5	Oxford, Bodleian, MS Junius 1	*c.* 1175–*c.* 1200	Verse
6	Paris, BnF, Latin 8898	*c.* 1180–*c.* 1190	Prose
7	Berlin, SBPK, MS theol. lat. fol. 323	*c.* 1100	Prose
8	London, BL, MS Harley 2777	*c.* 1150–*c.* 1200	Verse
9	Leiden, UB, SCA 69	*c.* 950–*c.* 1000	Prose
10	Paris, BnF, Latin 10477	1182	Prose
11	London, BL, MS Harley 3068	*c.* 1150–*c.* 1200	Prose
12	London, BL, MS Harley 2737, part i (fols 1–103)	*c.* 1200	Verse
13	Copenhagen, KB, GKS 2006 4°	*c.* 1175–*c.* 1200	Verse
14	Florence, Laurenziana, MS Plut. 34.13	*c.* 1100–*c.* 1150	Verse
15	St Gall, SB, Cod. Sang. 359	*c.* 922–*c.* 925	Prose
16	London, BL, MS Harley 5296	*c.* 1100–*c.* 1150	Verse
17	London, BL, MS Harley 110, fols 3–54	*c.* 975–*c.* 1025	Prose & Verse
18	London, BL, MS Harley 110, fols 1, 56 (fragments)	*c.* 1000–*c.* 1050	Prose

Contents	Relative width	Height (mm)	Width (mm)
Iymni (XXVII) Sangallenses in processionibus	0.31	255	80
'salter	0.35	526	186
Rule of Benedict	0.37	230	85
?ituale	0.39	360	140
)rrmulum (autograph)	0.39	500	195
:eremonial-pontifical of Soissons	0.39	368	145
ife of St Liudger	0.42	300	125
'irgil, *Aeneis*	0.42	285	120
:osmographia	0.43	140	60
abulae computi; calendar	0.43	290	125
oethius, *De consolatio*; Ephraem the Syrian; Sermons	0.43	255	110
)vid, *Metamorphoses*; Ovid, *Fasti*, excerpts	0.44	225	100
'irgil, *Aeneis*	0.44	236	105
Iorace, *Opera* (*Carm.*, *Epod.*, *Carm. Saec.*, *Ars*, *Sat.*, *Epist.*)	0.45	184	82
:antatorium	0.45	280	125
tatius, *Thebais*, glossed	0.46	250	115
rosper of Aquitaine, *Epigrammata*; Isidore, *Synonyma*	0.46	260	120
iradual	0.46	260	120

	Manuscript	Date	Verse or prose
19	Paris, BnF, Latin 9448	986	Prose
20	Geneva, Bibliothèque de Genève, MS lat. 37a	*c.* 900–*c.* 925	Prose
21	Paris, BnF, Latin 9449	1059	Prose
22	St Gall, SB, Cod. Sang. 549	*c.* 800	Prose
23	Copenhagen, KB, GKS 2014 4°	*c.* 1150	Verse
24	London, BL, MS Burney 273	*c.* 1100–*c.* 1150	Verse
25	London, BL, MS Harley 2608	*c.* 1125–*c.* 1175	Verse
26	London, BL, MS Burney 220	*c.* 1150–*c.* 1200	Verse
27	London, BL, MS Harley 2655	*c.* 1150–*c.* 1200	Verse
28	St Gall, SB, Cod. Sang. 380	*c.* 1050–*c.* 1060	Prose
29	Paris, BnF, Latin 8216	*c.* 1150–*c.* 1200	Verse
30	St Gall, SB, Cod. Sang. 833	*c.* 1100	Prose
31	London, BL, MS Royal 8 B XI	*c.* 950–*c.* 1000	Prose
32	Cambridge, Pembroke College, MS 302	*c.* 1050	Prose
33	London, BL, MS Harley 2652	*c.* 1100–*c.* 1150	Prose
34	Graz, Universitätsbibliothek, Cod. 735	1106–18	Prose
35	Cambridge, Peterhouse College, MS 229	*c.* 1150	Verse
36	London, BL, MS Burney 258	*c.* 1100–*c.* 1175	Verse
37	London, BL, MS Harley 2670	*c.* 1100	Prose
38	London, BL, MS Sloane 1621	*c.* 1050–*c.* 1100	Prose
39	The Hague, KB, MS 73 J 6	*c.* 1075–*c.* 1100	Prose
40	Vendôme, BM, MS 193	1129–32	Prose
41	Vienna, Österreichische Nationalbibliothek, Cod. 743	before 800	Prose
42	Copenhagen, KB, GKS 1995 4°	*c.* 1150–*c.* 1200	Prose
43	London, BL, MS Royal 6 A VI	*c.* 975–*c.* 1000	Prose
44	London, BL, MS King's 26	*c.* 1075–*c.* 1125	Verse
45	Durham, Cathedral Chapter Library, MS C.IV.29	*c.* 1100–*c.* 1200	Prose
46	London, BL, MS Harley 3534	*c.* 1100–*c.* 1125	Verse
47	London, BL, MS Harley 3859	*c.* 1100	Prose
48	Paris, BnF, NAL 1623	*c.* 1100–*c.* 1200	Prose
49	London, BL, MS Burney 357, part II (fols 15v–16r)	*c.* 1150–*c.* 1200	Prose

Contents	Relative width	Height (mm)	Width (mm)
Troper	0.47	320	150
Lectionary of St Gall	0.48	315	150
Troper	0.48	270	130
Life of St Marcellinus, with hymn at pp. 59–61	0.49	195	95
Ovid, *Tristia*; commentary	0.49	193	95
Virgil, *Aeneis*; Ps.-Virgil; Basil of Caesarea	0.50	240	120
Statius, *Thebais*	0.50	230	115
Ovid, *Epistolae ex Ponto*	0.50	200	100
Ovid, *Fasti*; calendar	0.50	210	105
Calendar, *computus*, troper, sequentiary	0.50	179	90
Horace, *Opera* (*Carm.*, *Epod.*, *Carm. Saec.*, *Ars*, *Epist.*, *Sat.*)	0.51	235	120
Porphyry, *Isagoge*	0.51	234	120
Paschasius Radbertus, *De corpore et sanguine domini*	0.51	222	114
Lectionary	0.52	193	101
Cicero, *Somnium Scipionis* and commentary; Plato, *Timaeus*; diagrams	0.52	210	110
Miscellany with historical and theological texts	0.53	190	100
Horace, *Opera* (*Carm.*, *Epod.*, *Carm. Saec.*, *Sat.*, *Epist.*)	0.53	240	127
Statius, *Thebais*, glossed, with *accessus*	0.53	245	130
Terence, *Comedies*	0.53	300	160
Roman *Pontificale*	0.54	205	110
Constantine the African, *Pantegni*	0.54	235	128
Gaufridus, *Epistolae*, sermons and other works	0.55	210	115
Commentary on Pauline Epistles	0.55	310	170
Terence, *Comedies*, with *accessus*	0.55	235	130
Aldhelm, *De laudibus virginitatis* (OE glosses); letter to Ehfrid	0.55	280	155
Ovid, *Metamorphoses*; *Tristia*	0.56	252	140
Extracts from three different glosses on Priscian, *Institutiones grammaticae*	0.56	233	130
Horace, *Opera* (*Carm.*, *Epod.*, *Carm. Saec.*, *Ars poetica*, *Serm.*)	0.56	205	115
Vegetius, *Epitome rei militaris*; other classical authors; Annals	0.57	265	150
Gloss on Priscian, *Institutiones grammaticae*, books i–xvi (fols 1–56) [= 'Glosule']	0.57	255	145
Polyphonic sequence	0.57	210	120

	Manuscript	Date	Verse or prose
50	London, BL, MS Burney 246	*c.* 1150–*c.* 1200	Verse
51	London, BL, MS Burney 357, part I (fols 1–15)	*c.* 1100–*c.* 1150	Prose
52	London, BL, MS Burney 357, part III (fols 17–24)	*c.* 1125–*c.* 1175	Prose
53	London, BL, MS Burney 285	*c.* 1100–*c.* 1150	Prose
54	London, BL, MS Burney 295	*c.* 1100–*c.* 1150	Prose
55	London, BL, MS Burney 344	*c.* 1150–*c.* 1200	Verse & Prose
56	The Hague, KB, MS 76 E 15	1178–83	Prose
57	Florence, Laurenziana, MS Plut. 66.21	*c.* 1075–*c.* 1100	Prose
58	Leiden, UB, BPL 43 (part II, fols 79–111)	*c.* 1100–*c.* 1200	Verse
59	London, BL, MS Harley 3023	*c.* 1050–*c.* 1100	Verse & Prose
60	London, BL, MS Harley 3032	*c.* 1050–*c.* 1100	Verse & Prose
61	St Gall, SB, Cod. Sang. 53	*c.* 895	Prose
62	Copenhagen, KB, GKS 2021 4°	*c.* 1100	Verse
63	London, BL, MS Arundel 356	*c.* 1050–*c.* 1100	Prose & Music
64	Cambridge, St John's College, MS D.19	1112–26	Prose
65	London, BL, MS Harley 2892	*c.* 1025–*c.* 1075	Prose
66	London, BL, MS Harley 2624	*c.* 1100–*c.* 1125	Prose
67	Leiden, UB, BUR Q 1	*c.* 1100	Verse
68	London, BL, MS Burney 238	*c.* 1125–*c.* 1150	Prose
69	London, BL, MS Harley 3097	*c.* 1100	Prose
70	Cologny, Fondation Martin Bodmer, Cod. Bodmer 89	*c.* 1150	Verse
71	London, BL, MS Lansdowne 383	*c.* 1125–*c.* 1150	Prose
72	London, BL, MS Arundel 39	*c.* 1100–*c.* 1150	Prose
73	Cambridge, Corpus Christi College, MS 146	1096–1112	Prose
74	Worcester, Cathedral Library, Q.8, part II	*c.* 1000–*c.* 1100	Verse
75	Auxerre, BM, MS 227	*c.* 1187	Prose
76	London, BL, MS Arundel 35	*c.* 1125–*c.* 1175	Prose
77	Leiden, UB, BPL 154 (part II)	*c.* 1100–*c.* 1150	Prose
78	Leiden, UB, BPL 154 (part I)	*c.* 1100–*c.* 1150	Prose
79	Paris, BnF, Latin 7029	*c.* 1075–*c.* 1100	Prose
80	London, BL, MS Harley 2621	*c.* 1150–*c.* 1200	Verse

Contents	Relative width	Height (mm)	Width (mm)
Sedulius and Turcius Rufus Asterius	0.57	210	120
Mico of Centula, *Opus prosodaicum*; Peter Damian	0.57	210	120
Hugh of St Victor, *Institutiones in decalogum legis* and *Soliloquium de arrha animae*	0.57	210	120
Anselm of Canterbury, *Epistola de sacrificio azymi et fermentati*; misc. theological texts	0.57	210	120
Anselm of Laon, misc. theological texts	0.57	210	120
Prosper of Aquitaine, *Epigrammata ex sententiis Augustini*; Ps.-Prosper	0.57	210	120
Jerome, *De viris illustribus*	0.57	297	170
Justinus, *Epitome historiarum Pompei Trogi*	0.57	235	135
Virgil, *Aeneis*, glossed	0.58	307	178
Prudentius; Fulbert of Chartres, etc.	0.58	215	125
Prudentius, *Peristephanon*; Fulbert of Chartres; Berengar of Tours	0.58	215	125
Gospels prepared for liturgical use	0.58	395	230
Lucan, *Pharsalia*	0.58	240	140
Various lunar and astronomical tracts, incl. *computus*	0.58	180	105
Ivo of Chartres, *De sacramentis*	0.58	236	138
Benedictional, with prayers ('Canterbury Benedictional')	0.58	265	155
Cicero, *De inventione*; Ps.-Cicero, *Rhetorica ad Herennium*	0.59	205	120
Lucan, *Pharsalia*	0.59	276	162
Master Guido, Gloss on Priscian; Hugh of St Victor, *Didascalicon*	0.59	170	100
Theological miscellany (including Jerome)	0.59	280	165
Horace, *Opera*, glossed	0.59	212	125
Shaftesbury Psalter	0.59	220	130
Epistles of Paul (prepared for gloss)	0.59	270	160
Supplementum ad pontificale	0.59	315	187
Statius, *Thebais*	0.60	260	155
Annals; historical texts devoted to monastery; *Chronicle*	0.60	260	155
William of Malmesbury, *Gesta regum Anglorum*	0.60	310	185
Commentary on Priscian, *Institutiones grammaticae*	0.60	207	124
Priscian, *Institutiones grammaticae* (excerpts); Bede, computation; *medica*	0.60	207	124
Medica (*Articella*)	0.60	200	120
Horace, *Opera* (*Ars*, *Epist.*)	0.60	215	130

Appendix F

Glossary of Scribes

The following identifications are designed to help readers remind themselves of the various scribes and manuscript references revealed through this book's analysis. For the precise pages where each is mentioned, please consult the Indices that follow. Readers unfamiliar with palaeographical or codicological technical terms might consult Michelle P. Brown, *Understanding Illuminated Manuscripts: A Guide to Technical Terms*, a version of which is now available on the British Library's website.[1]

Apuleius Rubricator: Monte Cassino scribe responsible for the distinctive *capitalis* and Caroline minuscule in Florence, Laurenziana, MS Plut. 68.2, fols 126^{r}–183^{v}, Apuleius, *Apologia*, *Metamorphoses* (The Golden Ass), and *Florida*. Hand also seen in:

1. Geneva, Bibliothèque de Genève, MS lat. 357, Beatus of Liebana;
2. Copenhagen, KB, GKS 1653 4°, *Medica*;
3. Aberdeen, UL, MS 106, fols 55^{r}–64^{r}, Alberic.

[1] The British Library version is found at <https://www.bl.uk/catalogues/illuminatedmanuscripts/glossary.asp> [accessed 19 October 2018].

Bodleian Juvenal Scribe: not trained at Monte Cassino, but he worked there. His rounded Beneventan minuscule and equally distinctive *capitalis* is seen in his 'name' manuscript, Oxford, Bodleian, Canon. Class. Lat 41, Juvenal. Hand also seen in:

1. Paris, BnF, NAL 1628, fols 19^{r}–26^{v}, *Isagoge*;
2. Eton, College Library, MS 150, *Theoduli Ecloga*, etc.;
3. Copenhagen, KB, GKS 1653 4°, *Medica*;
4. Monte Cassino, MS 351, Paulus Aegineta.

Geraldus: the main scribe who at Monte Cassino copied The Hague, KB, MS 73 J 6, *Theorica Pantegni*. Called Scribe A in discussions of that manuscript in this monograph. Geraldus's identity is revealed in his signature to the document Monte Cassino, Archivum, Aula II, Caps. CIII, Fasc. II, no. 10, dated June 1061. Hand also seen in:

1. Paris, BnF, NAL 1628, *Isagoge*, interlinear and marginal suppletions;
2. Copenhagen, KB, GKS 1653 4°, *Medica*;
3. Monte Cassino, MS 333, Maximus Confessor, the ancient *scholia* in the margins;
4. Monte Cassino, MS 580, *Lexicon prosodiacum*, in Beneventan and Caroline minuscule.

Hague Rubricator: wrote the original rubrics in The Hague, KB, MS 73 J 6, *Theorica Pantegni,* as well as Prologue Part C, where he inserted Atto/Theodemar's final rhetorical flourish. Called Scribe B in discussions of that manuscript in this monograph. Hand also seen in:

1. Aberdeen, UL, MS 106, fols 55^{r}–64^{r}, Augustine, *De doctrina Christiana*;
2. Padua, Biblioteca Universitaria, lat. 892, Constantine the African, translation of Isaac's *De febribus*.

Bibliography

Primary Sources

ʿAli ibn al-ʿAbbās al-Maǧūsī, *Kāmil al-ṣinaʿah al-ṭibbiyah* (Cairo?: Publisher unknown, 1877)

——, *Kāmil al-ṣināʿa al-ṭibbiyya*, ed. by Fuat Sezgin, Publications of the Institute for the History of Arabic-Islamic Science (Frankfurt am Main: Institute for the History of Arabic-Islamic Science at Johann Wolfgang Goethe University, 1985)

Amatus of Montecassino, *History of the Normans*, trans. by Prescott N. Dunbar, rev. by Graham A. Loud (Woodbridge: Boydell & Brewer, 2002)

Aristoteles Latinus: Codices, ed. by George Lacombe and others, 2 vols (Rome: Libreria dello Stato, 1939, 1945), with supplement, ed. by Lorenzo Minio-Paluello (Bruges: Desclée de Brouwer, 1961)

Chronica monasterii Casinensis, ed. by Hartmut Hoffmann, in *Monumenta Germaniae historica: Scriptores*, XXXIV (Hannover: Hahn, 1980)

Chronicon Hildesheimense, ed. by Georg H. Pertz, in *Monumenta Germaniae historica: Scriptores*, VII (Hannover: Hahn, 1846)

Constantine the African, *Summi in omni philosophia viri Constantini Africani medici operum reliqua* […], ed. and printed by Heinrichus Petrus (Basel: Heinrichus Petrus, 1539). Available online via Bibliothèque interuniversitaire de medicine (Paris) <http://www.bium.univ-paris5.fr/histmed/medica/cote?00128x02> [accessed 29 March 2011]

——, *L'arte universale della Medicina*, part I, ed. and trans. by Marco T. Malato and Umberto de Martini (Rome: Istituto di storia della medicina dell'Università di Roma, 1961)

Einhard, *The Life of Charlemagne*, trans. by Samuel Epes Turner (New York: Harper & Brothers, 1880). Available in Fordham University's Medieval Sourcebook <https://sourcebooks. fordham.edu/basis/einhard> [accessed 3 March 2019]

Il Regesto di Sant'Angelo in Formis, facsim. ed. of Reg. 4 (1137–66) conserved in the Biblioteca del Monumento nazionale di Montecassino (Naples: M. D'Auria, Pubblicazioni Cassinesi, 2002)

Iotsaldus, *Vita S. Odilonis*, in *Patrologiae cursus completus: series latina*, ed. by Jacques-Paul Migne, CXLII (Paris: Garnier, 1853), cols 897–940

Isaak ben Salomon Israeli, *Omnia opera Ysaac in hoc volumine contenta: cum quibusdam aliis opusculis*, trans. by Constantine the African (Lyon: Bartholomaeus Trot, 1515)

Lawrence of Amalfi, *Laurentius, monachus Casinensis Archiepiscopus Amalfitanus: Opera*, ed. by Francis Newton, in *Monumenta Germaniae historica: Quellen zur Geistesgeschichte des Mittelalters*, 7 (Weimar: Böhlau, 1973)

Liber Constantini De stomacho: El tratado 'Sobre el estómago' de Constantino el Africano. Estudio, edición critica y traducción, ed. by Enrique Montero Cartelle (Vallodolid: Ediciones Universidad de Vallodolid, 2016)

Martial, *Epigrams*, ed. and trans. by David R. Shackleton Bailey, Loeb Classical Library 94–96, 3 vols (Cambridge, MA: Harvard University Press, 1993)

Maximus Confessor, *Quaestiones ad Thalassium*, I: *Quaestiones I–LV, una cum latina interpretatione Iohannis Scotti Eriugenae)*, ed. by Carl Laga and Carlos Steel, Corpus Christianorum, Continuatio Mediaevalis, Series Graeca, 7 (Turnhout: Brepols, 1980)

Medieval Medicine: A Reader, ed. and trans. by Faith Wallis (Toronto: University of Toronto Press, 2010)

Nemesius, *Nemesii episcopi Premnon physicon sive, Peri fuseōs anthrōpou liber*, ed. by Karl Immanuel Burkhard (Leipzig: Teubner, 1917)

——, *On the Nature of Man*, ed. and trans. by Robert W. Sharples and Philip J. van der Eijk, Translated Texts for Historians, 49 (Liverpool: Liverpool University Press, 2008)

Peter Damian, *Letters of Saint Peter Damian, 1–30*, ed. and trans. by Owen J. Blum, Fathers of the Church, Mediaeval Continuation, 1 (Washington, D.C.: Catholic University of America Press, 1989)

——, *Die Briefe des Petrus Damiani*, ed. by Kurt Reindel, in *Monumenta Germaniae Historica: Die Briefen der deutschen Kaiserzeit*, IV.3 (Munich: Monumenta Germaniae Historica, 1993)

——, *Liber Gomorrhianus: Omesessualità ecclesiastica e riforma della Chiesa*, ed. by Eduardo D'Angelo (Alessandrine: Edizioni dell'Orso, 2001)

Peter the Deacon, *De viris illustribus Casinensibus*, in *Patrologiae cursus completus: series latina*, ed. by Jacques-Paul Migne, CLXXIII (Paris: Garnier, 1895), cols 1003–62c

——, *Ortus et vita iustorum cenobii Casinensis*, ed. by Robert H. Rodgers, Classical Studies, 10 (Berkeley: University of California Publications, 1971)

Phocas, *Carmen de vita Vergilii*, ed. by Alexander Riese, in *Anthologia Latina*, fasc. II (Leipzig: Teubner, 1870)

Sylvester II [Gerbert of Aurillac], *The Letters of Gerbert: With his Papal Privileges as Sylvester II*, ed. and trans. by Harriet Pratt Lattin (New York: Columbia University Press, 1961)

Theodorus Priscianus, *Theodori Prisciani Euporiston libri III, cum physicorum fragmento et additamentis pseudo-Theodoreis: Accedunt Vindiciani Afri quae feruntur reliquiae*, ed. by Valentin Rose (Leipzig: Teubner, 1894)

William of Conches, *Philosophia mundi*, ed. and trans. by Gregor Maurach with Heidemarie Telle (Pretoria: University of South Africa, 1980)

Secondary Works

Acocella, Nicola, 'La figura e l'opera di Alfano I di Salerno', *Rassegna storia salernitana*, 19 (1958), 1–74

Altmann, Alexander, and Samuel M. Stern, *Isaac Israeli: A Neoplatonic Philosopher of the Early Tenth Century: His Works Translated with Comments and an Outline of his Philosophy* (Chicago: University of Chicago Press, 2009)

d'Alverny, Marie-Thérèse, 'La sagesse et ses sept filles. Recherches sur les allégories de la philosophie et des arts libéraux du XIe au XIIe siècle', *Mélanges dédiés a la mémoire de Félix Grat*, i (Paris: Pecqueur-Grat, 1946), pp. 245–78

——, 'L'écriture de Bernard Itier et son évolution', *Medievalia et humanistica*, 14 (1962), 47–54

Anderson, Diane Warne, 'Lexicon Prosodiacum Casinense-Ottobonianum' (unpublished doctoral thesis, Duke University, 1986)

——, 'Medieval Teaching Texts on Syllable Quantities and the Innovations from the School of Alberic of Monte Cassino', in *Latin Grammar and Rhetoric: From Classical Theory to Medieval Practice*, ed. by Carol Dana Lanham (London: Bloomsbury Academic, 2002), pp. 180–210

'Articella', Medieval Manuscripts in the National Library of Medicine, <www.nlm.nih.gov/hmd/medieval/articella.html> [accessed 24 November 2016]

Beccaria, Augusto, *I codici di medicina del periodo presalernitano (secoli IX, X e XI)*, Storia e letteratura, raccolta di studi e testi, 53 (Rome: Edizioni di Storia e letteratura, 1956)

——, 'Sulle tracce di un antico canone latino di Ippocrate e di Galeno. i., ii., iii.', *Italia medioevale e umanistica*, 2 (1959), 1–56; *Italia medioevale e umanistica*, 4 (1961), 1–75; and *Italia medioevale e umanistica*, 14 (1971), 1–23

Becker, Gustav Heinrich, *Catalogi bibliothecarum antiqui* (Bonn: M. Cohen et filius, 1885)

Bischoff, Bernhard, *Latin Palaeography: Antiquity and the Middle Ages*, trans. by Dábhí O' Cróinín and David Ganz (Cambridge: Cambridge University Press, 1990)

Black, Winston, '"I Will Add What the Arab Once Taught": Constantine the African in Northern European Medical Verse', in *Herbs and Healers from the Ancient Mediterranean through the Medieval West: Essays in Honor of John Riddle*, ed. by Anne Van Arsdall and Timothy Graham (Aldershot: Ashgate, 2012), pp. 153–86

Bloch, Herbert, 'Monte Cassino's Teachers and Library in the High Middle Ages', in *La scuola nell'occidente latino dell'alto medioevo*, i (Spoleto: Presso la sede del centro, 1972), pp. 563–605

——, *Monte Cassino in the Middle Ages*, 2 vols (Cambridge, MA: Harvard University Press, 1986)

Boeren, Petrus C., Anne S. Korteweg, and G. Piket, *Catalogus van de liturgische handschriften van de Koninklijke Bibliotheek* (The Hague: Koninklijke Bibliotheek, 1988)

Boffey, Julia, and John J. Thompson, 'Anthologies and Miscellanies: Production and Choice of Texts', in *Book Production and Publishing in Britain, 1375–1475*, ed. by Jeremy Griffiths and Derek Pearsall (Cambridge: Cambridge University Press, 1989), pp. 279–315

Bos, Gerrit, 'Ibn al-Ǧazzār's *Risāla fī al-nisyān* and Constantine's *Liber de oblivione*', in *Constantine the African and 'Alī ibn al-'Abbās al-Maǧūsī: The 'Pantegni' and Related Texts*, ed. by Charles Burnett and Danielle Jacquart, Studies in Ancient Medicine, 10 (Leiden: Brill, 1994), pp. 203–23

Bowen, James, *A History of Western Education: Civilization of Europe, Sixth to Sixteenth Century*, II (London: St Martin's, 1975)

Bozzolo, Carla, and Ezio Ornato, *Pour une histoire du livre manuscrit au moyen-âge: Trois essais de codicologie quantitative* (Paris: CNRS, 1983)

Braga, Gabriella, 'Lorenzo d'Amalfi, un agiografo lettore dei classici nella Montecassino del secolo XI', in *Virgilio e il chiostro: Manoscritti di autori classici e civiltà monastica*, ed. by Mariano Dell'Omo (Rome: Fratelli Palombi, 1996), pp. 91–101

Brett, Michael, 'Ifriqiya as a Market for Saharan Trade from the Tenth to the Twelfth Century A.D.', *Journal of African History*, 10 (1969), 347–64

British Library, 'Treasures Known and Unknown: Tall Narrow Books', Catalogue of Illuminated Manuscripts <www.bl.uk/catalogues/illuminatedmanuscripts/TourKnownE.asp> [accessed 23 November 2016]

Brown, Michelle P., *Understanding Illuminated Manuscripts: A Guide to Technical Terms* (Malibu: J. Paul Getty Museum, 1994); online via the British Library at <https://www.bl.uk/catalogues/illuminatedmanuscripts/glossary.asp> [accessed 19 October 2018]

Brown, Virginia, '"Where Have All the Grammars Gone?" The Survival of Grammatical Texts in Beneventan Script', in *Manuscripts and Tradition of Grammatical Texts from Antiquity to the Renaissance: Proceedings of a Conference Held at Erice, 16–34 October 1997, as the 11th Course of International School for the Study of Written Records*, ed. by Mario De Nonno, Paolo De Paolis, and Louis Holtz, 2 vols (Cassino: Edizioni dell'Università degli Studi di Cassino, 2000), I, 389–414

de Bruin, Cebus C., '"Retractationes" with Reference to the Question Whether MS Brussels 2849–51 Is an Autograph', in *Essays Presented to G. I. Lieftinck*, III: *Neerlandica manuscripta, litterae textualis*, ed. by Johan P. Gumbert and Max J. M. de Haan (Amsterdam: Van Gendt, 1976), pp. 84–98

de Bruyne, Donatien, 'Le plus ancien catalogue des manuscrits de Notre-Dame de Paris', *Revue bénédictine*, 29 (1912), 481–85

Bulst-Thiele, Marie Luise, *Kaiserin Agnes*, Beiträge zur Kulturgeschichte des Mittelalters und der Renaissance, 52 (Leipzig: Teubner, 1933)

Burnett, Charles, 'The Chapter on the Spirits in the *Pantegni* of Constantine the African', in *Constantine the African and 'Alī ibn al-'Abbās al-Maǧūsī: The 'Pantegni' and Related Texts*, ed. by Charles Burnett and Danielle Jacquart, Studies in Ancient Medicine, 10 (Leiden: Brill, 1994), pp. 99–120

——, 'Give Him the White Cow: Notes and Note-Taking in the Universities in the Twelfth and Thirteenth Centuries', *History of Universities*, 14 (1995–96), 1–30

——, 'Encounters with Rāzī the Philosopher: Constantine the African, Petrus Alfonsi and Ramón Martí', in *Pensamiento medieval hispano: Homenaje a Horacio Santiago-Otero*, ed. by Jose María Soto Rábanos, 2 vols (Madrid: Consejo superior de investigaciones científicas, 1998), II, 973–92

——, 'Physics before the *Physics*: Early Translations from Arabic of Texts concerning Nature in MSS British Library, Additional 22719 and Cotton Galba E IV', *Medioevo: Rivista di storia della filosofia medievale*, 27 (2002), 53–109

Burnett, Charles, and Danielle Jacquart, eds, *Constantine the African and 'Alī ibn al-'Abbās al-Maǧūsī: The 'Pantegni' and Related Texts*, ed. by Charles Burnett and Danielle Jacquart, Studies in Ancient Medicine, 10 (Leiden: Brill, 1994)

——, 'Preface', in *Constantine the African and 'Alī ibn al-'Abbās al-Maǧūsī: The 'Pantegni' and Related Texts*, ed. by Charles Burnett and Danielle Jacquart, Studies in Ancient Medicine, 10 (Leiden: Brill, 1994), pp. vii–ix

Catalogues des manuscrits datés. Numerous volumes, editors, and publishers in an ongoing collection <http://www.palaeographia.org/cipl/cmd.htm> [accessed 8 December 2016]

Clanchy, Michael, *From Memory to Written Record, England 1066–1307*, 3rd edn (Hoboken: Wiley-Blackwell, 2013)

Cleaver, Laura, 'Grammar and her Children: Learning to Read in the Art of the Twelfth Century', *Marginalia*, 9 (2009) <www.marginalia.co.uk/journal/09education/cleaver.php> [accessed 24 November 2016]

Collins, Minta, *Medieval Herbals: The Illustrative Traditions*, British Library Studies in Medieval Culture (London: British Library, 2000)

'Constantinus Africanus', SISMEL's Mirabile: Archivio Digitale della Cultura Medievale <http://www.mirabileweb.it/calma/constantinus-africanus-n-1020-ca-m-1087/736> [accessed 10 June 2016]

Creutz, Rudolf, 'Erzbischof Alfanus I, ein frühsalernitanischer Arzt', *Studien und Mitteilungen zur Geschichte des Benediktiner-Ordens und seiner Zweige*, 47 (1929), 413–32

——, 'Nachtrag zu "Erzbischof Alfanus I, ein frühsalernitanischer Arzt"', *Studien und Mitteilungen zur Geschichte des Benediktiner-Ordens und seiner Zweige*, 48 (1930), 205–08

——, 'Additamenta zu Konstantinus Africanus und seinen Schülern Johannes und Atto', *Studien und Mitteilungen zur Geschichte des Benediktiner Ordens und seiner Zweige*, 50 (1932), 420–42

——, 'Der Frühsalernitaner Alfanus und sein bislang unbekannter "Liber de pulsibus": Zum Gedenken an die 850. Wiederkehr seines Todestages (7 Okt. 1085)', *Sudhoffs Archiv für Geschichte der Medizin und der Naturwissenschaften*, 29 (1936), 57–83

Cyrus, Cynthia J., *The Scribes for Women's Convents in Late Medieval Germany* (Toronto: University of Toronto Press, 2009)

Dales, Richard C., 'Marius "On the Elements" and the Twelfth-Century Science of Matter', *Viator*, 3 (1972), 191–218

Dalli, Charles, 'Bridging Europe and Africa: Norman Sicily's Other Kingdom', in *Bridging the Gaps: Sources, Methodology and Approaches to Religion in History*, ed. by Joaquim Carvalho (Pisa: Plus-Pisa University Press, 2008), pp. 77–93

Derolez, Albert, 'The Genesis of Hildegard of Bingen's *Liber divinorum operum*. The Codicological Evidence', in *Litterae textuales: Festschrift für G. I. Lieftinck*, ed. by Johan P. Gumbert and Max. J. M. de Haan, 4 vols (Amsterdam: Van Gendt, 1972), II, 23–33

——, *The Palaeography of Gothic Manuscript Books from the Twelfth to the Early Sixteenth Century*, Cambridge Studies in Palaeography and Codicology, 9 (Cambridge: Cambridge University Press, 2001)

Desilve, Julius, 'De schola Elnonensi Sancti Amandi a saeculo IX ad XII usque' (unpublished doctoral dissertation, Katholieke Universiteit Leuven, 1890)

De Wald, Ernest T., 'Notes on the Tuotilo Ivories in St Gall', *The Art Bulletin*, 15 (1933), 202–09

Dillon, Emma, *Medieval Music-Making and the Roman de Fauvel* (Cambridge: Cambridge University Press, 2002)

Dronke, Peter, *A History of Twelfth-Century Western Philosophy* (Cambridge: Cambridge University Press, 1992)

Duft, Johannes, and Rudolf Schnyder, *Die Elfenbein-Einbände der Stiftsbibliothek St Gallen* (Beuron: Beuroner Kunstverlag, 1984)

e-codices: Virtual Manuscript Library of Switzerland <www.e-codices.unifr.ch> [accessed 23 November 2016]

Eder, Christine Elisabeth, *Die Schule des Klosters Tegernsee im frühen Mittelalter im Spiegel der Tegernseer Handschriften* (Munich: Arbeo-Gesellschaft, 1972)

Escudier, Denis, 'Les manuscrits musicaux du Moyen Age (die XIe au XIIe siècle): Essai de typologie', *Codicologica*, 3 (1980), 34–45

Evans, Gillian Rosemary, *Old Arts and New Theology: The Beginnings of Theology as an Academic Discipline* (Oxford: Clarendon, 1980)

Everett, Nicholas, *The Alphabet of Galen: Pharmacy from Antiquity to the Middle Ages* (Toronto: University of Toronto Press, 2012)

Fagnoni, Anna Maria, 'Un cronista medievale al lavoro. Leone Ostiense e la prima redazione della Cronaca Cassineses. Problemi di analisi', *Scripta philologa*, 2 (1980), 51–129

von Falkenhausen, Vera, Nadia Jamil, and Jeremy Johns, 'The Twelfth-Century Documents of St George's of Tròccoli (Sicily)', *Journal of Arabic and Islamic Studies*, 16 (2016), 1–84b

Gamber, Klaus, *Codices liturgici latini antiquiores*, 2 vols (Freiburg: Universitätsverlag, 1968)

Gibson, Craig A., and Francis Newton, 'Pandulf of Capua's *De calculatione*: An Illustrated Abacus Treatise and Some Evidence for the Hindu-Arabic Numerals in Eleventh-Century South Italy', *Mediaeval Studies*, 57 (1995), 293–335

Gibson, Margaret T., 'The Study of the *Timaeus* in the Eleventh and Twelfth Centuries', *Pensamiento*, 25 (1969), 183–94

Gehl, Paul F., 'Vat. Ottobonianus lat. 1354: Apropos of Catalogue Notices and the History of Grammatical Pedagogy', *Revue d'histoire des textes*, 8 (1978), 303–97

Geyl, Arie, 'Zwei lateinische Handschriften aus dem 11ten Jahrhundert, respective von Gariopontus und Constantinus Afer', *Janus*, 13 (1909), 161–66

Glare, Peter G. W., ed., *Oxford Latin Dictionary* (Oxford: Oxford University Press, 1968)

Glauche, Günter, *Schullektüre im Mittelalter: Entstehung und Wandlungen des Lektürekanons bis 1200 nach den Quellen dargestellt* (Munich: Arbeo-Gesellschaft, 1970)

Glaze, Florence Eliza, 'The Perforated Wall: The Ownership and Circulation of Medical Books in Medieval Europe, c. 800–1200' (unpublished doctoral dissertation, Duke University, 2000); abstract in ProQuest Dissertation Abstracts International (2000–01, A 61/01)

——, 'Gariopontus and the Salernitans: Textual Traditions in the Eleventh and Twelfth Centuries', in *La 'Collectio Salernitana' di Salvatore De Renzi*, ed. by Danielle Jacquart and Agostino Paravicini Bagliani (Firenze: SISMEL Edizioni del Galluzzo, 2008), pp. 149–90

——, 'Prolegomena: Scholastic Openings to Gariopontus of Salerno's *Passionarius*', in *Between Text and Patient: The Medical Enterprise in Medieval and Early Modern Europe*, ed. by Florence Eliza Glaze and Brian K. Nance (Florence: SISMEL Edizioni del Galluzzo, 2011), pp. 57–86

——, 'Speaking in Tongues: Medical Wisdom and Glossing Practices in and around Salerno, c. 1040–1200', in *Herbs and Healers from the Ancient Mediterranean through the Medieval West: Essays in Honor of John M. Riddle*, ed. by Anne van Arsdall and Timothy Graham (Farnham: Ashgate, 2012), pp. 63–106

——, 'Salerno's Lombard Prince: Johannes Abbas de Curte as Medical Practitioner', *Early Science and Medicine*, 23 (2018), 177–216

——, 'Authority: Trusting the Text in the Early Middle Ages', in *The Cultural History of Medicine*, II: *The Middle Ages*, ed. by Iona McCleery (London: Bloomsbury Academic, forthcoming 2020)

——, *Medicine, Sister of Philosophy: Rational Medicine in the Latin West, c. 500–1200*, unpublished (in preparation)

Glenn, Jason, *Politics and History in the Tenth Century: The Work of Richer of Rheims* (Cambridge: Cambridge University Press, 2007)

Glick, Thomas F., 'Communication', in *Medieval Science, Technology and Medicine: An Encyclopedia*, ed. by Thomas F. Glick, Steven J. Livesey, and Faith Wallis (New York: Routledge, 2005), pp. 135–39

Grape-Albers, Heidi, *Spätantike Bilder aus der Welt des Arztes: Medizinische Bilderhandschriften der Spätantike und ihre mittelalterliche Überlieferung* (Wiesbaden: Pressler, 1977)

Green, Monica, 'The *De genecia* Attributed to Constantine the African', *Speculum*, 62 (1987), 299–323

——, 'The Re-Creation of *Pantegni*, *Practica*, Book VIII', in *Constantine the African and 'Alī ibn al-'Abbās al-Mağūsī: The 'Pantegni' and Related Texts*, ed. by Charles Burnett and Danielle Jacquart, Studies in Ancient Medicine, 10 (Leiden: Brill, 1994), pp. 121–60

——, 'Constantine the African', in *Medieval Science, Technology and Medicine: An Encyclopedia*, ed. by Thomas F. Glick, Steven J. Livesey, and Faith Wallis (New York: Routledge, 2005), pp. 145–47

Grier, James, *The Musical World of a Medieval Monk: Adémar de Chabannes in Eleventh-Century Aquitaine* (Cambridge: Cambridge University Press, 2006)

Gumbert, Johan P., *Die Utrechter Kartäuser und ihre Bücher im frühen fünfzehnten Jahrhundert* (Leiden: Brill, 1974)

——, 'The Sizes of Manuscripts: Some Statistics and Notes', in *Hellinga Festschrift/ Feestbundel/ Mélanges: Forty-Three Studies in Bibliography Presented to Prof. Dr Wytze Hellinga on the Occasion of his Retirement from the Chair of Neophilology in the University of Amsterdam at the End of the Year 1978*, ed. by Anthony R. A. Croiset van Uchelen (Amsterdam: Nico Israel, 1980), pp. 277–88

——, 'The Speed of Scribes', in *Scribi e colofoni: Le Sottoscrizioni di Copisti dalle origini all'Avvento della stampa, atti del seminario di Erice X Colloquio del Comite International de Paleographie Latine (23–28 ottobre 1993)*, ed. by Emma Condello and Giuseppe De Gregorio, Biblioteca del Centro per il Collegamento degli Studi Medievale e Umanistici in Umbria, 14 (Spoleto: Centro per il Collegamento degli Studi Medievale e Umanistici in Umbria, 1995), pp. 57–69

——, 'The Irish Priscian in Leiden', *Quaerendo*, 4 (1997), 280–99

Halleux, Robert, and Jacques Schamp, eds, *Les lapidaires grecs: Lapidaire Orphique, Kérygmes lapidaires d'Orphée, Socrate et Denys, lapidaire nautique, Damigéron-Évax (traduction latine)* (Paris: Les Belles Lettres, 1985)

de Hamel, Christopher, *The Book: A History of the Bible* (London: Phaidon, 2001)

Hanson, Ann Ellis, and Monica Green, 'Soranus of Ephesus: *Methodicorum princeps*', in *Wissenschaften: Medizin und Biologie*, Aufstieg und Niedergang der römischen Welt, II.37.2, ed. by Wolfgang Haase and Hildegard Temporini (Berlin: de Gruyter, 1994), pp. 968–1075

Haskins, Charles Homer, 'A List of Text-Books from the Close of the Twelfth Century', in *Studies in the History of Mediaeval Science* (Cambridge, MA: Harvard University Press, 1924), pp. 356–78

Hettinger, Anette, 'Zum Lebensgeschichte und zum Todesdatum des Constantinus Africanus', *Deutsches Archiv für Erforschung des Mittelalters Köln-Weimar-Wien*, 46 (1990), 517–29

Hoffmann, Hartmut, 'Der Kalender des Leo Marsicanus', *Deutsches Archiv für Erforschung des Mittelalters*, 21 (1965), 82–149

——, 'Studien zur Chronik von Montecassino', *Deutsches Archiv*, 29 (1973), 59–162

Holcomb, Melanie, ed., *Pen and Parchment: Drawing in the Middle Ages* (New Haven: Yale University Press, 2009)

Holtz, Louis, 'Le Parisinus Latinus 7530, synthèse cassinienne des arts libéraux', *Studi medievali*, 3rd ser., 16 (1975), 97–152

Holtzmann, Walther, 'Laurentius von Amalfi: Ein Lehrer Hildebrands', *Studi Gregoriani*, 1 (1947), 207–36

Huglo, Michel, 'The Cantatorium: From Charlemagne to the Fourteenth Century', in *The Study of Medieval Chant: Paths and Bridges, East and West. In Honor of Kenneth Levy*, ed. by Peter Jeffery (Cambridge: Boydell, 2001), pp. 89–103

Irving, Andrew J. M., '(Not) Identifying a Desiderian Evangelistary Fragment BAV Vat. Lat. 10644, f. 28r–31v', *Scriptorium*, 66 (2012), 109–55

Irving, Andrew J. M., and Brian Long, 'An Early Fragment of Constantine the African's Viaticum in Beneventan Script', *Bibliografia dei manoscritti in scrittura beneventana*, 24 (2016), 33–37

Iskandar, Albert Z., 'An Attempted Reconstruction of the Alexandrian Medical Curriculum', *Medical History*, 20 (1976), 235–58

Jacquart, Danielle, 'À l'aube de la renaissance médicale des XIe–XIIe siècles: L'"Isagoge Johannitii" et son traducteur', *Bibliothèque de l'École des Chartes*, 144 (1986), 209–40

——, 'Le sens donné par Constantin l'Africain à son œuvre: les chapitres introductifs en arabe et en latin', in *Constantine the African and 'Alī ibn al-'Abbās al-Maǧūsī: The 'Pantegni' and Related Texts*, ed. by Charles Burnett and Danielle Jacquart, Studies in Ancient Medicine, 10 (Leiden: Brill, 1994), pp. 71–89

——, 'La medicine entre théorique et pratique: Retour sur quelques définitions originelles', in *Handlung und Wissenschaft: Die Epistemologie der praktischen Wissenschaften im 13. und 14. Jahrhundert / Action and Science: The Epistemology of the Practical Sciences in the 13th and 14th Centuries*, ed. by Matthias Lutz-Bachman and Alexander Fidora, Wissenskultur und gesellschaftlicher Wander, 29 (Berlin: De Gruyter, 2008), pp. 33–42

Jacquart, Danielle, and Francoise Micheau, *La médecine arabe et l'occident médiéval* (Paris: Maisonneuve et Larose, 1990)

Jones, Peter Murray, *Medieval Medicine in Illuminated Manuscripts* (London: British Library, 1998)

Jordan, Mark, 'Medicine as Science in the Early Commentaries on Johannitius', *Traditio*, 43 (1987), 121–45

——, 'The Construction of a Philosophical Medicine: Exegesis and Argument in Salernitan Teaching on the Soul', *Renaissance Medical Learning* (1990), 42–61

——, 'The Fortune of Constantine's *Pantegni*', in *Constantine the African and 'Alī ibn al-'Abbās al-Maǧūsī: The 'Pantegni' and Related Texts*, ed. by Charles Burnett and Danielle Jacquart, Studies in Ancient Medicine, 10 (Leiden: Brill, 1994), pp. 286–302

Ker, Neil R., *Catalogue of Manuscripts Containing Anglo-Saxon* (Oxford: Clarendon, 1957; repr. 1990)

Kibre, Pearl, *Hippocrates Latinus: Repertorium of Hippocratic Writings in the Latin Middle Ages* (New York: Fordham University Press, 1985)

Kinney, Dale, 'A Late Antique Ivory Plaque and Modern Response', *American Journal of Archaeology*, 98 (1994), 457–80

Knight, Valerie, 'The *De podagra* (*On Gout*): A pre-Gariopontean Treatise Excerpted from the Latin Translation of the Greek *Therapeutica* by Alexander of Tralles' (unpublished doctoral thesis, University of Manchester, 2015)

Köhler, Theodor Wolfram, *'Homo animal nobilissimum': Konturen des spezifisch Menschlicher in der naturphilosophischen Aristoteleskommentierung des dreizehnten Jahrhunderts* (Leiden: Brill, 2008)

Kristeller, Paul Oskar, 'The School at Salerno: Its Development and its Contribution to the History of Learning', *Bulletin of the History of Medicine*, 17 (1945), 138–94

Kwakkel, Erik, *Dit sijn die Dietsche boeke die ons toebehoeren: De kartuizers van Herne en de productie van Middelnederlandse handschriften in de regio Brussel (1350–1400)*, Miscellanea Neerlandica, 27 (Leuven: Peeters, 2002)

——, 'The Cultural Dynamics of Medieval Book Production', in *Manuscripten en miniaturen: Studies aangeboden aan Anne S. Korteweg bij haar afscheid van de Koninklijke Bibliotheek*, ed. by Jos Biemans and others, Bijdragen voor de geschiedenis van de Nederlandse boekhandel, 8 (Zutphen: Walburg Pers, 2007), pp. 243–52

——, 'Lost but Not Forgotten: References to a Remarkable Middle Dutch *Legenda aurea* Manuscript', in *Signs on the Edge: Space, Text and Margins in Medieval Manuscripts*, ed. by Rolf H. Bremmer Jr and Sarah Larratt Keefer (Leuven: Peeters, 2007), pp. 261–87

——, 'Behind the Scenes of a Revision: Michael Scot and the Oldest Manuscript of his *Abbreviatio Avicenne*', *Viator*, 40 (2009), 107–32

——, 'Commercial Organization and Economic Innovation', in *The Production of Books in England 1350–1500*, ed. by Alexandra Gillespie and Daniel Wakelin (Cambridge: Cambridge University Press, 2011), pp. 173–91

——, 'Biting, Kissing and the Treatment of Feet', in *Turning over a New Leaf: Change and Development in the Medieval Book*, ed. by Erik Kwakkel, Rosamond McKitterick, and Rodney Thomson (Leiden: Leiden University Press, 2012), pp. 79–126; 206–08

——, 'Discarded Parchment as Writing Support in English Manuscript Culture', *English Manuscript Studies 1100–1700*, 17 (2012), 239–61

——, '"Dit boek heeft niet de vereiste breedte": Afwijkende bladdimensies in de elfde en twaalfte eeuw', in *Jaarboek voor Nederlandse boekgeschiedenis*, XIX, ed. by Goran Proot and others (The Hague: Koninklijke Bibliotheek, 2012), pp. 33–49

——, 'Decoding the Material Book: Cultural Residue in Medieval Manuscripts', in *The Medieval Manuscript Book: Cultural Approaches*, ed. by Michael Van Dussen and Michael Johnson (Cambridge: Cambridge University Press, 2015), pp. 60–76

——, 'Manuscripts of the Latin Classics 800–1200: An Introduction', in *Manuscripts of the Latin Classics 800–1200*, ed. by Erik Kwakkel (Leiden: Leiden University Press, 2015), pp. 13–21

——, 'The Margin as Editorial Space: Upgrading *Dioscorides alphabeticus* in Eleventh-Century Monte Cassino', in *The Annotated Book in the Early Middle Ages: Practices of Reading and Writing*, ed. by Irene van Renswoude and Mariken Teeuwen, Utrecht Studies in Medieval Literacy (Turnhout: Brepols, 2018), pp. 357–74

Langslow, David R., *The Latin Alexander Trallianus: The Text and Transmission of a Late Latin Medical Book*, Journal of Roman Studies Monograph, 10 (London: Society for the Promotion of Roman Studies, 2006)

——, 'The *Epistula* in Ancient Scientific and Technical Literature, with Special Reference to Medicine', in *Ancient Letters: Classical and Late Antique Epistolography*, ed. by Ruth Morello and Andrew D. Morrison (Oxford: Oxford University Press, 2007), pp. 211–54

Lanham, Carol D., 'Alberic of Monte Cassino', in *Medieval Italy: An Encyclopedia*, I, ed. by Christopher Kleinhenz (New York: Routledge, 2004), pp. 8–9

Larpi, Luca, 'Early Medieval Medici in Italian Charters, *s.* IX–XI', Society for the Social History of Medicine Conference, Oxford University, 10–12 July 2014 <https://manchester.academia.edu/LucaLarpi> [accessed 2 January 2017]

Leclercq, Jean, *The Love of Learning and the Desire for God: A Study of Monastic Culture*, trans. by Catharine Misrahi, 3rd edn (New York: Fordham University Press, 1998)

Leiser, Gary, 'Medical Education in Islamic Lands from the Seventh to the Fourteenth Century', *Journal of the History of Medicine and Allied Sciences*, 38 (1983), 48–75

Lemaire, Jacques, *Introduction à la codicologie* (Louvain: Université catholique de Louvain, Institut d'études médiévales, 1989)

Lendinara, Patrizia, 'Instructional Manuscripts in England: The Tenth and Eleventh Century Codices', in *Form and Content of Instruction in Anglo-Saxon England in the Light of Contemporary Manuscript Evidence: Papers Presented at the International Conference, Udine, 6–8 April 2006*, ed. by Patrizia Lendinara, Loredana Lazzari, and Maria Amalia D'Aronco (Turnhout: Brepols, 2007), pp. 59–113

Lentini, Anselmo, and Faustino Avagliano, *I carmi di Alfano I Arcivescovo di Salerno* (Montecassino: Monaci di Montecassino, 1974)

Light, Laura, 'The Bible and the Individual: The Thirteenth-Century Paris Bible', in *The Practice of the Bible in the Middle Ages: Production, Reception, and Performance in Western Christianity*, ed. by Susan Boynton and Diane J. Reilly (New York: Columbia University Press, 2011), pp. 228–46

Lohrmann, Dietrich, *Das Register Papst Johannes' VIII (872–82): Neue Studien zur Abschrift Reg. Vat. I, zum verlorenen Originalregister und zum Diktat der Briefe*, Bibliothek des Deutschen Historischen Instituts in Rom, 30 (Tübingen: Niemeyer, 1968)

Long, Brian, and Andrew J. M. Irving, 'An Early Fragment of Constantine the African's *Viaticum* in Beneventan Script', *Bibliografia dei manoscritti in scrittura Beneventana*, 24 (2016), 81–85

Lorch, Richard, 'The Science of Weights', in *Medieval Science, Technology and Medicine: An Encyclopedia*, ed. by Thomas F. Glick, Steven J. Livesey, and Faith Wallis (New York: Routledge, 2005), pp. 513–14

Loud, Graham, *The Age of Robert Guiscard: Southern Italy and the Norman Conquest* (Harlow: Longman, 2000)

Lowe, Elias A., *'Scriptura Beneventana': Facsimiles of South Italian and Dalmatian Manuscripts from the Sixth to the Fourteenth Century* (Oxford: Clarendon, 1929)

——, 'A New List of Beneventan Manuscripts', in *Collectanea Vaticana in honorem Anselmi M. Cardinalis Albareda a Biblioteca Apostolica edita*, II, Studi e Testi, 220 (Vatican City: Biblioteca Apostolica Vaticana, 1962), pp. 211–44

——, *The Beneventan Script: A History of the South Italian Minuscule*, 2nd edn, prepared and enlarged by Virginia Brown (Rome: Edizioni di storia e letteratura, 1980)

MacKinney, Loren C., 'Medical Ethics and Etiquette in the Early Middle Ages: The Persistence of Hippocratic Ideals', *Bulletin of the History of Medicine*, 26 (1952), 1–31

Magistrale, Francesco, *Cultura grafica e circolazione libraria a Bari in età medievale* (Bari: Graphis, 1997)

Maurach, Gregor, 'Johannicius: Isagoge ad Techne Galieni', *Sudhoffs Archiv*, 67 (1983), 148–74

McGinn, Bernard, *Three Treatises on Man: A Cistercian Anthropology*, Cistercian Fathers Series, 24 (Kalamazoo: Cistercian Publications, 1977)

McKitterick, Rosamond, 'Glossaries and Other Innovations in Carolingian Book Production', in *Turning over a New Leaf: Change and Development in the Medieval Book*, ed. by Erik Kwakkel, Rosamond McKitterick, and Rodney Thomson (Leiden: Leiden University Press, 2012), pp. 21–76

McNeill, John, '*Veteres statuas emit Rome*: Romanesque Attitudes to the Past', in *Romanesque and the Past: Retrospection in the Art and Architecture of Romanesque Europe*, ed. by John McNeill and Richard Plant (Leeds: Maney, 2013), pp. 1–24

McVaugh, Michael R., 'Bedside Manners in the Middle Ages', *Bulletin of the History of Medicine*, 71 (1997), 201–23

Micheau, Françoise, ''Ali ibn al-'Abbās al-Magūsī et son mileu', in *Constantine the African and 'Alī ibn al-'Abbās al-Mağūsī: The 'Pantegni' and Related Texts*, ed. by Charles Burnett and Danielle Jacquart, Studies in Ancient Medicine, 10 (Leiden: Brill, 1994), pp. 1–15

Metcalf, Alex, *Muslims and Christians in Norman Sicily: Arabic-Speakers and the End of Islam* (Abingdon: RoutledgeCurzon, 2003)

Metropolitan Museum of Art, 'Drawing and the Learned Tradition: Philosophy and the Seven Liberal Arts', in Pen and Parchment: Drawing in the Middle Ages <www.blog.metmuseum.org/penandparchment/exhibition-images/cat250ar5_49c/> [accessed 24 November 2016]

Meyvaert, Paul, 'The Exegetical Treatises of Peter the Deacon and Eriugena's Latin Rendering of the *Ad Thalassium* of Maximus the Confessor', *Sacris erudiri*, 14 (1963), 130–48

——, 'Eriugena's Translation of the *Ad Thalassium* of Maximus: Preliminaries to an Edition of This Work', in *The Mind of Eriugena*, ed. by John J. O'Meara and Ludwig Bieler (Dublin: Irish University Press, 1973), pp. 77–88

de Meÿier, Karel A., *Codices Vossiani latini*, II: *Codices in quarto* (Leiden: Leiden University Press, 1975)

Minnis, Alastair J., *Medieval Theory of Authorship: Scholastic Literary Attitudes in the Later Middle Ages*, 2nd edn (Aldershot: Wildwood House, 1988)

Minnis, Alastair J., and Alexander B. Scott, *Medieval Literary Theory and Criticism, c. 1100–c. 1375: The Commentary Tradition* (Oxford: Oxford University Press, 1988)

Munk Olsen, Birger, *L'Étude des auteurs classiques latins aux XIe et XIIe siècles*, 3 vols (Paris: Centre national de la recherche scientifique, 1982–89)

——, 'The Production of Classics in the Eleventh and Twelfth Centuries', in *Medieval Manuscripts of the Latin Classics: Production and Use*, ed. by Claudine A. Chavannes-Mazel and Margaret McFadden Smith (Los Altos Hills: Anderson-Lovelace, 1996), pp. 1–18

Nees, Lawrence, 'Early Carolingian Manuscripts and Ivories', in *Les manuscrits carolingiens: Actes du colloque de Paris, Bibliothèque nationale de France, le 4 mai 2007,* ed. by Marie-Pierre Laffitte and Jean-Pierre Caillet, Bibliologia, 27 (Turnhout: Brepols, 2009), pp. 159–84

Newman, Barbara, ed., *Voice of the Living Light: Hildegard of Bingen and her World* (Berkeley: University of California Press, 1998)

Newton, Francis, 'Tibullus in Two Grammatical Florilegia of the Middle Ages', *Transactions and Proceedings of the American Classical Association*, 93 (1962), 253–86

——, 'Leo Marsicanus and the Dedicatory Text and Drawing in Monte Cassino 99', *Scriptorium*, 33 (1979), 181–205 and pls 20–21

——, 'One Scriptorium, Two Scripts: Beneventan, Caroline, and the Problem of Marston 112', *Beinecke Studies in Early Manuscripts: Yale University Library Gazette*, Supplementary, 66 (1991), 118–33

——, 'Constantine the African and Monte Cassino: New Elements and the Text of the *Isagoge*', in *Constantine the African and 'Alī ibn al-'Abbās al-Maǧūsī: The 'Pantegni' and Related Texts*, ed. by Charles Burnett and Danielle Jacquart, Studies in Ancient Medicine, 10 (Leiden: Brill, 1994), pp. 16–47

——, *The Scriptorium and Library at Monte Cassino, 1058–1105* (Cambridge: Cambridge University Press, 1999)

——, '"Expolitio" per l'Umanesimo: la formazione classica dei monaci cassinesi nell'XI secolo', in *Il monaco, il libro, la biblioteca: Atti del Convegno Cassino-Montecassino, 5–8 settembre 2000*, ed. by Oronzo Pecere (Cassino: Università degli studi di Cassino, 2003), pp. 169–79, pls pp. 224–35

——, 'Fifty Years of Beneventan Studies', *Archiv für Diplomatik: Schriftgeschichte Sigel- und Wappenkunde*, 50 (2004), 327–45

——, 'Arabic Medicine and Other Arabic Cultural Influences in Southern Italy in the Time of Constantinus Africanus (saec. XI^{2})', in *Between Text & Patient: The Medical Enterprise in Medieval and Early Modern Europe*, ed. by Florence Eliza Glaze and Brian K. Nance (Florence: SISMEL Edizioni del Galluzzo, 2011), pp. 25–55

——, 'Un *codex Casinensis nobilissimus* di testi classici: Il Vat. Ottobon. lat. 1406 e il suo contesto storico e artistico', in *Libri e testi Lavori in corso a Cassino: Atti del Seminario internazionale Cassino, 30–31 gennaio 2012*, ed. by Roberta Casavecchia and others (Cassino: Università degli Studi di Cassino e del Lazio meridionale, Dipartimento di Lettere e Filosofia, 2013), pp. 185–212

O'Boyle, Cornelius, *The Art of Medicine: Medical Teaching at the University of Paris* (Leiden: Brill, 1998)

——, 'Gesturing in the Early Universities', *Dynamis: Acta hispanica ad medicinae scientiarumque historiam illustrandam*, 20 (2000), 250–81

O'Connor, Flannery, 'Parker's Back', in *The Complete Stories* (New York: Farrar, Straus and Giroux, 1971), pp. 510–30

Orofino, Giulia, *I codici decorati dell'Archivio di Montecassino*, 3 vols (Rome: Istituto poligrafico e zecca dello Stato, Libreria dello Stato, 1994–2006)

——, 'Miniatura a Montecassino. 1071–1087', in *Miniatura a Montecassino: L'età desideriana* (Cassino: Università degli Studi di Cassino e del Lazio meridionale — Dipartimento di Lettere e Filosofia, 2013)

Overgaauw, Eef A., 'Where Are the Colophons? On the Frequency of Datings in Late-Medieval Manuscripts', in *Sources for the History of Medieval Books and Libraries*, ed. by Rita Schlusemann, Joseph M. M. Hermans, and Margriet Hoogvliet (Groningen: Egbert Forsten, 1999), pp. 81–93

Palazzo, Éric, *A History of Liturgical Books from the Beginning to the Thirteenth Century* (Collegeville: The Order of St Benedict, 1998)

Palmer, Nigel F., and Klaus Speckenback, *Träume und Kräuter: Studien zur Petroneller 'Circa instans'-Handschrift und zu den deutschen Traumbüchern des Mittelalters* (Cologne: Böhlau, 1990)

Pilsworth, Claire, *Healthcare in Early Medieval Northern Italy: More to Life than Leeches* (Turnhout: Brepols, 2014)

Pormann, Peter, and Emilie Savage-Smith, *Medieval Islamic Medicine* (Washington, D.C.: Georgetown University Press, 2007)

Radding, Charles M., and Antonio Ciaralli, *The 'Corpus iuris civilis' in the Middle Ages: Manuscripts and Transmission from the Sixth Century to the Juristic Revival*, Studies in Intellectual History, 147 (Leiden: Brill, 2006)

Radding, Charles M., and Francis Newton, *Theology, Rhetoric, and Politics in the Eucharistic Controversy, 1078–1079: Alberic of Monte Cassino against Berengar of Tours* (New York: Columbia University Press, 2003)

Ramseyer, Valerie, *The Transformation of a Religious Landscape: Medieval Southern Italy 850–1150* (Ithaca: Cornell University Press, 2006)

Rand, Edward Kennard, and Leslie Webber Jones, *The Earliest Book of Tours: With Supplementary Descriptions of Other Manuscripts of Tours*, Studies on the Script of Tours, 2 (Cambridge, MA: Medieval Academy of America, 1934)

Reindel, Kurt, 'Studien zur Überlieferung des Werke des Petrus Damiani', *Deutsches Archiv*, 15 (1959), 23–102

Reynolds, Suzanne, '"Let Him Read the Satires of Horace": Reading, Literacy and Grammar in the Twelfth Century', in *The Practice and Representation of Reading in England*, ed. by James Raven, Helen Small, and Naomi Tadmor (Cambridge: Cambridge University Press, 1996), pp. 22–40

——, 'Glossing Horace: Using the Classics in the Medieval Classroom', in *Medieval Manuscripts of the Latin Classics: Production and Use*, ed. by Claudine A. Chavannes-Mazel and Margaret McFadden Smith (Los Altos Hills: Anderson-Lovelace, 1996), pp. 103–17

Robinson, Pamela, 'The Format of Books — Books, Booklets and Rolls', in *The Cambridge History of the Book in Britain: 1100–1400*, ed. by Nigel Morgan and others (Cambridge: Cambridge University Press, 2008), pp. 41–54

Ronca, Italo, 'The Influence of the *Pantegni* on William of Conches' *Dragmaticon*', in *Constantine the African and 'Alī ibn al-'Abbās al-Mağūsī: The 'Pantegni' and Related Texts*, ed. by Charles Burnett and Danielle Jacquart, Studies in Ancient Medicine, 10 (Leiden: Brill, 1994), pp. 266–85

Rosenthal, Franz, *The Classical Heritage in Islam*, trans. by Emile Marmorstein and Jenny Marmorstein (New York: Routledge, 1975)

Roth, Otto, *Klinische Terminologie* (Erlangen: Verlag von Eduard Besold, 1889)

Schuler, Stefan, '*Medicina secunda philosophia*: Die Einordnung der Medizin als Hauptdisziplin und die Zusammenstellung ihrer Quellen im *Speculum maius* des Vinzenz von Beauvais', *Frühmittelalterliche Studien*, 33 (1999), 169–251

Schum, Wilhelm, *Beschreibendes Verzeichniss der Amplonianischen Handschriften-Sammlung zu Erfurt* (Berlin: Weidmann, 1887). Available online: <http://bilder.manuscripta-mediaevalia.de/> [accessed 29 November 2016]

Schwaiger, Georg, 'Gelasius II', in *The Papacy: Galus-Proxies*, ed. by Philippe Levillain (New York: Routledge, 2002), pp. 625–26

Schwarzmaier, Hansmartin, 'Der *Liber vitae* von Subiaco. Die Klöster Farfa und Subiaco in ihrer geistigen und politischen Umwelt während der letzten Jahrzehnte des 11. Jahrhunderts', *Quellen und Forschungen aus italienischen Archiven und Bibliotheken*, 48 (1968), 80–147

Shogimen Takashi, and Cary J. Nederman, 'The Best Medicine? Medical Education, Practice and Metaphor in John of Salisbury's *Policraticus* and *Metalogicon*', *Viator*, 42 (2011), 55–73

Simon, Isidore, 'L'ethique médicale (Moussar ha-Rofim) d'Isaac Israeli', *Révue de l'histoire de la médecine Hébraique*, 26 (1973), 151–56

Singer, Charles, 'A Legend of Salerno: How Constantine Brought the Art of Medicine to the Christians', *Bulletin of the Johns Hopkins Hospital*, 28 (1917), 64–69

Smith, Romney David, 'Calamity and Transition: Re-Imagining Italian Trade in the Eleventh-Century Mediterranean', *Past & Present*, 228 (2015), 15–56

Strohmaier, Gotthard, 'Constantine's Pseudo-Classical Terminology and its Survival', in *Constantine the African and 'Alī ibn al-'Abbās al-Maǧūsī: The 'Pantegni' and Related Texts*, ed. by Charles Burnett and Danielle Jacquart, Studies in Ancient Medicine, 10 (Leiden: Brill, 1994), pp. 90–98

Sudhoff, Karl, 'Die medizinischen Schriften, welche Bischof Bruno von Hildesheim 1161 in seiner Bibliothek besass, und die Bedeutung des Konstantin von Afrika im 12. Jahrhundert', *Archiv für Geschichte der Medizin*, 9 (1915/16), 348–56

Talbert, Richard J. A., ed., *Barrington Atlas of the Greek and Roman World* (Princeton: Princeton University Press, 2000)

Taylor, Andrew, 'The Myth of the Minstrel Manuscript', *Speculum*, 66 (1991), 43–73

Thomson, Rodney M., '"Liber marii de elementis": The Work of a Hitherto Unknown Salernitan Master?', *Viator*, 3 (1972), 179–90

Thomson, Rodney M., and others, 'Technology of Production of the Manuscript Book', in *The Cambridge History of the Book in Britain*, II: *1100–1400*, ed. by Nigel Morgan and Rodney M. Thomson (Cambridge: Cambridge University Press, 2014), pp. 75–109

Thorndike, Lynn, *A History of Magic and Experimental Science*, I (New York: Columbia University Press, 1923)

Torrell, Jean-Pierre, *Saint Thomas Aquinas*, 2 vols (Washington, D.C.: The Catholic University of America Press, 2005)

Tristano, Caterina, 'Scrittura beneventana e scrittura carolina in manoscritti dell'Italia meridionale', *Scrittura e civiltà*, 3 (1979), 89–150

Ullmann, Manfred, *Die Medizin im Islam*, Handbuch der Orientalistik, 6 (Leiden: Brill, 1970)

——, *Islamic Medicine* (Edinburgh: Edinburgh University Press, 1978)

Vázquez de Benito, María de la Concepción, *Libro de la introduccion al arte de la medicina o 'Isagoge' de Abū Bakr Muhammad b. Zakarīyā al-Rāzī* (Salamanca: Universidad de Salamanca, 1979)

Victor, Stephen, 'A Study of Johannes de Muris' Autograph of the *De arte mesurandi*', *Isis*, 61 (1970), 389–95

Voigts, Linda Ehrsam, 'The Significance of the Name *Apuleius* to the *Herbarium Apulei*', *Dumbarton Oaks Papers*, 52 (1978), 214–27

——, 'Scientific and Medical Books', in *Book Production and Publishing in Britain, 1375–1475*, ed. by Jeremy Griffiths and Derek Pearsall (Cambridge: Cambridge University Press, 1989), pp. 345–402

Wack, Mary, *Lovesickness in the Middle Ages: The 'Viaticum' and its Commentaries* (Philadelphia: University of Pennsylvania Press, 1990)

——, ''Alī ibn al-'Abbās al-Mağūsī and Constantine on Love, and the Evolution of the *Practica Pantegni*', in *Constantine the African and 'Alī ibn al-'Abbās al-Mağūsī: The 'Pantegni' and Related Texts*, ed. by Charles Burnett and Danielle Jacquart, Studies in Ancient Medicine, 10 (Leiden: Brill, 1994), pp. 161–202

Ward, John O., 'Lawrence of Amalfi and the Boundary between the Oral and the Written in Eleventh-Century Europe', in *What Nature Does Not Teach: Didactic Literature in the Medieval and Early-Modern Periods*, ed. by Juanita Feros Ruys, Disputatio, 15 (Turnhout: Brepols, 2008), pp. 305–43

Willard, Henry M., 'Codex Casinensis 580T, Lexicon Prosodiacum saec. XI', in *Casinensia*, I (Monte Cassino, 1929), pp. 297–304

Wlaschky, Montschil, '*Sapientia artis medicinae*: Ein frühmittelalterliches Kompendium der Medizin', *Kyklos*, 1 (1928), 103–13

World Digital Library, 'Medical Questions', U.S. Library of Congress, 29 September 2017 <https://www.wdl.org/en/item/17838/> [accessed 16 February 2018]

Yawn, Lila, 'The Italian Giant Bibles', in *The Practice of the Bible in the Middle Ages: Production, Reception, and Performance in Western Christianity*, ed. by Susan Boynton and Diane J. Reilly (New York: Columbia University Press, 2011), pp. 126–56

Index of Manuscripts

General Index

Speculum Sanitatis: Studies in Medieval and Early Modern Medical Culture (500–1800)

All volumes in this series are evaluated by an Editorial Board, strictly on academic grounds, based on reports prepared by referees who have been commissioned by virtue of their specialism in the appropriate field. The Board ensures that the screening is done independently and without conflicts of interest. The definitive texts supplied by authors are also subject to review by the Board before being approved for publication. Further, the volumes are copyedited to conform to the publisher's stylebook and to the best international academic standards in the field.